Prostate Imaging

Editors

NICOLA SCHIEDA
ANDREI S. PURYSKO

RADIOLOGIC CLINICS OF NORTH AMERICA

www.radiologic.theclinics.com

Consulting Editor
FRANK H. MILLER

January 2024 • Volume 62 • Number 1

ELSEVIER

1600 John F. Kennedy Boulevard ● Suite 1800 ● Philadelphia, Pennsylvania, 19103-2899

http://www.theclinics.com

RADIOLOGIC CLINICS OF NORTH AMERICA Volume 62, Number 1
January 2024 ISSN 0033-8389, ISBN 13: 978-0-443-18356-0

Editor: John Vassallo (j.vassallo@elsevier.com)
Developmental Editor: Isha Singh

Radiologic Clinics of North America (ISSN 0033-8389) is published bimonthly by Elsevier Inc., 360 Park Avenue South, New York, NY 10010-1710. Months of issue are January, March, May, July, September, and November. Periodicals postage paid at New York, NY and additional mailing offices. Subscription prices are USD 561 per year for US individuals, USD 100 per year for US students and residents, USD 643 per year for Canadian individuals, USD 754 per year for international individuals, USD 100 per year for Canadian students/residents, and USD 315 per year for international students/residents. For institutional access pricing please contact Customer Service via the contact information below. To receive student and resident rate, orders must be accompanied by name of affiliated institution, date of term and the signature of program/residency coordinatior on institution letterhead. Orders will be billed at individual rate until proof of status is received. Foreign air speed delivery is included in all *Clinics* subscription prices. All prices are subject to change without notice. **POSTMASTER:** Send address changes to *Radiologic Clinics of North America*, Elsevier Health Sciences Division, Subscription Customer Service, 3251 Riverport Lane, Maryland Heights, MO63043. **Customer Service: Telephone: 1-800-654-2452** (U.S. and Canada); **1-314-447-8871** (outside U.S. and Canada). **Fax: 1-314-447-8029. E-mail: journalscustomerservice-usa@ elsevier.com (for print support); journalsonlinesupport-usa@elsevier.com (for online support)**.

Reprints. For copies of 100 or more of articles in this publication, please contact the Commercial Reprints Department, Elsevier Inc., 360 Park Avenue South, New York, New York 10010-1710. Tel.: +1-212-633-3874; Fax: +1-212-633-3820; E-mail: reprints@elsevier.com.

Radiologic Clinics of North America also published in Greek Paschalidis Medical Publications, Athens, Greece.

Radiologic Clinics of North America is covered in *MEDLINE/PubMed (Index Medicus), EMBASE/Excerpta Medica, Current Contents/Life Sciences, Current Contents/Clinical Medicine, RSNA Index to Imaging Literature, BIOSIS, Science Citation Index,* and *ISI/BIOMED.*

Contributors

CONSULTING EDITOR

FRANK H. MILLER, MD, FACR, FSAR, FSABI
Lee F. Rogers, MD Professor of Medical
Education, Chief, Body Imaging Section,
Medical Director, MRI, Professor, Department
of Radiology, Northwestern Memorial Hospital,
Northwestern University Feinberg School of
Medicine, Chicago, Illinois, USA

EDITORS

NICOLA SCHIEDA, MD, FRCPC
Director, Abdominal and Pelvic MR Imaging
and Prostate Imaging, Associate Professor,
Department of Radiology, University of Ottawa,
Department of Medical Imaging, The Ottawa
Hospital, Ottawa, Ontario, Canada

ANDREI S. PURYSKO, MD, FSAR
Section of Abdominal Imaging and Nuclear
Radiology, Department of Diagnostic
Radiology, Glickman Urological and Kidney
Institute, Cleveland Clinic, Cleveland, Ohio,
USA

AUTHORS

JORGE ABREU-GOMEZ, MD
Joint Department of Medical Imaging, University
Health Network, Mount Sinai Hospital,
Women's College Hospital, University of
Toronto, Toronto, Ontario, Canada

DANIEL A. ADAMO, MD
Assistant Professor of Radiology, Mayo Clinic,
Rochester, Minnesota, USA

SANDEEP ARORA, MBBS
Associate Professor of Radiology and
Biomedical Imaging, Yale University, New
Haven, Connecticut, USA

TRISTAN BARRETT, MD, FRCR
Associate Professor, Department of Radiology,
University of Cambridge, Department of
Radiology, Cambridge University Hospitals NHS
Foundation Trust, Cambridge, United Kingdom

**THARAKESWARA KUMAR BATHALA, MD,
MS**
Division of Diagnostic Imaging, The University
of Texas MD Anderson Cancer Center,
Houston, Texas, USA

SILVIA D. CHANG, MD
Associate Professor, Department of Radiology,
University of British Columbia, Radiologist,
Vancouver General Hospital, Vancouver,
Canada

DANIEL N. COSTA, MD
Associate Professor, Departments of
Radiology and Urology, The University of
Texas Southwestern Medical Center, Dallas,
Texas, USA

LARISSA BASTOS COSTA, MD
Radiology and Nuclear Medicine Department,
Hospital Sirio Libanes and Americas Group,
São Paulo, Brazil

FELIPE DE GALIZA BARBOSA, MD
Radiology and Nuclear Medicine Department,
Hospital Sirio Libanes and Americas Group,
São Paulo, Brazil

JEEBAN PAUL DAS, MD
Department of Radiology, Memorial Sloan
Kettering Cancer Center, New York, New York,
USA

MAARTEN DE ROOIJ, MD
Department of Medical Imaging, Radboud University Medical Center, Nijmegen, the Netherlands

AILIN DEHGHANPOUR, MD
Radiology Resident, Department of Radiological Sciences, Oncology and Pathology, Sapienza University, Policlinico Umberto I, Rome, Italy

ADRIANO BASSO DIAS, MD
Joint Department of Medical Imaging, University Medical Imaging Toronto, University Health Network, Mount Sinai Hospital, Women's College Hospital, University of Toronto, Toronto, Ontario, Canada

CAMERON ENGLMAN, MD
Department of Radiology, University College London Hospital NHS Foundation Trust, Division of Surgery and Interventional Science, University College London, London, United Kingdom

FIONA M. FENNESSY, MD, PhD
Associate Professor, Department of Radiology, Brigham and Women's Hospital, Harvard Medical School, Boston, Massachusetts, USA

ANDREI GAFITA, MD
The Russell H. Morgan Department of Radiology and Radiological Science, Johns Hopkins School of Medicine, Baltimore, Maryland, USA

PRISCILLA ROMANO GASPAR, MD
Nuclear Medicine Department, Hospital Vitória (Americas Group), Hospital de Força Aérea do Galeão, Rio de Janeiro, Brazil

SANGEET GHAI, MD
Joint Department of Medical Imaging, University Medical Imaging Toronto, University Health Network, Mount Sinai Hospital, Women's College Hospital, University of Toronto, Toronto, Ontario, Canada

PEJMAN GHANOUNI, MD, PhD
Associate Professor of Radiology and by courtesy of Neurosurgery, Urology and Obstetrics and Gynecology, Stanford University, Stanford, California, USA

FRANCESCO GIGANTI, MD, PhD
Department of Radiology, University College London Hospital NHS Foundation Trust, Division of Surgery and Interventional Science, University College London, London, United Kingdom

BERNADETTE MARIE GREENWOOD, MSc, RT(R)(MR)(ARRT)
Chief Research Officer, HALO Diagnostics, Indian Wells, California, USA; PhD Candidate, Radboud Research Institute, Nijmegen, the Netherlands

RAJAN T. GUPTA, MD
Departments of Radiology and Surgery, Duke University Medical Center, Duke Cancer Institute Center for Prostate and Urologic Cancers

MASOOM A. HAIDER, MD, FRCPC
Lunenfeld-Tanenbaum Research Institute, Joint Department of Medical Imaging, Sinai Health System, Princess Margaret Hospital, University of Toronto, Toronto, Ontario, Canada

KEN-PIN HWANG, PhD
Division of Diagnostic Imaging, The University of Texas MD Anderson Cancer Center, Houston, Texas, USA

LATRICE A. JOHNSON, BS
Molecular Imaging Branch, National Cancer Institute, National Institutes of Health, Bethesda, Maryland, USA

PRANEETH KALVA, BS
The University of Texas Southwestern Medical School, Dallas, Texas, USA

KANG-LUNG LEE, MD
Department of Radiology, Addenbrooke's Hospital, University of Cambridge, Cambridge, United Kingdom; Department of Radiology, Taipei Veterans General Hospital, School of Medicine, National Yang Ming Chiao Tung University, Taipei, Taiwan

CHRISTOPHER LIM, MD
Department of Medical Imaging, Sunnybrook Health Sciences Centre, University of Toronto, Toronto, Ontario, Canada

YUE LIN, AB
Molecular Imaging Branch, National Cancer Institute, National Institutes of Health, Bethesda, Maryland, USA

DANIEL J.A. MARGOLIS, MD
Department of Radiology, Weill Cornell
Medical College, New York, New York, USA

CAROLINE M. MOORE, MD, FRCS
Division of Surgery and Interventional Science,
University College London, Department of
Urology, University College London Hospital
NHS Foundation Trust, London, United
Kingdom

RENATA MOREIRA, MD
Radiology and Nuclear Medicine Department,
Casa de Saúde São José, Rio de Janeiro,
Brazil

JORGE D. OLDAN, MD
Department of Radiology, The University of
North Carolina at Chapel Hill, Chapel Hill, North
Carolina, USA

VALERIA PANEBIANCO, MD
Department of Radiological Sciences,
Oncology and Pathology, Sapienza University,
Policlinico Umberto I, Rome, Italy

MARTINA PECORARO, MD
Department of Radiological Sciences,
Oncology and Pathology, Sapienza University,
Policlinico Umberto I, Rome, Italy

MARTIN G. POMPER, MD, PhD
The Russell H. Morgan Department of
Radiology and Radiological Science, Johns
Hopkins School of Medicine, Baltimore,
Maryland, USA

DEBORA Z. RECCHIMUZZI, MD
Department of Radiology, The University of
Texas Southwestern Medical Center, Dallas,
Texas, USA

STEVEN P. ROWE, MD, PhD
The Russell H. Morgan Department of
Radiology and Radiological Science, Johns
Hopkins School of Medicine, Baltimore,
Maryland, USA

MOHAMMAD S. SADAGHIANI, MD
The Russell H. Morgan Department of
Radiology and Radiological Science, Johns
Hopkins School of Medicine, Baltimore,
Maryland, USA

NICOLA SCHIEDA, MD, FRCPC
Director, Abdominal and Pelvic MR
Imaging and Prostate Imaging, Associate
Professor, Department of Radiology,
University of Ottawa, Department of Medical
Imaging, The Ottawa Hospital, Ottawa,
Ontario, Canada

SARA SHEIKHBAHAEI, MD, MPH
The Russell H. Morgan Department of
Radiology and Radiological Science, Johns
Hopkins School of Medicine, Baltimore,
Maryland, USA

LILJA B. SOLNES, MD, MBA
The Russell H. Morgan Department of
Radiology and Radiological Science, Johns
Hopkins School of Medicine, Baltimore,
Maryland, USA

BENJAMIN SPILSETH, MD, MBA
Associate Professor, Department of Radiology,
University of Minnesota Medical School,
Minneapolis, Minnesota, USA

AVERY SPITZ, RN
Sidney Kimmell Comprehensive Cancer
Center, Johns Hopkins School of Medicine,
Baltimore, Maryland, USA

DEVAKI SHILPA SUDHA SURASI, MD, CMQ
Division of Diagnostic Imaging, The University
of Texas MD Anderson Cancer Center,
Houston, Texas, USA

BARIS TURKBEY, MD
Molecular Imaging Branch, National Cancer
Institute, National Institutes of Health,
Bethesda, Maryland, USA

RUDOLF A. WERNER, MD
Department of Nuclear Medicine, University
Hospital Würzburg, Würzburg, Germany

SUNGMIN WOO, MD, PhD
Department of Radiology, Memorial Sloan
Kettering Cancer Center, New York, New York,
USA

JEFFREY YOUNG, BS, CNMT
Radiotheranostics Manager, Johns Hopkins
Hospital, Baltimore, Maryland, USA

Contents

Prostate MR imaging quality has improved dramatically over recent times, driven by
advances in hardware, software, and improved functional imaging techniques. MRI
now plays a key role in prostate cancer diagnostic work-up, but outcomes of the
MRI-directed pathway are heavily dependent on image quality and optimization.
MR sequences can be affected by patient-related degradations relating to motion
and susceptibility artifacts which may enable only partial mitigation. In this Review,
we explore issues relating to prostate MRI acquisition and interpretation, mitigation
strategies at a patient and scanner level, PI-QUAL reporting, and future directions in
image quality, including artificial intelligence solutions.

Prostate magnetic resonance imaging (MRI) is increasingly being used to diagnose
and stage prostate cancer. The Prostate Imaging and Data Reporting System (PI-
RADS) version 2.1 is a consensus-based reporting system that provides a standardized and reproducible method for interpreting prostate MRI. This primer provides
an overview of the PI-RADS system, focusing on its current role in clinical interpretation. It discusses the appropriate use of PI-RADS and how it should be applied by
radiologists in clinical practice to assign and report PI-RADS assessments. We also
discuss the changes from prior versions and published validation studies on PI-
RADS accuracy and reproducibility.

The aim of this article is to review the technical and clinical considerations encountered with PI-RADS 3 lesions, which are equivocal for clinically significant Prostate
Cancer (csPCa) with detection rates ranging between 10% and 35%. The number
of PI-RADS 3 lesions reported vary according to several factors including MRI quality and radiologist training/expertise among the most influential. PI-RADS v.2.1 updated definitions for scores 2 and 3 in the PZ and scores 1 and 2 in the TZ is
reviewed. The role of DWI role is highlighted in the assessment of the TZ with the
possibility of upgrading score 2 lesions to score 3 based on DWI score. Given the
increased utilization for prostate MRI, biparametric MRI can be considered as an alternative for low-risk patients where there is a need to rule out csPCa acknowledging
this technique may increase the number of indeterminate cases going for biopsies.
Management of patients with equivocal lesions at mpMRI and factors influencing biopsy decision process remain as an unmet need and additional studies using molec-
ular/imaging markers as well as artificial intelligence tools are needed to further
address their role in proper patient selection for biopsy.

treatment alternative to traditional whole-gland therapies, such as radical prostatectomy or radiation therapy. This is especially true in men with localized, low- to intermediate-risk prostate cancer. Although long-term oncologic data remain limited, the authors describe several MR imaging-guided therapeutic options for the treatment of prostate cancer, including cryoablation, laser ablation, transrectal high-intensity focused ultrasound, and transurethral ultrasound ablation.

Detection of prostate cancer recurrence after whole-gland treatment with curative intent is critical to identify patients who may benefit from local salvage therapy. Among the different imaging modalities used in clinical practice, MR imaging is the most accurate in identifying local prostate cancer recurrence; indeed, it is an excellent technique for local recurrence detection superior to PET/CT, even at low PSA, but provides no information about extra-pelvic lymph nodes or bone metastasis. In 2021, a group of experts developed the Prostate Imaging for local Recurrence Reporting scoring system to standardize acquisition, interpretation, and reporting of prostate cancer recurrence.

Prostate-specific membrane antigen PET (PSMA-PET) has emerged as a powerful imaging tool for prostate cancer primary staging, biochemical recurrence, and advanced disease assessment. This article offers a concise overview of the benefits and challenges associated with PSMA-PET for prostate cancer evaluation. The article highlights the advantages of PSMA-PET over conventional imaging, such as its higher sensitivity and specificity for detecting metastases, and the potential for guiding personalized treatment decisions. However, it also explores the limitations and potential pitfalls for interpretation. Overall, the article aims to provide valuable insights for clinicians and diagnostic imaging physicians in clinical practice.

The discovery and clinical development of radiolabeled small-molecule ligands targeting prostate-specific membrane antigen (PSMA) has had a profound influence on the field of nuclear medicine. Such agents have been successfully deployed for both imaging and therapeutic applications. In particular, PSMA radioligand therapy (PRLT) has been shown to be a life-prolonging therapy for men with metastatic, castration-resistant prostate cancer and has also brought nuclear medicine physicians and nuclear radiologists into the forefront of direct patient care. In this review, we will discuss the clinical study data regarding the efficacy and toxicities related to PRLT, outline the key personnel that any center offering PRLT should have, offer salient clinical examples, and provide an overview of future directions for PRLT. As PRLT continues to evolve as a treatment modality, it is paramount that nuclear medicine physicians and nuclear radiologists understand the clinical context, management implications, and practical aspects so as to best deliver high-value care to patients.

Adriano Basso Dias and Sangeet Ghai

Prostate cancer (PCa) is the most common non-cutaneous cancer diagnosed in males. Multiparametric Magnetic Resonance Imaging (mpMRI) with targeted biopsy can detect PCa and is currently the recommended initial test in men at risk for PCa. Micro-Ultrasound (MicroUS) is a novel high-resolution 29-MHz ultrasound with ~three times greater resolution of conventional transrectal ultrasound (TRUS) resolution. Preliminary data suggest improved accuracy of ultrasound for targeted prostate biopsy. A growing body of evidence has become available supporting MicroUS as a potentially time and cost saving modality for PCa detection, with early results suggesting comparable accuracy to mpMRI. Additionally, microUS allows real-time visualization for accurate targeted biopsy. It is not yet clear whether MicroUS should be used on its own or in combination with mpMRI for prostate cancer detection. The ongoing OPTIMUM randomized controlled trial will help to establish the role of MicroUS in the diagnostic algorithm for the detection of clinically significant (cs)-PCa. Early data also indicate this imaging modality may have a role in local staging (eg, extracapsular extension prediction) and active surveillance of PCa. MicroUS has also the potential to add value to biparametric (bp) MRI, and may represent a promising tool for guidance of focal therapy in the near future.

RADIOLOGIC CLINICS OF NORTH AMERICA

SERIES OF RELATED INTEREST

Advances in Clinical Radiology
Available at: https://www.advancesinclinicalradiology.com/
Magnetic Resonance Imaging Clinics
Available at: https://www.mri.theclinics.com/
Neuroimaging Clinics
Available at: www.neuroimaging.theclinics.com
PET Clinics
Available at: www.pet.theclinics.com

THE CLINICS ARE AVAILABLE ONLINE!
Access your subscription at:
www.theclinics.com

PROGRAM OBJECTIVE
The objective of the *Radiologic Clinics of North America* is to keep practicing radiologists and radiology residents up to date with current clinical practice in radiology by providing timely articles reviewing the state of the art in patient care.

TARGET AUDIENCE
Practicing radiologists, radiology residents, and other healthcare professionals who provide patient care utilizing radiologic findings.

LEARNING OBJECTIVES
Upon completion of this activity, participants will be able to:
1. Describe the potential pitfalls associated with prostate MRI interpretation.
2. Discuss the advantages, disadvantages and compare principles of different modalities available for guidance of targeted prostate biopsy.
3. Recognize emerging user-friendly systems designed to improve accuracy and reproducibility of radiologists approaching prostate cancer recurrence in clinical practice.

ACCREDITATION
The Elsevier Office of Continuing Medical Education (EOCME) is accredited by the Accreditation Council for Continuing Medical Education (ACCME) to provide continuing medical education for physicians.

The EOCME designates this journal-based CME activity for a maximum of 12 *AMA PRA Category 1 Credit*(s)™. Physicians should claim only the credit commensurate with the extent of their participation in the activity.

All other healthcare professionals requesting continuing education credit for this enduring material will be issued a certificate of participation.

DISCLOSURE OF CONFLICTS OF INTEREST
The EOCME assesses conflict of interest with its instructors, faculty, planners, and other individuals who are in a position to control the content of CME activities. All relevant conflicts of interest that are identified are thoroughly vetted by EOCME for fair balance, scientific objectivity, and patient care recommendations. EOCME is committed to providing its learners with CME activities that promote improvements or quality in healthcare and not a specific proprietary business or a commercial interest.

The planning committee, staff, authors, and editors listed below have identified no financial relationships or relationships to products or devices they or their spouse/life partner have with commercial interest related to the content of this CME activity:
Jorge Abreu-Gomez, MD; Daniel A. Adamo, MD; Tristan Barrett, MBBS, MD, BSc; Tharakeswara Kumar Bathala, MD, MS; Silvia D. Chang, MD; Daniel N. Costa, MD; Larissa Bastos Costa, MD; Jeeban Paul Das, MD; Felipe de Galiza Barbosa, MD; Maarten de Rooij, MD, PhD; Ailin Dehghanpour, MD; Adriano Basso Dias, MD; Cameron Englman, MD; Fiona Fennessy, MD, PhD; Andrei S. Gafita, MD; Priscilla Romano Gaspar, MD; Francesco Giganti, MD, PhD; Rajan T. Gupta, MD; Masoom Haider, MD; Ken-Pin Hwang, PhD; Latrice Johnson; Praneeth Kalva; Kothainayaki Kulanthaivelu, BCA, MBA; Kang-Lung Lee, MD; Christopher Lim, MD, FRCPC; Yue Lin; Michelle Littlejohn; Daniel J.A. Margolis, MD; Caroline M. Moore, MBBS; Renata Moreira, MD; Jorge Oldan, MD; Valeria Panebianco, MD; Martina Pecoraro, MD; Andrei Saraiva Purysko, MD; Debora Z. Recchimuzzi, MD; Mohammad S. Sadaghiani, MD; Nicola Schieda, MD, FRCPC; Sara Sheikhbahaei, MD, MPH; Lilja Bjork Solnes, MD, MBA; Benjamin Spilseth, MD MBA; Avery Spitz, RN, MSN Baris Turkbey, MD; Rudolf Werner, MD; Sungmin Woo, MD, PhD; Jeffrey Young, BS,CNMT, RT(CT)(ARRT)

The planning committee, staff, authors, and editors listed below have identified financial relationships or relationships to products or devices they or their spouse/life partner have with commercial interest related to the content of this CME activity:
Sandeep Arora, MBBS: Researcher: Profound Medical

Sangeet Ghai, MD: Researcher: Exact Imaging

Pejman Ghanouni, MD, PhD: Advisor: SonALAsense, Profound Medical, Insightec; Ownership Interest: SonALAsense; Consultant: HistoSonics

Bernadette Marie Greenwood: Employee/Executive Role/Ownership Interest: Halo Precision Diagnostics

Martin G. Pomper, MD, PhD: Royalties/Patent Beneficiary/Researcher: Lantheus

Steven P. Rowe, MD, PhD: Consultant/Researcher: Lantheus

Devaki Shilpa Sudha Surasi, MD, CMQ: Researcher: Blue Earth Diagnostics

UNAPPROVED/OFF-LABEL USE DISCLOSURE
The EOCME requires CME faculty to disclose to the participants:
1. When products or procedures being discussed are off-label, unlabelled, experimental, and/or investigational (not US Food and Drug Administration [FDA] approved); and

2. Any limitations on the information presented, such as data that are preliminary or that represent ongoing research, interim analyses, and/or unsupported opinions. Faculty may discuss information about pharmaceutical agents that is outside of FDA-approved labelling. This information is intended solely for CME and is not intended to promote off-label use of these medications. If you have any questions, contact the medical affairs department of the manufacturer for the most recent prescribing information.

TO ENROLL

To enroll in the *Radiologic Clinics of North America* Continuing Medical Education program, call customer service at 1-800-654-2452 or sign up online at http://www.theclinics.com/home/cme. The CME program is available to subscribers for an additional annual fee of USD 340.00.

METHOD OF PARTICIPATION

In order to claim credit, participants must complete the following:
1. Complete enrolment as indicated above.
2. Read the activity.
3. Complete the CME Test and Evaluation. Participants must achieve a score of 70% on the test. All CME Tests and Evaluations must be completed online.

CME INQUIRIES/SPECIAL NEEDS

For all CME inquiries or special needs, please contact elsevierCME@elsevier.com.

Preface
Prostate Cancer Imaging

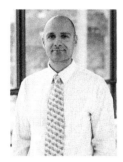   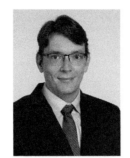

Nicola Schieda, MD, FRCPC   Andrei S. Purysko, MD, FSAR
Editors

Prostate cancer remains a critical health concern, affecting millions of men worldwide. Prostate cancer screening, diagnosis, and treatment have evolved significantly in the past few years. Specifically, there have been remarkable advancements in medical imaging, transforming how we detect, diagnose, and manage this complex disease. In this special issue of the *Radiologic Clinics of North America*, we delve into cutting-edge techniques and breakthroughs in prostate cancer imaging, focusing on prostate MR imaging, prostate-specific membrane antigen (PSMA) PET, and microultrasound.

Prostate MR imaging is an established tool clinicians use to diagnose, stage, and to some extent, prognosticate prostate cancer. The articles in this issue cover the basics of image acquisition and interpretation, specifically including an approach to image quality, a summary of the Prostate Imaging and Reporting Data System (PI-RADS) version 2.1, staging of prostate cancer with MR imaging, and recognition and avoidance of imaging pitfalls. Emerging topics include the management of PI-RADS category 3 lesions, the application of MR imaging for patients enrolled in or being considered for active surveillance, and in men with suspected biochemical recurrence after therapy. The

latest advancements in MR imaging–guided prostate cancer treatments are also discussed.

The emergence of PSMA PET imaging has revolutionized the management of prostate cancer, providing unprecedented sensitivity for the detection and staging of this disease. PSMA-targeted radiotracers enable the visualization of prostate cancer lesions, even at low PSA levels, guiding biopsy decisions, assisting in accurate staging, and facilitating therapeutic planning. This issue features articles exploring PSMA PET's role in different clinical scenarios, such as initial diagnosis, biochemical recurrence, and restaging after therapy. Furthermore, we discuss the ongoing research on theranostic applications of PSMA-targeted radionuclide therapy.

Microultrasound is an exciting addition to the armamentarium of prostate cancer imaging and diagnosis, offering high-resolution imaging with real-time capabilities enabling immediate, precise biopsy and enhanced detection of clinically significant prostate cancer compared with conventional ultrasound. The article in this issue highlights the potential of microultrasound in improving the accuracy of prostate cancer diagnosis, particularly in combination with MR imaging and fusion techniques. In addition, this issue discusses the

Radiol Clin N Am 62 (2024) xv–xvi
https://doi.org/10.1016/j.rcl.2023.07.004
0033-8389/24/© 2023 Published by Elsevier Inc.

approach to prostate biopsy in general, using ultrasound and MR imaging fusion, and "what the radiologist needs to know" in this domain.

We are honored to present this special issue, which brings together a diverse group of renowned experts in the field of prostate cancer imaging. Their expertise and groundbreaking research contribute to the expanding knowledge base in this rapidly evolving field. We hope the articles presented herein will inspire further research, facilitate clinical decision making, and improve patient outcomes.

We extend our sincere gratitude to the authors, reviewers, and editorial staff who have diligently contributed to developing this special issue. Their dedication and commitment to advancing prostate cancer imaging have made this publication possible.

We invite you to immerse yourself in the wealth of knowledge contained within these pages. We hope this special issue will serve as a valuable resource for radiologists, urologists, oncologists, and all health care professionals involved in the care of patients with prostate cancer.

Nicola Schieda, MD, FRCPC
Department of Radiology
University of Ottawa
1053 Carling Avenue
K1Y 0E9. C1 Radiology
Ottawa, ON, Canada

Andrei S. Purysko, MD, FSAR
Section of Abdominal Imaging and
Nuclear Radiology Department
Diagnostic Radiology, and
Glickman Urological and
Kidney Institute Cleveland Clinic
9500 Euclid Avenue
Cleveland, OH 44195, USA

E-mail addresses:
nschieda@toh.ca (N. Schieda)
puryska@ccf.org (A.S. Purysko)

Update on Optimization of Prostate MR Imaging Technique and Image Quality

Tristan Barrett, MBBS, MD[a],*, Kang-Lung Lee, MD[a,b,c],
Maarten de Rooij, MD[d], Francesco Giganti, MD[e,f]

KEYWORDS

- Prostate ● MR image quality ● PI-QUAL ● Artifacts

KEY POINTS

- High-quality prostate MR imaging is a pre-requisite for accurately identifying lesions, with lower image quality is associated with increased uncertainty in MRI decision-making
- Compliance with Prostate Imaging-Reporting and Data System (PI-RADS) technical parameters helps improve image quality but does not guarantee this
- Patient-related degradations independently influence quality and potentially only allow for partial mitigation via rectal preparation, spasmolytics, novel diffusion techniques, or metal-reduction sequences
- Historically prostate MR image quality this has been reported in a non-uniform and inconsistent manner; Prostate Imaging Quality (PI-QUAL) represents the first attempt at standardization
- AI solutions can be applied for image-reconstruction to increase signal-to-noise ratios; future developments may enable on-table monitoring of image quality and real-time adjustment of parameters

INTRODUCTION

The first MRI study of the prostate gland was performed by Steyn and Smith in 1982[1]; however, MR imaging only became clinically feasible with the introduction of endorectal coils and higher strength imaging at 1.5 T in the mid-1990s.[2] Since then, the image quality of prostate MR imaging has improved dramatically due to advances in MR hardware, including introduction of multichannel array coils, and consistent high-quality diffusion-weighted imaging (DWI), and dynamic contract-enhanced (DCE) sequences, with faster imaging acquisitions.[3,4] Higher image quality has resulted in MR imaging playing a key role in the diagnostic pathway of prostate cancer, enabling a reduction in the number of unnecessary biopsy procedures by 27% to 49%, with a concurrent reduction in the detection of insignificant disease, while maintaining similar detection rates of clinically significant prostate cancer (csPCa).[5–9] However, the diagnostic ability of prostate MR imaging is significantly affected by image quality; high-quality prostate MR imaging is a prerequisite for accurately identifying lesions,[10] while lower image quality is associated with increased uncertainty in MR imaging decision-making.[11] The Prostate Imaging-Reporting and Data System (PI-RADS) recommendations, last updated in 2019,[12] are designed to limit variation in quality by providing

[a] Department of Radiology, Addenbrooke's Hospital and University of Cambridge, Cambridge, UK; [b] Department of Radiology, Taipei Veterans General Hospital, Taipei, Taiwan; [c] School of Medicine, National Yang Ming Chiao Tung University, Taipei, Taiwan; [d] Department of Medical Imaging, Radboud University Medical Center, Nijmegen, Netherlands; [e] Department of Radiology, University College London Hospital NHS Foundation Trust, London, UK; [f] Division of Surgery and Interventional Science, University College London, London, UK
* Corresponding author.
E-mail address: tristan.barrett@nhs.net

Radiol Clin N Am 62 (2024) 1–15
https://doi.org/10.1016/j.rcl.2023.06.006
0033-8389/24/© 2023 Elsevier Inc. All rights reserved.

minimum technical requirements for the acquisition of prostate MR imaging sequences. Despite this, prostate MR imaging quality shows considerable heterogeneity between scanners and centers,[13–15] and compliance to the guidelines alone does not guarantee optimal image quality.[13,14] Moreover, patient-related degradations such as from rectal spasm, bulk motion, and pelvic metalwork can independently affect image quality with potential for only partial mitigation.[4,13,16] A recent joint European Society of Urogenital Radiology (ESUR) and European Association of Urology Section of Urologic Imaging (ESUI) consensus document recommends that image quality should be routinely reported for all prostate MR imaging studies,[17] with the Prostate Imaging Quality (PI-QUAL) scoring system representing the first attempt to standardize such an approach.[18]

In this review, we explore issues relating to the acquisition and interpretation of prostate MR imaging, mitigation strategies that can be employed at a patient and scanner level, PI-QUAL reporting, and future directions aimed at improving image quality, including artificial intelligence (AI) solutions.

QUALITY IN THE PROSTATE CANCER DIAGNOSTIC PATHWAY

Quality is important throughout the prostate cancer diagnostic pathway, from image acquisition and reporting through to performance of biopsy and pathologic interpretation. However, high-quality MR imaging is the first and most crucial step along the pathway and will heavily influence all downstream events.[16] Image quality is determined by several factors, including resolution, signal-to-noise ratio (SNR), contrast, and the presence of artifacts.[19] Quality can be impacted by technical parameters, hardware and software considerations, and patient-related factors. Moreover, image interpretation made by radiologists can also influence clinical decision-making and ultimately impact the quality of the prostate cancer diagnostic pathway.[4,16]

Patient-related quality factors

Several patient-related factors may influence prostate MR imaging quality and interpretation, such as motion artifact due to bulk patient movement or rectal spasm and susceptibility artifact secondary to rectal gas or pelvic metalwork. However, aside from hyperventilation in patients with anxiety or claustrophobia, it is unusual to encounter respiratory motion artifact given the low pelvic location of the prostate, and artifact related to post-biopsy hemorrhage[20] is now rarely seen with the use of MR imaging prior to biopsy.

Imaging technique-based factors

When optimizing MR image quality there is a trade-off between SNR, resolution, and scan time with these 3 key components collectively known as the "MR imaging triangle." Improving one component of the triangle may compromise the other 2, for instance, increased SNR can be obtained with lower resolution and/or with an increase in scan time (**Fig. 1**).[19,21] SNR is theoretically linearly related to the magnetic field strength; thus, 3T provides twice that of 1.5 T. The PI-RADS steering committee express a preference for 3T prostate MR imaging where available; however, they state that 1.5 T systems if optimized are diagnostically acceptable for prostate MR imaging. Notably, 1.5 T scanning is mandatory if patients have implants or devices considered conditional only for imaging at 1.5 T (ie, prohibited at 3T). In such scenarios, good quality 1.5 T prostate MR imaging can be performed.[22] The choice of receiver coil is between an endorectal coil (ERC) or phased-array surface coil, with studies generally showing that an ERC improves SNR on both T2-weighted images (T2WI) and DWI.[23–26] However, the presence of an ERC may stimulate bowel peristalsis and induce ghosting artifacts in the phase encoding direction, which may be further amplified by poor coil positioning[23] and will also increase the cost, time, and associated discomfort

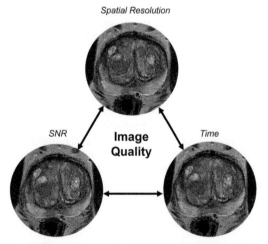

Spatial Resolution

SNR   **Image Quality**   Time

Fig. 1. MR imaging triangle. A 68 year old patient, PSA 8.11 ng/mL on active surveillance for low-risk prostate cancer with no MR imaging visible lesion. Increased voxel size (top image) improves spatial resolution. Increasing matrix size from 512 × 512 to 1024 × 1024 with a higher acquired phase resolution of 0.4 × 0.5 mm compared to 0.4 × 0.7 (left image) leads to more noise with the image and lower SNR. Reduced scan time from 4:43 to 3:27 (right image) results in lower SNR.

of MR imaging.[4] On balance, the PI-RADS committee recommends that an ERC be reserved for use with older 1.5 T MR imaging systems, or where adequate SNR cannot otherwise be achieved with use of a surface coil.[12]

The PI-RADS document proposes minimum technical standards for the acquisition of each individual multiparametric (mp) MR imaging sequence, including in-plane spatial resolution, repetition time, time-to-echo, and slice thickness and gap on all sequences, along with optimal choices for DWI *b*-values (**Table 1**). Nevertheless, some ambiguity exists. The optimal field of view (FOV) is stated for T2WI (12–20 cm) and DWI (16–22 cm), but DCE simply recommends covering the entire prostate and seminal vesicles. In our experience, a larger FOV and lower spatial resolution is required for surface coil imaging at 1.5 T.[27] For DCE, the minimal total observation time should be 2 minutes; however, the start point is not clearly defined as being at the time of contrast medium administration or when contrast arrives in the prostate. It is important to note that full adherence to these recommendations does not guarantee good quality imaging,[13,14] and improvements can be achieved with (slight) parameter deviations in particular situations.[28–30]

There is an ongoing debate as to the added value of gadolinium contrast in mpMR imaging and whether a noncontrast biparametric (bp) MR imaging approach is sufficient.[31,32] Prospective multicenter trials addressing this question are currently recruiting[33,34]; however, it should be noted that there is a benefit of DCE as a "safety net" for both lesion detection and for overall image quality (**Fig. 2**). DCE is a more robust sequence than echo-planar DWI, with a lower degree of susceptibility artifacts[35] and can remain diagnostic when T2WI and DWI are compromised. Notably, a PI-RADS committee update states that bpMR imaging should only be used if high-quality imaging, expert interpretation, and availability of patient recall or on-table monitoring have all been established.[36]

Radiologist-based factors

The wide application of the PI-RADS scoring system has aided standardization; however, there remains a moderate degree of inter-reader variability with reported κ values ranging from 0.42 to 0.92,[37–41] and with significant variation in the positive predictive value of MR imaging, even among established centers.[42] Certification for interpretation is a potential quality control method for reducing inter-reader variability and enhancing outcomes, but requires a multifaceted approach incorporating peer learning, accrual of continuing medical education credits, multidisciplinary meeting participation, and radiology-pathology feedback mechanisms.[16,43] The American College of Radiology recommends reporting a minimum of 150 prostate MR imagings unassisted or 100 under direct supervision before reporting independently[44]; however, real-world data suggest reading of 200 to 300 cases is required to overcome the initial reporting learning curve.[45,46] Recent UK and European consensus documents have outlined proposals for certification[47,48]; however, a German process initiated in 2018 offers the only currently available qualification for prostate MR imaging interpretation.[49]

Common artifacts affecting prostate MR imaging

Movement during image acquisition, including bulk patient motion, small bowel peristalsis, or rectal spasm, can result in a phase shift in k-space, leading to the creation of motion artifact on images. If the motion is periodic, there may be the appearance of more discrete "ghosting" artifacts. Several strategies can be employed to reduce motion artifact, including physical stabilization and employing sequences that are more resilient to motion due to their use of parallel and/or partial Fourier imaging for reduced scan time[50,51] (**Table 2**). Additionally, changing the phase- and frequency-encoding directions can act to shift the direction of artifact away from areas of diagnostic interest.[52]

Rectal distension is known to negatively correlate with image quality,[53] with secondary spasm causing motion artifact predominantly on T2WI and DCE and, if air is present at the recto-prostatic interface, susceptibility artifact on DWI (**Fig. 3**). Clearly an empty rectum will mitigate against both types of artifacts and PI-RADS recommends that patients should evacuate the rectum just prior to MR imaging.[12] More invasive preparation methods have also been assessed including dietary restrictions, enema, rectal gel, catheter decompression, and anti-spasmodic agents.[54–59] However, the current evidence is inconclusive, and the published literature has rarely evaluated the potential impact on eventual prostate cancer diagnosis.[60] PI-RADS therefore does not recommend additional preparation steps, noting further potential disadvantages such as increased costs, enema-induced peristalsis, and contraindications or drug reactions with anti-spasmodic agents.[61]

Susceptibility artifact occurs due to variations in the magnetic properties between different tissues in the body, with resultant magnetic field inhomogeneities distorting the MR signal. Metallic

Table 1
Technical requirements for multiparametric prostate MR imaging according (PI-RADS v. 2.1 guidelines)

	Imaging Planes	Slice Thickness	FOV	In-Plane Dimension	Pulse Sequence	Specific Recommendations	
T2WI	Same used for DWI and DCE	3 mm No gap	12–20 cm[a]	≤ 0.7 mm (phase) x ≤ 0.4 mm (frequency)	FSE/TSE	Axial plane: either straight axial to the patient or in an oblique axial plane matching the long axis of the prostate	At least one additional orthogonal plane (sagittal and/or coronal)	3D axial as an adjunct to 2D acquisitions
DWI	Same used for T2WI and DCE	≤ 4 mm No gap	16–22 cm	≤ 2.5 mm (phase and frequency)	Free-breathing spin echo EPI Spectral fat saturation	*Low b value:* 50–100 s/mm²	*Intermediate b value:* 800–1000 s/mm²	*High b value:* • Dedicated (≥1400 s/mm²) • Synthesized (from other b-values)
DCE	Same used for T2WI and DWI	3 mm No gap	No specific recommendations[a]	≤ 2 mm (phase and frequency)	T1W GRE *Fat suppression and/or subtractions*	*Temporal resolution ≤ 15 s*	*GBCA:* 0.1 mmol/kg *Injection rate:* 2-3 cc/s *Observation rate > 2 min*	2D or 3D with 3D acquisitions preferred

DCE, dynamic contrast enhanced; DWI, diffusion-weighted imaging; EPI, echo planar imaging; FOV, field of view; FSE, fast spin echo; GBCA, gadolinium-based contrast agent; GRE, gradient echo; T1WI, T2-weighted imaging; TSE, turbo spin echo.
[a] To encompass the entire prostate gland and seminal vesicles.

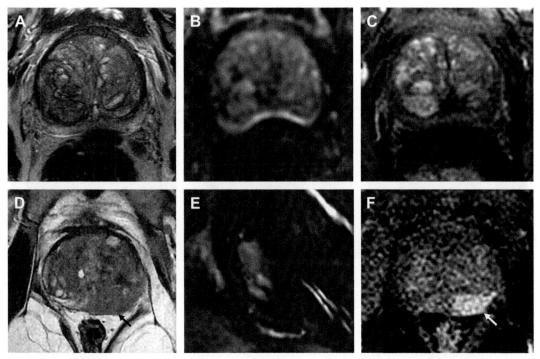

Fig. 2. DCE as a "safety net" for quality. (*A–C*) A 65 year old man, PSA 14.79 ng/mL. T2WI (*A*) is of good quality, DWI (*B*) poor quality due to susceptibility artifact, but DCE (*C*), is of good quality, overall PI-QUAL score 4, with the study able to both rule in and rule out csPCa. MR imaging reported as negative, systematic biopsy performed due to high PSA, with all cores negative. (*D–F*) An 81 year old patient, PSA 18.1 ng/mL. T2WI (*D*) shows a left-sided lesion with T3a features, DWI (*E*) is nondiagnostic due to left THR, DCE (*F*) confirms early enhancement in the lesion, PI-QUAL score 4. MR imaging reported as PI-RADS 5, biopsy on left side shows Gleason 4 + 3 = 7.

Table 2 Common artifacts and potential solutions of prostate MR imaging			
Artifact		**More Susceptible Sequence**	**Mitigating Strategies**
Motion		T2WI +++ DWI + DCE ++	Physical: Stabilization Pharmaceutical: Anti-spasmodics Sequence related: Faster scanning (parallel imaging, DLR, partial Fourier imaging) Radial acquisition (eg, PROPELLER/BLADE) Swapping phase- and frequency axes
Susceptibility	Metal	T2WI + DWI +++ DCE +	1.5 T scanning Fat-suppressed DWI Metal reduction sequences Increase receiver bandwidth Parallel image Swapping phase- and frequency axes Radial acquisition
	Air	DWI +++	Non-EPI DWI techniques Bowel preparation techniques Prone imaging
Wraparound (aliasing)		T2WI + DWI ++ DCE +	Increasing the FOV Swapping phase- and frequency axes Using surface coils
Chemical shift		DCE +	Increase receiver bandwidth Fat-suppression sequences Use of subtraction images

DCE, dynamic contract-enhanced; DLR, deep-learning-based reconstruction; DWI, diffusion-weighted imaging; EPI, echo planar imaging; FOV, field of view; T2WI, T2-weighted images.

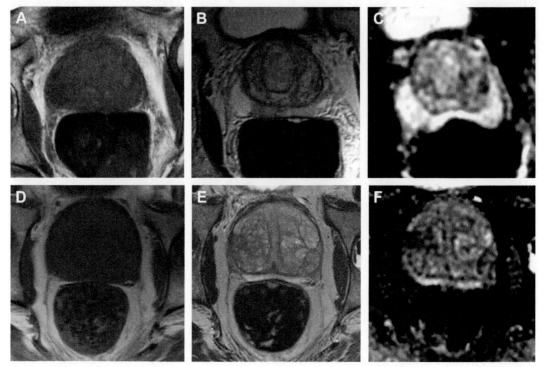

Fig. 3. Rectal distension associated artifact. (*A–C*) Patient with anteriorly located rectal air, better appreciated on T1WI (*A*), less apparent on T2 (*B*), with associated susceptibility artifact warping the posterior prostate on ADC maps (*C*). (*D–F*) Patient with rectal distension due to fecal loading, with no air level seen on T1 (*D*) or T2WI (*E*), and no artifact on ADC maps (*F*).

objects including hip protheses are a common cause of magnetic susceptibility causing signal loss, a "halo" effect, or distortion in the surrounding tissues. The severity of metalwork-related susceptibility artifact depends on the size, location, and composition of the prosthesis[4] and may be reduced by scanning at the lower field strength of 1.5 T (**Fig. 4**); however, evidence on this matter is conflicting.[62] Specific metal-reduction sequences can also be employed, for instance techniques that oversample the central portion of k-space, enabling artifacts to be corrected in the reconstruction process, reducing the susceptibility artifact seen on echo-planar imaging (EPI) DWI or the motion artifact on turbo-spin echo T2 sequences.[63–65] Alternatively, T2-mapping has also shown promise as a more robust substitute for EPI-DWI derived ADC maps for providing quantitative imaging data in patients with hip replacements.[66] Air-tissue interfaces also induce susceptibility artifact and are particularly problematic on EPI DWI sequences in the presence of rectal gas. The severity can vary from mild signal pile up at the posterior midline of the prostate, to moderate inhomogeneity causing anteroposterior displacement of the

prostate gland, through to more severe inhomogeneity producing a "warping" of the prostatic outline (**Fig. 5**).[51,67–69] Air-related susceptibility artifact can be mitigated by scanning patients in a supine position, displacing the air away from the recto-prostatic interface; however, to date improvements have not been objectively demonstrated in the literature and, in clinical practice, scheduling restrictions may be a limiting factor given the additional time needed to perform such sequences. Blooming artifact is a type of susceptibility artifact due to presence of paramagnetic substances and are particularly encountered on MR imaging sequences such as gradient echo DCE; small metallic implants in the prostate such a brachytherapy seeds or fiducial markers can demonstrate similar effects.

Acquiring DCE sequences without fat suppression is generally required when there is severe metal artifact in the pelvis; however, it can also make interpretation more challenging, due to reduced conspicuity of enhancement and presence of chemical shift artifact.[51] The chemical shift phenomenon is observed when water and lipid protons are present in the same voxel, as the protons in fat are shielded to a greater extent to those

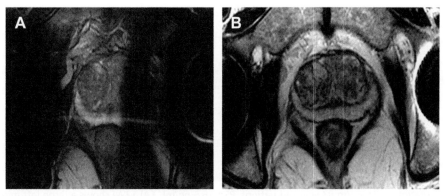

Fig. 4. THR associated artifact magnified at 3T. A 67 year old man, PSA 4.8 ng/mL. Patient has bilateral THRs, with marked artifact noted on T2WI performed at 3T (A). Repeat imaging the same day at 1.5 T (B) shows minimal susceptibility artifact and diagnostic T2 imaging.

in water, resulting in a noticeable difference in their resonant frequencies. Using fat-suppression techniques or increasing receiver bandwidth can mitigate against this artifact (Fig. 6). When fat suppression fails due to pelvic metal hardware, acquiring a subtraction series from the non-fat suppressed DCE series can be beneficial if images are adequately co-registered.

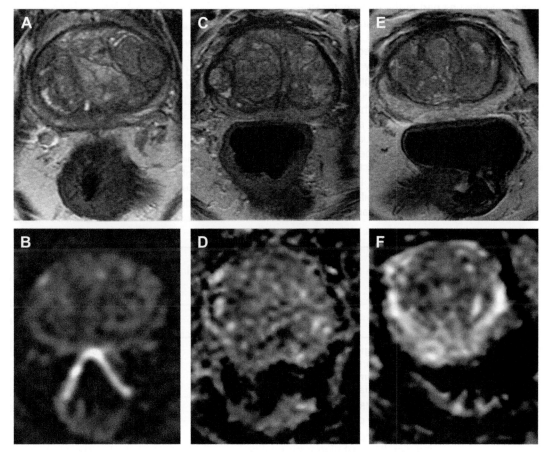

Fig. 5. Susceptibility artifact on DWI. (A, B) Mild signal pile-up at the posterior midline of the prostate on b-1400 DWI (B), with no distortion compared with T2 (A). (C, D) Moderate inhomogeneity causing anteroposterior displacement of the prostate gland <5 mm on ADC map (D) compared with T2 (C). (E, F) Severe susceptibility artifact producing a "warping" of the prostatic outline on ADC maps (E) compared with T2 (E).

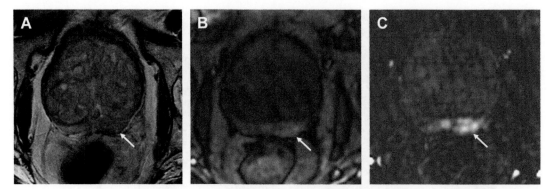

Fig. 6. Fat saturation on DCE. An 83 year old patient, PSA 16.5 ng/mL. (*A*) T2WI shows a large left mid PZ lesion with features of T3a disease (*arrow*). (*B*) DCE acquired without fat saturation and with associated chemical shift imaging (CSI) artifact on the gradient echo T1 sequence shows early enhancement, DCE "positive". (*C*) Subtraction imaging performed on the same DCE sequence minimizes the CSI and "black boundary" artifact, with increased conspicuity and CNR of the early enhancement within the lesion.

STANDARDIZED REPORTING OF IMAGE QUALITY: PROSTATE IMAGING QUALITY

The PI-QUAL scoring system was developed from imaging acquired as part of the multicenter PRE-CISION trial[6] and represents the first attempt to standardize reporting of prostate MR imaging quality. The PI-QUAL score is based on a 1 to 5 scale that indicates the adequacy of the diagnostic quality of prostate MR imaging and mandates a multiparametric examination (**Table 3**). PI-QUAL scores of 1 or 2 indicate that 2 or all sequences (ie, T2WI, DWI, and DCE) are below the minimum standard of diagnostic quality and clinically significant lesions cannot be ruled in or out. A PI-QUAL score of 3 implies that the scan is of sufficient diagnostic quality, but it is only possible to rule in all clinically significant lesions. PI-QUAL scores of 4 or 5 mean that all 3 sequences are of sufficient diagnostic quality to both rule in and rule out clinically significant lesions. The original PI-QUAL document also includes a dedicated scoring sheet that allows the evaluation of the technical parameters for each single MR sequence. A total of 20 technical parameters are evaluated across the 3 sequences, with visual assessment including clear delineation of prostatic and periprostatic structures on T2WI, identification of vessels on DCE, adequacy of ADC maps, and the absence of artifacts on all 3 sequences.[70] Growing evidence is being published on the role of the PI-QUAL score in different clinical settings and cohorts and suggests that higher PI-QUAL scores may improve the efficiency of diagnostic pathway of prostate cancer by reducing false-positive MR imaging calls and unnecessary biopsies.

Table 3
Evaluation form for scoring the quality of multiparametric MR imaging using the PI-QUAL v.1

PI-QUAL v.1 Score	Criteria	Clinical Implications: All Significant Lesions Could Be Ruled in	Ruled out
1	All mpMR imaging sequences are below the minimum standard for diagnostic quality	X	X
2	Only 1 mpMR imaging sequence is of acceptable diagnostic quality		
3	At least 2 mpMR imaging sequences taken together are of diagnostic quality	✔	X
4	Two or more mpMR imaging sequences are independently of diagnostic quality	✔	✔
5	All mpMR imaging sequences are of optimal diagnostic quality		

(*Adapted from* Ref.[17])

Brembilla and colleagues[71] investigated the impact PI-QUAL scores on the diagnostic performance in a targeted biopsy cohort of 300 patients. They observed a higher proportion of PI-RADS 3 lesions in scans with suboptimal (51%) compared with those with optimal (PI-QUAL 4–5) quality (33%). For suboptimal scans, the positive predictive value was lower compared with PI-QUAL $\geq$ 4 (35% vs 48%; P = 0.09), as was the detection rate of clinically significant prostate cancer ($\geq$Grade Group 2) in both PI-RADS 3 and PI-RADS 4 to 5 lesions (15% vs 23% and 56% vs 63%, respectively). The authors also observed that overall MR imaging quality increased over time and concluded that scan quality affects the diagnostic performance of prostate MR imaging, as scans of suboptimal quality were associated with lower positive predictive values for clinically significant prostate cancer.

Windisch and colleagues [72] compared upstaging of localized disease on mpMR imaging to locally invasive disease in radical prostatectomy specimens ($\geq$pT3a) in relation to PI-QUAL in a multicenter setting. The authors found that scans scoring PI-QUAL $\geq$ 3 were associated with a lower rate of upstaging (19% vs 35%; P = 0.02), greater detection of T3a and T3b disease on mpMR imaging (17% vs 2.5%; P = 0.016), a higher rate of PI-RADS 5 lesions (47% vs 27.5%; P = 0.002), and a higher number of PI-RADS $\geq$ 3 lesions (34.7% vs 15%; P = 0.012) when compared with scans scoring PI-QUAL 1 and 2. On multivariate analysis, PI-QUAL 1 and 2 scans were associated with more frequent upstaging at radical prostatectomy (odds ratio 3.4; P = 0.01). They concluded that PI-QUAL 1 and 2 scans were significantly associated with a higher rate of upstaging from organ-confined disease on MR Imaging to locally advanced disease on pathology, lower detection rates for PI-RADS 5 lesions and extraprostatic extension, and a lower number of suspicious lesions.

Hötker and colleagues[73] evaluated PI-QUAL to assess factors that limit the diagnostic accuracy of prostate MR imaging. The study included 4 readers with different levels of experience who independently reviewed 295 scans and assigned scores for subjective image quality (1–5; 1: poor, 5: excellent), the PI-QUAL score, and the prostate signal intensity homogeneity score (PSHS) scoring system. Both PI-QUAL and the PSHS scoring system showed good results in assessing the effect of image quality on detection rates of csPCa and the authors concluded that both scoring systems should be included in the prostate MR reports as they focus on different aspects of image quality.

The first inter-reader assessment of PI-QUAL between 2 experts in prostate MR showed a strong agreement for each single PI-QUAL score (κ = 0.85, with percent agreement = 84%).[74] Notably, the agreement for diagnostic quality for each sequence was highest for T2-WI (89%), followed by DCE (91%) and DWI (78%) sequences. However, subsequent studies demonstrated only moderate agreement between 2 independent readers, with Cohen's kappa coefficients ranging between 0.42 and 0.55.[11,75,76] This suggests that defining scan quality can be subjective in nature, and readers are likely to disagree on what entails optimal prostate MR image quality.

Prostate Imaging Quality Version 2

The current version of PI-QUAL serves as a starting point for the standardized evaluation of prostate MR imaging image quality. However, PI-QUAL can only fulfill its purpose if the scoring system has an impact on the diagnostic MR imaging-driven pathway. Like the PI-RADS guidelines, PI-QUAL is envisioned to be a "living document" that evolves with increasing clinical experience and scientific data.[77] An international working group with representatives from the European Society of Urogenital Radiology (ESUR) and EAU Section of Urologic Imaging (ESUI), among others, is working on an updated version of PI-QUAL to address its current limitations. There are 3 main concerns related to the first version of PI-QUAL.

The first limitation is the clinical implication that is automatically derived from the observed PI-QUAL score. A PI-QUAL score of 4 or 5 implicates that image quality is good enough to rule in and rule out all significant lesions, whereas this is not possible when an examination is assessed as PIQ-UAL $\leq$ 2. However, a large tumor-suspicious lesion can be detected even on a PI-QUAL 1 or 2 study (**Fig. 7**), while a small clinically significant tumor can be missed even with good-quality imaging (PI-QUAL 4–5), which a known limitation of MR imaging.[78,79] Although it is important to give recommendations on the clinical implication, these examples show that deriving these automatically from the observed PI-QUAL score may not be helpful in all clinical scenarios. A 2-step approach seems to be more appropriate: the first step should involve an assessment that evaluates image quality as objectively as possible, independent from the diagnostic findings. The second step determines the clinical impact of the observed image quality, taking into consideration the diagnostic findings, the clinical context, and the patient history. This 2-step approach should ideally be taken by the reporting radiologist and, if necessary, should also involve the opinion of the other members of the multidisciplinary team.

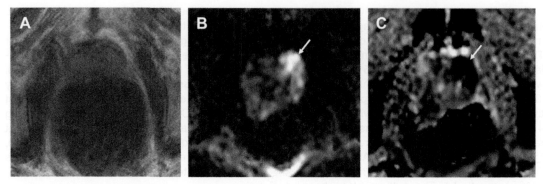

Fig. 7. PI-QUAL score 1 but able to rule in csPCa. A 76 year old man, PSA 27.22 ng/mL. (*A*) Claustrophobic patient with bulk motion, and additional rectal loading with spasm making T2WI nondiagnostic. (*B, C*) DWI shows susceptibility artifact but identifies a clear lesion on the left mid anterior TZ/PZ (*arrows*) with high signal on b-1400 (*B*) and low ADC (*C*). Study abandoned without DCE due to patient tolerance. PI-QUAL equivalent score 1 (allowing for no DCE acquisition). High probability lesion reported (ie, "rule in" ability of the study was preserved), targeted biopsy showed Gleason 4 + 4 = 8 lesion in the left anterior mid gland.

The potential outcome of this (multidisciplinary) decision could for instance be to repeat (a part of) the MR examination, take no further action, or proceed straight to biopsy.

The second limitation that will be addressed in future iterations of PI-QUAL refers to the technical recommendations derived from the PI-RADS v2.1 guidelines. Adoption of PI-QUAL v1 may be hindered due to the complexity of the 20 technical parameters it contains. Conformity will not necessarily guarantee good quality, and acquiring T2WI with an in-plane resolution of 0.7 × 0.5 mm rather than 0.7 × 0.4 mm will have minimal effect on quality, particularly when juxtaposed to the presence significant motion artifact at visual assessment. For widespread adoption, PI-QUAL needs to be as straightforward as possible. Therefore, in future iterations of PI-QUAL, suboptimal image quality should be identified if noncompliant with only basic rather than detailed technical PI-RADS parameters.

The final factor to consider is that in future versions of PI-QUAL one should be able to apply the scoring system on bpMR imaging. The current version of PI-QUAL applies to mpMR imaging only, but due to rising interest in bpMR imaging, especially in low prevalence (screening) situations, the PI-QUAL system should be amended to allow for both bpMR imaging and mpMR imaging quality scoring.

After addressing these limitations, PI-QUAL will strengthen its role as a reliable quality assessment tool and safeguard the quality of MR imaging at the start of the diagnostic pathway. Future reproducibility and generalizability studies are required to evaluate its inter- and intra-reader agreement to establish PI-QUAL as the international standard for assessment of prostate MR image quality.

FUTURE IMPROVEMENTS IN MR IMAGE QUALITY

Future improvements in magnet hardware and coil design alongside novel sequence development and software updates, including AI solutions, would be expected to improve image quality. According to the current PI-RADS guidelines, high b-value ($b \geq 1400$ s/mm^2) DWI can be obtained either as an acquired or calculated sequence. Calculated b-values offer higher SNR by avoiding the noise penalty of acquiring DWI at higher b-values with longer echo times, and clearly save on scanning time, thus breaking the "MR imaging triangle". Several articles have suggested that using calculated high b-value DWI can result in higher image quality and improved image contrast.[80–83] Single-shot EPI has been widely used in acquiring clinical DWI due to its rapid acquisition capabilities. However, it is important to acknowledge some of the limitations associated with single-shot EPI, which include vulnerability to susceptibility artifacts, ghosting artifacts from poor fat suppression of the anterior abdominal wall, relatively low SNR, and blurring. Novel DWI techniques can potentially improve the image quality of DWI. One such technique involves using reverse polarity gradient methods, where images at $b = 0$ s/mm^2 are acquired using both forward and reverse phase encode trajectories. By calculating a deformation field map, the entire diffusion data set can be corrected for distortion.[84–86] Additionally, multi-shot EPI has been proposed as an alternative to single-shot EPI, aiming to enhance the quality of acquired images. Several segmented techniques have been devised for multi-shot EPI, such as MUSE by GE Healthcare and RESOLVE by

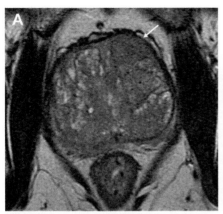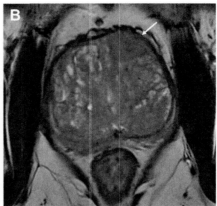

Fig. 8. DLR denoising showing an oversmoothed TZ lesion. A 73 year old, PSA 10.38 ng/mL, gland volume 105 cm³. (A) Original FRFSE T2-weighted image shows a 15 × 12 mm BPH nodule in the left anterior TZ which is mostly encapsulated (*arrow*); PI-RADS score 2. (B) T2 image with application of high DLR resulting in a "smoothed" homogeneous, moderately hypointense appearance to the nodule and with no margination; PI-RADS score 3. Systematic transperineal biopsy performed, with all cores benign.

Siemens and can achieve improved SNR, reduced susceptibility artifacts, and minimized blurring within an acceptable scanning time.[87] DWI sequences with reduced FOV are more routinely available in clinical practice and have been shown to improve image distortion at the recto-prostatic interface by allowing for higher spatial resolution and a shorter echo-train length in the phase-encoding direction.[88,89] Deep learning-based reconstruction (DLR) is a commercially available AI technique that has shown promise in maintaining/enhancing image quality while substantially reducing acquisition time.[90–95] DLR is a post-processing step that applies a "de-noising" algorithm, therefore allowing for deliberate acquisition of "noisy" images, which can either enable quicker scans times or sequences with reduced slice thickness. The reduction in scan time offered by DLR can enhance accessibility to prostate MR imaging, improve patient comfort, and mitigate against motion artifacts.[4,96] However, it is worth noting that DLR software typically provides differing levels of denoising, and applying higher levels may risk "over smoothing" images which and lead to false positive results, particularly in the TZ (Fig. 8). Therefore, effective implementation of DLR into clinical practice requires evaluation of the optimal scanning parameters in conjunction with the optimal DLR denoising level.

AI applications may also have a future role in the assessment of MR image quality. Manually verifying the Digital Imaging and Communications in Medicine (DICOM) headers of prostate MR imaging studies for compliance with PI-RADS technical parameters is arduous, ideally suited to a software tool that can perform this quickly and automatically. Likewise, PI-QUAL scoring is time-consuming and semi-automated workflows to reduce the time have been proposed, however, these remain subjective with only moderate inter-reader agreement.[97] There is a clear need for a software solution that can evaluate prostate MR image quality in a simpler and more objective way. Cipollari and colleagues[98] developed a convolutional neural network-based analysis tool that could accurately classify prostate MR imaging quality into a binary category of "low" or "high" quality compared to expert radiologist opinion. Nevertheless, more complex software that can evaluate multi-category PI-QUAL scoring is yet to be developed. An AI-based tool to assess image quality offers several advantages including time savings and standardization. Future iterations may enable integration into the MR imaging system with automatic assessments of image quality, flagging any sequences that require repeat acquisition and potentially suggesting relevant parameter changes. Advice on the need for contrast injection may also be feasible to decide if DCE acquisition is necessary for lesion detection or as a safety net for the overall quality of the study. Such an application may minimize the need for patient recalls, a decision often made at a much later time point, when reporting.

SUMMARY

Prostate MR imaging is now integral to the prostate cancer diagnostic pathway, driven by hardware and software developments improving image quality, with all downstream aspects of the diagnostic work-up being reliant on the first step of MR imaging acquisition. PI-RADS provides a menu of minimal technical parameters; however, adherence alone does not guarantee high-quality imaging and will not account for patient-related factors. AI solutions can currently be applied as a post-processing step for increasing SNR, and future developments may enable on-table monitoring of image quality and identification of sequences that require repeating or parameter adjustments. The PI-QUAL system represents the first attempt to provide an objective assessment of image quality and PI-QUAL version 2 will aim to further improve on this process; however, further validation is required to ensure its clinical effectiveness.

ACKNOWLEDGMENTS

This research was supported by the NIHR Cambridge Biomedical Research Centre, United Kingdom (NIHR203312). The views expressed are those of the authors and not necessarily those of the NIHR or the Department of Health and Social Care. The authors also acknowledge support from Cancer Research UK, United Kingdom (Cambridge Imaging Centre grant number C197/A16465), the Engineering and Physical Sciences Research Council Imaging Centre in Cambridge and Manchester, and the Cambridge Experimental Cancer Medicine Centre. F Giganti is a recipient of the 2020 Young Investigator Award (20YOUN15) funded by the Prostate Cancer Foundation, United States/CRIS Cancer Foundation. F Giganti reports consulting fees from Lucida Medical LTD outside of the submitted work. The authors would like to thank Dimitri Alexander Kessler for his MR physics input.

DISCLOSURE

All authors declare no conflict of interests and competing interests relevant to the manuscript.

FUNDING

FG is a recipient of the 2020 Young Investigator Award (20YOUN15) funded by the Prostate Cancer Foundation / CRIS Cancer Foundation. FG reports consulting fees from Lucida Medical LTD outside of the submitted work.

REFERENCES

1. Steyn JH, Smith FW. Nuclear magnetic resonance imaging of the prostate. Br J Urol 1982;54(6):726–8.
2. Schnall MD, Lenkinski RE, Pollack HM, et al. Prostate: MR imaging with an endorectal surface coil. Radiology 1989;172(2):570–4.
3. Edelman RR. The history of MR imaging as seen through the pages of radiology. Radiology 2014; 273(2 Suppl):S181–200.
4. Lin Y, Yilmaz EC, Belue MJ, et al. Prostate MRI and image Quality: It is time to take stock. Eur J Radiol 2023;161:110757.
5. Ahmed HU, El-Shater Bosaily A, Brown LC, et al. Diagnostic accuracy of multi-parametric MRI and TRUS biopsy in prostate cancer (PROMIS): a paired validating confirmatory study. Lancet 2017;389(10071): 815–22.
6. Kasivisvanathan V, Rannikko AS, Borghi M, et al. MRI-Targeted or Standard Biopsy for Prostate-Cancer Diagnosis. N Engl J Med 2018;378(19): 1767–77.
7. Rouviere O, Puech P, Renard-Penna R, et al. Use of prostate systematic and targeted biopsy on the basis of multiparametric MRI in biopsy-naive patients (MRI-FIRST): a prospective, multicentre, paired diagnostic study. Lancet Oncol 2019;20(1):100–9.
8. van der Leest M, Cornel E, Israel B, et al. Head-to-head comparison of transrectal ultrasound-guided prostate biopsy versus multiparametric prostate resonance imaging with subsequent magnetic resonance-guided biopsy in biopsy-naive men with elevated prostate-specific antigen: a large prospective multicenter clinical study. Eur Urol 2019;75(4):570–8.
9. Drost FH, Osses D, Nieboer D, et al. Prostate magnetic resonance imaging, with or without magnetic resonance imaging-targeted biopsy, and systematic biopsy for detecting prostate cancer: a cochrane systematic review and meta-analysis. Eur Urol 2020;77(1):78–94.
10. Padhani AR, Barentsz J, Villeirs G, et al. PI-RADS steering committee: the PI-RADS multiparametric MRI and MRI-directed biopsy pathway. Radiology 2019;292(2):464–74.
11. Karanasios E, Caglic I, Zawaideh JP, et al. Prostate MRI quality: clinical impact of the PI-QUAL score in prostate cancer diagnostic work-up. Br J Radiol 2022;95(1133):20211372.
12. Turkbey B, Rosenkrantz AB, Haider MA, et al. prostate imaging reporting and data system version 2.1: 2019 update of prostate imaging reporting and data system version 2. Eur Urol 2019;76(3):340–51.
13. Burn PR, Freeman SJ, Andreou A, et al. A multicentre assessment of prostate MRI quality and compliance with UK and international standards. Clin Radiol 2019;74(11):894 e19.
14. Sackett J, Shih JH, Reese SE, et al. Quality of prostate MRI: Is the PI-RADS Standard Sufficient? Acad Radiol 2021;28(2):199–207.
15. Giganti F, Kasivisvanathan V, Kirkham A, et al. Prostate MRI quality: a critical review of the last 5 years and the role of the PI-QUAL score. Br J Radiol 2022;95(1131):20210415.
16. Barrett T, de Rooij M, Giganti F, et al. Quality checkpoints in the MRI-directed prostate cancer diagnostic pathway. Nat Rev Urol 2023;20(1):9–22.
17. de Rooij M, Israel B, Barrett T, et al. Focus on the quality of prostate multiparametric magnetic resonance

imaging: synopsis of the ESUR/ESUI recommendations on quality assessment and interpretation of images and radiologists' training. Eur Urol 2020; 78(4):483–5.

18. Giganti F, Allen C, Emberton M, et al. Prostate imaging quality (PI-QUAL): a new quality control scoring system for multiparametric magnetic resonance imaging of the prostate from the PRECISION trial. Eur Urol Oncol 2020;3(5):615–9.

19. Weigel M. Image quality. Presented at. Paris, France: ISMRM; 2018. https://cds.ismrm.org/protected/18M Proceedings/PDFfiles/E1309.html.

20. Barrett T, Vargas HA, Akin O, et al. Value of the hemorrhage exclusion sign on T1-weighted prostate MR images for the detection of prostate cancer. Radiology 2012;263(3):751–7.

21. Kale SC, Chen XJ, Henkelman RM. Trading off SNR and resolution in MR images. NMR Biomed 2009; 22(5):488–94.

22. Abreu-Gomez J, Isupov I, McInnes M, et al. Multiparametric magnetic resonance imaging of the prostate at 1.5-Tesla without endorectal coil: Can it be used to detect clinically significant prostate cancer in men with medical devices that are contraindicated at 3-Tesla? Can Urol Assoc J 2021;15(3): E180–3.

23. Ullrich T, Kohli MD, Ohliger MA, et al. Quality Comparison of 3 Tesla multiparametric MRI of the prostate using a flexible surface receiver coil versus conventional surface coil plus endorectal coil setup. Abdom Radiol (NY) 2020;45(12):4260–70.

24. O'Donohoe RL, Dunne RM, Kimbrell V, et al. Prostate MRI using an external phased array wearable pelvic coil at 3T: comparison with an endorectal coil. Abdom Radiol (NY) 2019;44(3):1062–9.

25. Mazaheri Y, Vargas HA, Nyman G, et al. Diffusion-weighted MRI of the prostate at 3.0 T: comparison of endorectal coil (ERC) MRI and phased-array coil (PAC) MRI-The impact of SNR on ADC measurement. Eur J Radiol 2013;82(10):e515–20.

26. de Rooij M, Hamoen EH, Witjes JA, et al. Accuracy of magnetic resonance imaging for local staging of prostate cancer: a diagnostic meta-analysis. Eur Urol 2016;70(2):233–45.

27. Abreu-Gomez J, Shabana W, McInnes MDF, et al. Regional Standardization of Prostate Multiparametric MRI Performance and Reporting: Is There a Role for a Director of Prostate Imaging? AJR Am J Roentgenol 2019;213(4):844–50.

28. Leest MV, Israel B, Engels RRM, et al. Reply to Arnaldo Stanzione, Massimo Imbriaco, and Renato Cuocolo's Letter to the Editor re: Marloes van der Leest, Bas Israel, Eric Bastiaan Cornel, et al. High Diagnostic Performance of Short Magnetic Resonance Imaging Protocols for Prostate Cancer Detection in Biopsy-naive Men: The Next Step in Magnetic

Resonance Imaging Accessibility. Eur Urol 2019;76: 574–81.

29. Are We Meeting Our Standards? Stringent Prostate Imaging Reporting and Data System Acquisition Requirements Might be Limiting Prostate Accessibility. Eur Urol 2020;77(3):e58–581.

30. Papoutsaki MV, Allen C, Giganti F, et al. Standardisation of prostate multiparametric MRI across a hospital network: a London experience. Insights Imaging 2021;12(1):52.

31. Zawaideh JP, Sala E, Shaida N, et al. Diagnostic accuracy of biparametric versus multiparametric prostate MRI: assessment of contrast benefit in clinical practice. Eur Radiol 2020;30(7):4039–49.

32. Kuhl CK, Bruhn R, Kramer N, et al. Abbreviated biparametric prostate MR imaging in men with elevated prostate-specific antigen. Radiology 2017;285(2): 493–505.

33. Asif A, Nathan A, Ng A, et al. Comparing biparametric to multiparametric MRI in the diagnosis of clinically significant prostate cancer in biopsy-naive men (PRIME): a prospective, international, multicentre, non-inferiority within-patient, diagnostic yield trial protocol. BMJ Open 2023;13(4):e070280.

34. Imperial Prostate 7 - Prostate Assessment Using Comparative Interventions - Fast Mri and Image-fusion for Cancer (IP7-PACIFIC). Available at: https:// clinicaltrials.gov/ct2/show/NCT05574647. Accessed May 24, 2023.

35. Belue MJ, Yilmaz EC, Daryanani A, et al. Current Status of Biparametric MRI in Prostate Cancer Diagnosis: Literature Analysis. Life 2022;12(6). https:// doi.org/10.3390/life12060804.

36. Schoots IG, Barentsz JO, Bittencourt LK, et al. PI-RADS Committee position on MRI without contrast medium in biopsy-naive men with suspected prostate cancer: narrative review. AJR Am J Roentgenol 2021;216(1):3–19.

37. Bhayana R, O'Shea A, Anderson MA, et al. PI-RADS Versions 2 and 2.1: interobserver agreement and diagnostic performance in peripheral and transition zone lesions among six radiologists. AJR Am J Roentgenol 2021;217(1):141–51.

38. Brancato V, Di Costanzo G, Basso L, et al. Assessment of DCE Utility for PCa Diagnosis Using PI-RADS v2.1: Effects on Diagnostic Accuracy and Reproducibility. Diagnostics (Basel) 2020;10(3). https://doi.org/10.3390/diagnostics10030164.

39. Wen J, Ji Y, Han J, et al. Inter-reader agreement of the prostate imaging reporting and data system version v2.1 for detection of prostate cancer: A systematic review and meta-analysis. Front Oncol 2022; 12:1013941.

40. Lee CH, Vellayappan B, Tan CH. Comparison of diagnostic performance and inter-reader agreement between PI-RADS v2.1 and PI-RADS v2: systematic

review and meta-analysis. Br J Radiol 2022; 95(1131):20210509.

41. Smith CP, Harmon SA, Barrett T, et al. Intra- and interreader reproducibility of PI-RADSv2: A multireader study. J Magn Reson Imaging 2019;49(6): 1694–703.

42. Bazargani S, Bandyk M, Balaji KC. Variability of the Positive Predictive Value of PI-RADS for Prostate MRI across 26 Centers: What about the Negatives? Radiology 2021;298(1):E57.

43. Barrett T, Ghafoor S, Gupta RT, et al. Prostate MRI qualification: AJR Expert Panel Narrative Review. AJR Am J Roentgenol 2022;219(5):691–702.

44. Tan N, Lakshmi M, Hernandez D, et al. Upcoming American College of Radiology prostate MRI designation launching: what to expect. Abdom Radiol (NY) 2020;45(12):4109–11.

45. Gatti M, Faletti R, Calleris G, et al. Prostate cancer detection with biparametric magnetic resonance imaging (bpMRI) by readers with different experience: performance and comparison with multiparametric (mpMRI). Abdom Radiol (NY) 2019;44(5):1883–93.

46. Gaziev G, Wadhwa K, Barrett T, et al. Defining the learning curve for multiparametric magnetic resonance imaging (MRI) of the prostate using MRI-transrectal ultrasonography (TRUS) fusion-guided transperineal prostate biopsies as a validation tool. BJU Int 2016;117(1):80–6.

47. de Rooij M, Israel B, Tummers M, et al. ESUR/ESUI consensus statements on multi-parametric MRI for the detection of clinically significant prostate cancer: quality requirements for image acquisition, interpretation and radiologists' training. Eur Radiol 2020; 30(10):5404–16.

48. Barrett T, Padhani AR, Patel A, et al. Certification in reporting multiparametric magnetic resonance imaging of the prostate: recommendations of a UK consensus meeting. BJU Int 2021;127(3):304–6.

49. German Radiological Society Website. Certification mpMRI of the prostate. www.ag-uro.drg.de/de-DE/4285/zertifizierung/.

50. Wood ML, Henkelman RM. MR image artifacts from periodic motion. Med Phys 1985;12(2):143–51.

51. Zhuo J, Gullapalli RP. AAPM/RSNA physics tutorial for residents: MR artifacts, safety, and quality control. Radiographics 2006;26(1):275–97.

52. Zaitsev M, Maclaren J, Herbst M. Motion artifacts in MRI: A complex problem with many partial solutions. J Magn Reson Imaging 2015;42(4):887–901.

53. Caglic I, Hansen NL, Slough RA, et al. Evaluating the effect of rectal distension on prostate multiparametric MRI image quality. Eur J Radiol 2017;90:174–80.

54. Arnoldner MA, Polanec SH, Lazar M, et al. Rectal preparation significantly improves prostate imaging quality: Assessment of the PI-QUAL score with visual grading characteristics. Eur J Radiol 2022; 147:110145.

55. Coskun M, Mehralivand S, Shih JH, et al. Impact of bowel preparation with Fleet's enema on prostate MRI quality. Abdom Radiol (NY) 2020;45(12):4252–9.

56. Slough RA, Caglic I, Hansen NL, et al. Effect of hyoscine butylbromide on prostate multiparametric MRI anatomical and functional image quality. Clin Radiol 2018;73(2):216 e9.

57. Caglic I, Barrett T. Optimising prostate mpMRI: prepare for success. Clin Radiol 2019;74(11):831–40.

58. Purysko AS, Mielke N, Bullen J, et al. Influence of Enema and Dietary Restrictions on Prostate MR Image Quality: A Multireader Study. Acad Radiol 2022;29(1):4–14.

59. Reischauer C, Cancelli T, Malekzadeh S, et al. How to improve image quality of DWI of the prostate-enema or catheter preparation? Eur Radiol 2021; 31(9):6708–16.

60. Prabhakar S, Schieda N. Patient preparation for prostate MRI: A scoping review. Eur J Radiol 2023;162: 110758.

61. Barrett T, Rajesh A, Rosenkrantz AB, et al. PI-RADS version 2.1: one small step for prostate MRI. Clin Radiol 2019;74(11):841–52.

62. Boschheidgen M, Ullrich T, Blondin D, et al. Comparison and prediction of artefact severity due to total hip replacement in 1.5 T versus 3 T MRI of the prostate. Eur J Radiol 2021;144:109949.

63. Czarniecki M, Caglic I, Grist JT, et al. Role of PROPELLER-DWI of the prostate in reducing distortion and artefact from total hip replacement metalwork. Eur J Radiol 2018;102:213–9.

64. Czyzewska D, Sushentsev N, Latoch E, et al. T2-PROPELLER Compared to T2-FRFSE for Image Quality and Lesion Detection at Prostate MRI. Can Assoc Radiol J 2022;73(2):355–61.

65. Meier-Schroers M, Marx C, Schmeel FC, et al. Revised PROPELLER for T2-weighted imaging of the prostate at 3 Tesla: impact on lesion detection and PI-RADS classification. Eur Radiol 2018;28(1):24–30.

66. Sathiadoss P, Schieda N, Haroon M, et al. Utility of Quantitative T2-Mapping Compared to Conventional and Advanced Diffusion Weighted Imaging Techniques for Multiparametric Prostate MRI in Men with Hip Prosthesis. J Magn Reson Imaging 2022;55(1):265–74.

67. Hargreaves BA, Worters PW, Pauly KB, et al. Metal-induced artifacts in MRI. AJR Am J Roentgenol 2011;197(3):547–55.

68. Lee EM, Ibrahim EH, Dudek N, et al. Improving MR Image Quality in Patients with Metallic Implants. Radiographics 2021;41(4):E126–37.

69. Gill AB, Czarniecki M, Gallagher FA, et al. A method for mapping and quantifying whole organ diffusion-weighted image distortion in MR imaging of the prostate. Sci Rep 2017;7(1):12727.

70. Giganti F, Kirkham A, Kasivisvanathan V, et al. Understanding PI-QUAL for prostate MRI quality: a practical primer for radiologists. Insights Imaging 2021;12(1):59.

71. Brembilla G, Lavalle S, Parry T, et al. Impact of prostate imaging quality (PI-QUAL) score on the detection of clinically significant prostate cancer at biopsy. Eur J Radiol 2023;164:110849.

72. Windisch O, Benamran D, Dariane C, et al. Role of the prostate imaging quality PI-QUAL score for prostate magnetic resonance image quality in pathological upstaging after radical prostatectomy: a multicentre european study. Eur Urol Open Sci 2023;47:94–101.

73. Hotker AM, Njoh S, Hofer LJ, et al. Multi-reader evaluation of different image quality scoring systems in prostate MRI. Eur J Radiol 2023;161:110733.

74. Giganti F, Dinneen E, Kasivisvanathan V, et al. Inter-reader agreement of the PI-QUAL score for prostate MRI quality in the NeuroSAFE PROOF trial. Eur Radiol 2022;32(2):879–89.

75. Girometti R, Blandino A, Zichichi C, et al. Inter-reader agreement of the Prostate Imaging Quality (PI-QUAL) score: a bicentric study. Eur J Radiol 2022;150:110267.

76. Potsch N, Rainer E, Clauser P, et al. Impact of PI-QUAL on PI-RADS and cancer yield in an MRI-TRUS fusion biopsy population. Eur J Radiol 2022;154:110431.

77. de Rooij M, Barentsz JO, PI-QUAL v. 1: the first step towards good-quality prostate MRI. Eur Radiol 2022; 32(2):876–8.

78. Serrao EM, Barrett T, Wadhwa K, et al. Investigating the ability of multiparametric MRI to exclude significant prostate cancer prior to transperineal biopsy. Can Urol Assoc J 2015;9(11–12):E853–8.

79. Schouten MG, van der Leest M, Pokorny M, et al. Why and where do we miss significant prostate cancer with multi-parametric magnetic resonance imaging followed by magnetic resonance-guided and transrectal ultrasound-guided biopsy in biopsy-naive men? Eur Urol 2017;71(6):896–903.

80. Kordbacheh H, Seethamraju RT, Weiland E, et al. Image quality and diagnostic accuracy of complex-averaged high b value images in diffusion-weighted MRI of prostate cancer. Abdom Radiol (NY) 2019;44(6):2244–53.

81. Jendoubi S, Wagner M, Montagne S, et al. MRI for prostate cancer: can computed high b-value DWI replace native acquisitions? Eur Radiol 2019; 29(10):5197–204.

82. Rosenkrantz AB, Chandarana H, Hindman N, et al. Computed diffusion-weighted imaging of the prostate at 3 T: impact on image quality and tumour detection. Eur Radiol 2013;23(11):3170–7.

83. Bittencourt LK, Attenberger UI, Lima D, et al. Feasibility study of computed vs measured high b-value (1400 s/mm(2)) diffusion-weighted MR images of the prostate. World J Radiol 2014;6(6):374–80.

84. Rakow-Penner RA, White NS, Margolis DJA, et al. Prostate diffusion imaging with distortion correction. Magn Reson Imaging 2015;33(9):1178–81.

85. Holland D, Kuperman JM, Dale AM. Efficient correction of inhomogeneous static magnetic field-induced distortion in echo planar imaging. Neuroimage 2010; 50(1):175–83.

86. Digma LA, Feng CH, Conlin CC, et al. Correcting B(0) inhomogeneity-induced distortions in whole-body diffusion MRI of bone. Sci Rep 2022;12(1):265.

87. Wu W, Miller KL. Image formation in diffusion MRI: a review of recent technical developments. J Magn Reson Imaging 2017;46(3):646–62.

88. Korn N, Kurhanewicz J, Banerjee S, et al. Reduced-FOV excitation decreases susceptibility artifact in diffusion-weighted MRI with endorectal coil for prostate cancer detection. Magn Reson Imaging 2015;33(1):56–62.

89. Lawrence EM, Zhang Y, Starekova J, et al. Reduced field-of-view and multi-shot DWI acquisition techniques: Prospective evaluation of image quality and distortion reduction in prostate cancer imaging. Magn Reson Imaging 2022;93:108–14.

90. Ueda T, Ohno Y, Yamamoto K, et al. Deep learning reconstruction of diffusion-weighted MRI improves image quality for prostatic imaging. Radiology 2022;303(2):373–81.

91. Johnson PM, Tong A, Donthireddy A, et al. Deep Learning Reconstruction Enables Highly Accelerated Biparametric MR Imaging of the Prostate. J Magn Reson Imaging 2022;56(1):184–95.

92. Wang X, Ma J, Bhosale P, et al. Novel deep learning-based noise reduction technique for prostate magnetic resonance imaging. Abdom Radiol (NY) 2021; 46(7):3378–86.

93. Kim EH, Choi MH, Lee YJ, et al. Deep learning-accelerated T2-weighted imaging of the prostate: Impact of further acceleration with lower spatial resolution on image quality. Eur J Radiol 2021;145:110012.

94. Gassenmaier S, Afat S, Nickel MD, et al. Accelerated T2-weighted TSE imaging of the prostate using deep learning image reconstruction: a prospective comparison with standard T2-weighted TSE imaging. Cancers 2021;13(14). https://doi.org/10.3390/cancers13143593.

95. Gassenmaier S, Afat S, Nickel D, et al. Deep learning-accelerated T2-weighted imaging of the prostate: reduction of acquisition time and improvement of image quality. Eur J Radiol 2021;137:109600.

96. Gassenmaier S, Kustner T, Nickel D, et al. Deep learning applications in magnetic resonance imaging: has the future become present? Diagnostics 2021;11(12). https://doi.org/10.3390/diagnostics11122181.

97. Giganti F, Lindner S, Piper JW, et al. Multiparametric prostate MRI quality assessment using a semi-automated PI-QUAL software program. Eur Radiol Exp 2021;5(1):48.

98. Cipollari S, Guarrasi V, Pecoraro M, et al. Convolutional neural networks for automated classification of prostate multiparametric magnetic resonance imaging based on image quality. J Magn Reson Imaging 2022;55(2):480–90.

Interpretation of Prostate Magnetic Resonance Imaging Using Prostate Imaging and Data Reporting System Version 2.1: A Primer

Benjamin Spilseth, MD, MBA[a],*, Daniel J.A. Margolis, MD[b],
Rajan T. Gupta, MD[c,d], Silvia D. Chang, MD[e]

KEYWORDS

- Prostate MRI • PI-RADS • Prostate cancer • Cancer detection • Staging

KEY POINTS

- PI-RADS v2.1 application requires making assessments ranging from 1 to 5 on T2WI and DWI and binary assessments on DCE images.
- These assessments are then used to generate an overall assessment that is based primarily on the DWI assessment in the peripheral zone and the T2WI assessment on the transition zone.
- Lesion identification for further characterization involves finding foci that differ from background and have suspicious features on any sequence, not only the dominant sequence used for characterization.
- PI-RADS v2.1 clarifies anterior fibromuscular stroma lesion assessments, which should be performed according to the zone where the cancer most likely arose.
- Increased or asymmetric early enhancement or signal on high b-value DWI series is key to identifying cancer in the central zone.

INTRODUCTION

In the past decade, prostate MRI has proven itself to be of immense value in identifying and targeting malignancy[1] and has appropriately seen incredible growth in usage and interest as it has become incorporated into management models for prostate cancer.[2] As usage grew, it became clear that a standard terminology was needed to describe the findings, and the PI-RADS framework has been extremely successful in filling that need, now becoming by far the most common method of reporting prostate MRI results.[3] Originally developed in 2011 in an initiative by the European Society of Urogenital Radiology,[4] it has since gone through additional iterations with the most recent version 2.1 guidelines developed in 2019 through an international collaboration with the American College of Radiology and the AdMeTech foundation.[5,6] The latest iteration covers many

The authors report *no disclosure* which directly pertain to the content of the article.
[a] Department of Radiology, University of Minnesota Medical School, MMC 292420, Delaware Street, Minneapolis, MN 55455, USA; [b] Weill Cornell Medical College, Department of Radiology, 525 East 68th Street, Box 141, New York, NY 10068, USA; [c] Department of Radiology, Duke University Medical Center, Duke Cancer Institute Center for Prostate & Urologic Cancers, DUMC Box 3808, Durham, NC 27710, USA; [d] Department of Surgery, Duke University Medical Center, Duke Cancer Institute Center for Prostate & Urologic Cancers, DUMC Box 3808, Durham, NC 27710, USA; [e] Department of Radiology, University of British Columbia, Vancouver General Hospital, 899 West 12th Avenue, Vancouver B.C., Canada V5M 1M9
* Corresponding author. University of Minnesota, Department of Radiology, MMC 292420, Delaware Street, Minneapolis, MN 55455.
E-mail address: Spil0042@umn.edu

aspects of prostate MRI, including technical parameters, interpretation and reporting guidance, and preferred terminology. The goal of this article is to provide an overview of PI-RADS v2.1, including the key details needed for anyone to begin applying the system, as well as its current role, limitations, and documented validity. We hope for this to serve as the ideal first resource for those unfamiliar with PI-RADS, as well as a useful resource for advanced users to aid adherence to the guidelines.

PROSTATE IMAGING AND DATA REPORTING SYSTEM VERSION 2.1

At its core, the PI-RADS assessment system is designed to risk stratify observations made on prostate MRI. The goal is to identify the risk of clinically significant prostate cancer (csPCa), defined as a tumor with Gleason score $\geq 3 + 4$ (grade group ≥ 2), tumor volume ≥ 0.5 mL, or invasive tumor behavior such as extraprostatic extension (EPE). To achieve this, PI-RADS uses a scale extending from 1 to 5, with an increased risk of significant cancer with higher numerical assessments as later in discussion:

PI-RADS 1 – Very low risk (csPCa is highly unlikely to be present).

PI-RADS 2 – Low risk (csPCa is unlikely to be present).

PI-RADS 3 – Intermediate risk (the presence of csPCa is equivocal).

PI-RADS 4 – High risk (csPCa is likely to be present).

PI-RADS 5 – Very high risk (csPCa is highly likely to be present).

To arrive at a final PI-RADS risk assessment, individual assessments are first made on T2-weighted imaging (T2WI) and diffusion-weighted imaging (DWI) sequences using a 1-5 scale, as well as on dynamic contrast-enhanced (DCE) sequences in a binary manner (ie, positive vs. negative). The method of making these zonal-specific cancer risk assessments will be covered in detail, as well as the algorithm for using them to arrive at a final PI-RADS overall assessment.

In addition to this core purpose, PI-RADS attempts to guide prostate MRI performance and interpretation in many other ways, including providing detailed technical image acquisition parameters, volume measurement guidance, and a detailed sector map for locating findings. In this article, we focus on interpretation and reporting components, as the technical parameters are discussed elsewhere in this issue.

PI-RADS is appropriate for use in most settings where cancer detection, staging, or monitoring is performed, though there are situations when it does not apply. It requires T2WI sequences in the axial plane and at least one additional orthogonal plane (sagittal or coronal). It should generally be performed with DWI and DCE as well, though if at least one of these sequences is performed, a modified PI-RADS algorithm can be used.

In patients with prior hormonal or radiation therapy, the appearance of prostate malignancy changes substantially, and PI-RADS is not designed for use in these settings. Similarly, after prostatectomy, PI-RADS algorithms do not apply, and early contrast enhancement is much more important for determining the likelihood of disease recurrence. In regions of the prostate subjected to focal therapy, PI-RADS is also not validated and interpretation will depend on the type of therapy, timing after therapy, and careful inspection of changes at the site of prior treatment.

PROSTATE IMAGING AND DATA REPORTING SYSTEM INTERPRETATION
Relevant anatomy

The prostate anatomy is best visualized on the T2WI series, often referred to as the anatomic series. In PI-RADS, the prostate is divided into thirds: the cranially situated base abutting the bladder and proximal urethra; the midgland; and the apex, which surrounds the distal prostatic urethra extending to the external urethral sphincter (US). Prostate volume is an important metric and should be included in MRI reports. PI-RADS v2.1 specifically outlines the method of reporting, which is done using transverse measurements obtained on axial images, and longitudinal and anterior-posterior (AP) dimensions measured on sagittal images (Fig. 1). Volume is then reported in cc using the modified ellipsoid formula: (transverse x longitudinal x AP) * 0.52.

The prostate is not a homogeneous organ, and is typically characterized by zonal anatomy consisting of the peripheral, transition, and central zones as well as the anterior fibromuscular stroma (AFS). Each of these is easily identified on MR (Figs. 2 and 3) and characterized differently in the PI-RADS framework.[7] The aptly named peripheral zone (PZ) is located in the outermost prostate and is seen circumferentially at the apex and in the posterior and lateral aspects at the base. The PZ encompasses 70% of the prostate in younger males, and is the location of 70-80% of prostatic malignancies.[8,9] It is characterized by its homogeneous intense T2W signal extending from the surgical capsule centrally to the prostatic capsule peripherally, both of which are fibrous bands of tissue that are dark on T2WI. Inside the surgical

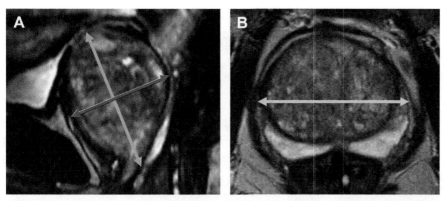

Fig. 1. *Volume measurements.* (*A*) Sagittal T2WI. PI-RADS v2.1 specifies that the craniocaudal (blue *arrows*) and AP (*red arrows*) be measured in the mid sagittal plane. (*B*) The transverse measurement should be performed on the axial T2WI slice where it is largest (*green arrows*).

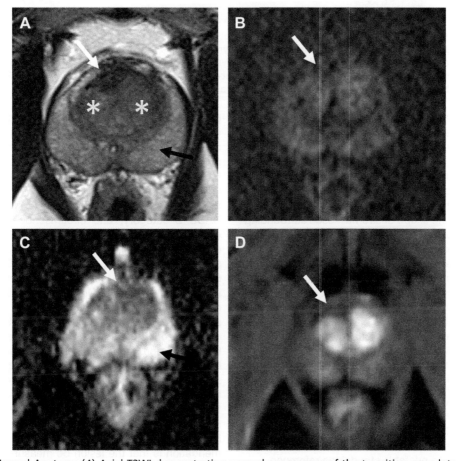

Fig. 2. Normal Anatomy (*A*) Axial T2WI demonstrating normal appearance of the transition zone lateral lobes (*asterisks*) and the homogeneous T2 hyperintense signal in the PZ (*black arrow*). The AFS anteriorly (*white arrow*) is homogenously hypointense. It appears slightly asymmetric in this case, but this is confirmed as normal on other sequences. (*B*) DWI sequence with a b value of 1400 s/mm2 demonstrates no hyperintense regions relative to background. Note the normal low signal intensity of the AFS. (*C*) ADC map demonstrating bright peripheral zone (*black arrow*) and no regions with markedly decreased signal. The normal mild to moderately decreased signal in the AFS is demonstrated (*white arrow*). (*D*) T1WI following the administration of IV gadolinium demonstrates absence of enhancement in the AFS (*white arrow*) and no focal enhancing lesions.

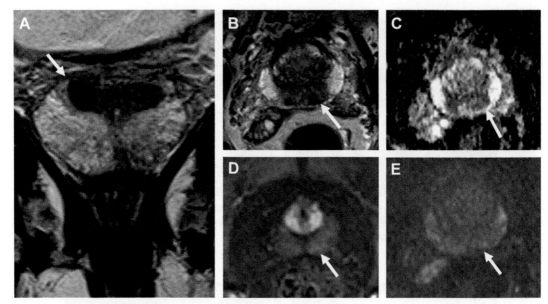

Fig. 3. Normal Central Zone. (*A*) Coronal T2WI demonstrating normal appearance of central zone with its triangular appearance at the prostate base. It may be mildly asymmetric. (*B–E*) Axial images at the base of the prostate through the central zone demonstrate low signal on T2WI (*B*) and on ADC map (*C*). Note that it does not have enhancement on post contrast T1WI (*D*) and there is no increased signal on high b value (2000 sec/mm2) DWI (*E*). These are the key factors that confirm this to be normal anatomy.

capsule lies the transition zone (TZ), which surrounds the proximal urethra and is the location for the benign prostatic hypertrophy changes that affect most older males. Approximately 20% of malignancy arises from within the TZ. Additionally, cancer can rarely but importantly be identified in the central zone (CZ), which is identified as an inverted cone shape of stromal tissue surrounding the ejaculatory ducts that is darker on T2WI than the adjacent peripheral zone. It extends from the base to the verumontanum in the midgland. Lastly, the AFS is a collection of smooth muscle at the anterior aspect of the prostate that is most prominent near the base, where it mixes with periurethral muscle fibers at the bladder neck, and it too can be involved with malignancy.

Prostate imaging and data reporting system assessments

The following sections detail the process of applying PI-RADS to the various prostate zones. The full criteria used for generating the PI-RADS assessments are listed in **Table 1**, which is intended as a printable standalone reference.

Peripheral zone

In general, prostate cancer can be easily identified in the peripheral zone on T2WI as hypointense observations against the more hyperintense glandular backdrop. However, many non-malignant processes can lead to decreased T2 signal, including prostatitis, atrophy, fibrosis, and hemorrhage. Malignancy is often more well-defined and more hypointense, whereas the other entities are more likely to be wedge-shaped or linear with less distinct margins.[10] It is for this reason that these descriptors are used in the likely benign PI-RADS 2 category, and circumscribed (ie, well defined) moderate homogeneously low signal is designated in the likely malignant PI-RADS 4 and 5 designations (**Fig. 4**). Note that PI-RADS 4 and 5 abnormalities have the same imaging characteristics, but PI-RADS 5 is either ≥ 1.5 cm or it demonstrates invasive behavior. Invasive behavior includes the extension of an abnormality across different zones or AFS as well as the extension beyond the prostate. The size measurement can be challenging as prostate MRI is known to substantially underestimate the size of lesions relative to prostatectomy, especially in small lesions and those with lower PI-RADS scores.[11] The best series for measurement is not entirely clear in the literature, and the PI-RADS consensus recommendation is that the lesion be measured on the Apparent Diffusion Coefficient (ADC) map for PZ lesions, while TZ lesions are measured on T2WI sequences. If these sequences are compromised or distorted, then the measurement should be in the plane where it is best visualized. If the lesion is larger or better visualized on the coronal or sagittal image, that should be used and described

Table 1
PI-RADS v2.1 assessment schema by sequence and zone

T2WI - Peripheral Zone	
1	Uniform hyperintense signal intensity(normal)
2	Linear or wedge-shaped hypointensity *OR* Diffuse mild hypointensity, usually indistinct margin
3	Heterogeneous signal intensity *OR* Non-circumscribed, rounded, moderate hypointensity Includes others that do not qualify as 2, 4, or 5
4	Circumscribed, homogenous moderate hypointense focus confined to prostate *AND* <1.5 cm in greatest dimension
5	Same as 4 but $\geq$ 1.5 cm in greatest dimension or definite extraprostatic extension/invasive behavior
T2WI -Transition Zone	
1	Normal appearing TZ *OR* A round or oval completely encapsulated nodule ("typical nodule")
2	A mostly encapsulated nodule *OR* A homogeneous circumscribed nodule without encapsulation *OR* A homogeneous mildly hypointense area between nodules
3	Heterogeneous signal intensity with obscured margins Includes others that do not qualify as 2, 4, or 5
4	Lenticular or non-circumscribed, homogeneous, moderately hypointense, and <1.5 cm in greatest dimension
5	Same as 4, but $\geq$1.5 cm in greatest dimension or definite extraprostatic extension/invasive behavior
DWI - Any Zone	
1	Normal on ADC and high b-value DWI
2	Linear/wedge shaped hypointense on ADC *and/or* Linear/wedge shaped hyperintense on high b-value DWI
3	Focally (discrete and different from the background) hypointense on ADC *and/or* Focally hyperintense on high b-value DWI May be markedly hypointense on ADC or markedly hyperintense on high b-value DWI, but not both
4	Focally markedly hypointense on ADC *AND* Markedly hyperintense on high b-value DWI <1.5 cm in greatest dimension
5	Same signal characteristic as 4 *AND* $\geq$1.5 cm in greatest dimension or definite extraprostatic extension/invasive behavior
DCE - Any Zone	
Negative	No early or contemporaneous enhancement *OR* Diffuse multifocal enhancement NOT corresponding to a focal finding on T2W and/or DWI *OR* Focal enhancement corresponding to a lesion demonstrating features of BPH on T2WI (Includes extruded BPH in the PZ)
Positive	Focal enhancement earlier than or contemporaneous with adjacent normal prostatic tissues *AND* Corresponds to suspicious finding on T2W and/or DWI

in the report. The greatest dimension should be reported, and additional dimensions or lesion volumes are optional.

Identifying csPCa on T2WI alone is typically not achievable with acceptable accuracy,[12] and DWI is a critical sequence in PZ evaluation. Many studies have demonstrated increased sensitivity and specificity when incorporating DWI into diagnostic algorithms.[12,13] As such, DWI has earned a role in PI-RADS v2.1 as the "dominant" sequence for the peripheral zone, due to its ability to differentiate malignancy from its key mimickers, and is the main determinant of the overall PI-RADS assessment (**Fig. 5**).

DWI signal corresponds to the degree of random motion of water molecules within a voxel, and prostate malignancy is known to lead to restricted motion of water. This, in turn, yields an

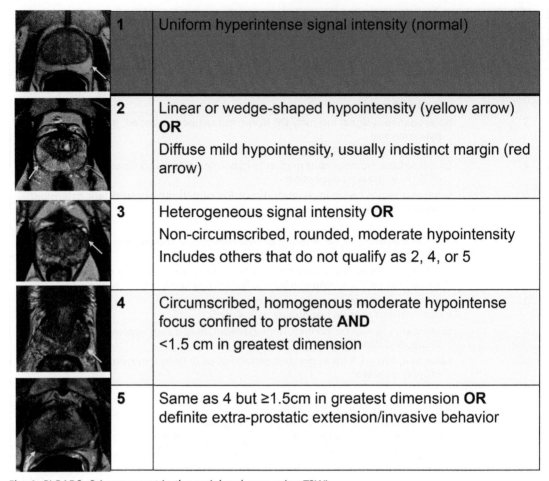

	1	Uniform hyperintense signal intensity (normal)
	2	Linear or wedge-shaped hypointensity (yellow arrow) **OR** Diffuse mild hypointensity, usually indistinct margin (red arrow)
	3	Heterogeneous signal intensity **OR** Non-circumscribed, rounded, moderate hypointensity Includes others that do not qualify as 2, 4, or 5
	4	Circumscribed, homogenous moderate hypointense focus confined to prostate **AND** <1.5 cm in greatest dimension
	5	Same as 4 but ≥1.5cm in greatest dimension **OR** definite extra-prostatic extension/invasive behavior

Fig. 4. PI-RADS v2.1 assessment in the peripheral zone using T2WI.

increased signal on DWI sequences and a corresponding decreased signal in ADC maps for areas of malignancy. PI-RADS compliant MRI protocols include conventional DWI sequences obtained with at least 2 b values (generally 50–100 sec/mm2 and 800–1000 sec/mm2) that allow the construction of an ADC map. Additionally, a high b-value image must be created with a b value of at least 1400 sec/mm2. This can be created by extrapolating the b-value data used to create the ADC map or by directly acquiring a separate high b-value DWI sequence.

The criteria for PI-RADS assessment on DWI is detailed in **Fig. 6**. In the assessment of DWI score, markedly increased signal on the high b-value DWI and markedly decreased signal on the ADC map are both needed for lesions to be considered PI-RADS 4 or 5. Currently, due to the fact that ADC and DWI values and display settings are not standardized or calibrated between scanners, it can be challenging to establish broadly generalizable quantitative values for differentiating malignant

and benign lesions. Therefore, accurate PI-RADS assessment requires reader experience to appropriately set the window and level of ADC and DWI series so that the degree to which a lesion demonstrates increased or decreased signal relative to background normal prostate can be accurately determined.

The criteria in PI-RADS v2.1 are similar to v2, with one relatively minor difference. The verbiage was changed to clarify that "linear/wedged shaped" areas of signal abnormality on DWI or ADC that are typical of benign entities such as prostatitis should now be characterized as PI-RADS 2 (**Fig. 7**).

The final sequence used in generating a numerical assessment is DCE. Prostate adenocarcinoma leads to neovascularization and therefore often early, intense enhancement of tumors is seen relative to the remainder of the gland. Many studies have demonstrated that incorporating DCE sequences into interpretation can increase sensitivity of cancer detection.[14–16] However, the added

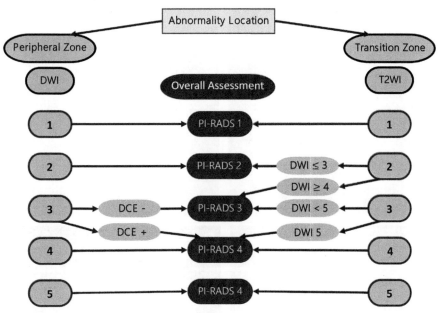

Fig. 5. PI-RADS v2.1 overall assessment schema. Note that the overall assessment is primarily determined according to the DWI series in the peripheral zone with DCE serving a minor tiebreaker role. If DCE is absent or inadequate, the PZ is determined entirely by the DWI series. In the TZ, the T2WI primarily determines the overall assessment with DWI serving to upgrade some lesions to PI-RADS 3 or 4.

value over DWI and T2WI sequences is small, and as such, in PI-RADS v2.1, DCE images are assessed as positive or negative and given less weight than other sequences, only being used as a "tiebreaker" sequence in specific scenarios.[17] There is extensive literature surrounding the different patterns of enhancement, and many different advanced pharmacokinetic models have been tested for csPCa identification, but at this point, there is no conclusive evidence that any of these approaches perform better than a simple binary subjective approach, and they may hamper reproducibility.[17,18] Therefore, PI-RADS v2.1 recommends a subjective approach, and any curve analysis or advanced pharmacokinetics should only be used as an adjunct to source data review.

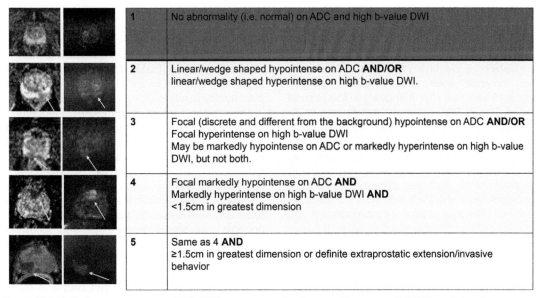

1	No abnormality (i.e. normal) on ADC and high b-value DWI
2	Linear/wedge shaped hypointense on ADC **AND/OR** linear/wedge shaped hyperintense on high b-value DWI.
3	Focal (discrete and different from the background) hypointense on ADC **AND/OR** Focal hyperintense on high b-value DWI May be markedly hypointense on ADC or markedly hyperintense on high b-value DWI, but not both.
4	Focal markedly hypointense on ADC **AND** Markedly hyperintense on high b-value DWI **AND** <1.5cm in greatest dimension
5	Same as 4 **AND** ≥1.5cm in greatest dimension or definite extraprostatic extension/invasive behavior

Fig. 6. PI-RADS v2.1 assessment on DWI. DWI assessments in the transition zone AND/OR peripheral zone.

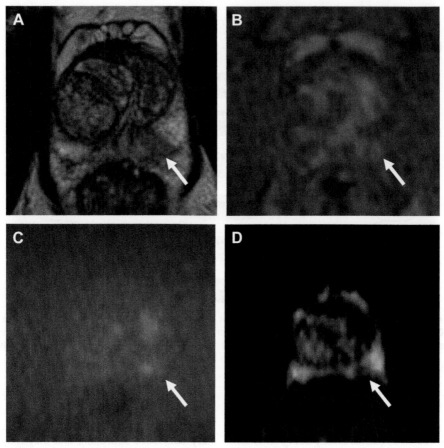

Fig. 7. *Prostatitis* (*A*) Axial T2WI demonstrates a wedge-shaped region of hypointense signal in the peripheral zone of the left prostate. Note the somewhat hazy margins and streaky appearance. (*B*) There is corresponding focal early enhancement on DCE images. (*C*) High b value DWI and (*D*) ADC map show wedge-shaped moderate diffusion restriction. In PI-RADS v2, the moderated diffusion restriction (PI-RADS 3) and early enhancement would lead to an overall assessment of PI-RADS 4 despite the typical and characteristic features of prostatitis. Changes in PI-RADS v2.1 clarify that linear/wedge shaped DWI signal such as this is best characterized as PI-RASD 2. In this case, template biopsy revealed prostatitis and no malignancy.

The DCE sequence should be assessed in a binary fashion by identifying the initial 1-2 datasets when contrast enters the prostate, typically around 10 seconds after it appears in the femoral arteries. The PI-RADS document defines a DCE-positive lesion as "one where enhancement is focal, earlier or contemporaneous with the enhancement of adjacent normal prostatic tissues, and corresponds to a finding on T2W and/or DWI sequences." We find this phrasing can cause some confusion, and the following is our interpretation of PI-RADS and how we incorporate it into our practice: For a lesion to be positive, it needs to have focal enhancement above adjacent normal prostatic tissues (**Fig. 8**). This needs to occur before the remainder of the prostate enhances, or at the same time. Any other pattern of enhancement is negative. Delayed focal enhancement is

not considered a positive DCE scan. Similarly, early enhancement that is diffuse and not isolated to the approximate location of the T2WI and DWI abnormality is negative.

Though not included in the PI-RADS algorithm, non-contrast T1-weighted images (T1WI) should also be obtained and reviewed. Hemorrhage is easily identifiable as marked T1 hyperintensity, typically in the peripheral zone.[19] It is important to characterize the location of hemorrhage, as it can mimic malignancy as it appears as T2 hypointense and shows mild diffusion restriction.[19] Hemorrhage is present in nearly all patients following prostate biopsy for 6 weeks, gradually dissipating thereafter but persisting to some degree beyond 12 weeks in as high as 85% of patients.[20] However, T1WI hemorrhage should not lead to a diagnostic dilemma as it typically persists only in the

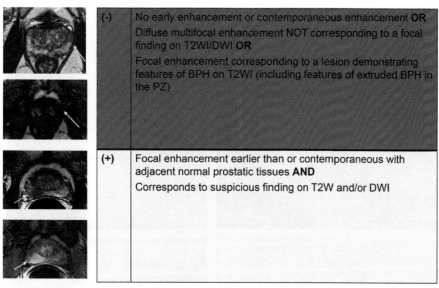

(-)	No early enhancement or contemporaneous enhancement **OR** Diffuse multifocal enhancement **NOT** corresponding to a focal finding on T2WI/DWI **OR** Focal enhancement corresponding to a lesion demonstrating features of BPH on T2WI (including features of extruded BPH in the PZ)	
(+)	Focal enhancement earlier than or contemporaneous with adjacent normal prostatic tissues **AND** Corresponds to suspicious finding on T2W and/or DWI	

Fig. 8. PI-RADS v2.1 assessment with DCE. Assessments are the same in the transition zone AND/OR peripheral zone.

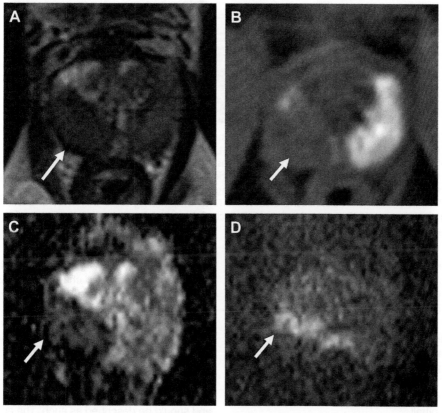

Fig. 9. Hemorrhage exclusion sign. (*A*) Axial T2WI demonstrating diffuse hypointensity throughout the majority of the peripheral zone, with only a small area of normal hyperintense signal anteriorly on the right. On these T2WIs alone, areas of malignancy are impossible to identify, though note the right side is slightly darker than the left, suggesting malignancy over hemorrhage. (*B*) T1WI before contrast demonstrates marked hyperintensity of the left PZ compatible with post biopsy hemorrhage. (*C*) ADC and (*D*) high b value DWI confirm restricted diffusion in the right peripheral zone where Gleason 4 + 4 prostate adenocarcinoma was identified. Note the sparing of hemorrhage in this region of malignancy, which is known as the "hemorrhage exclusion sign."

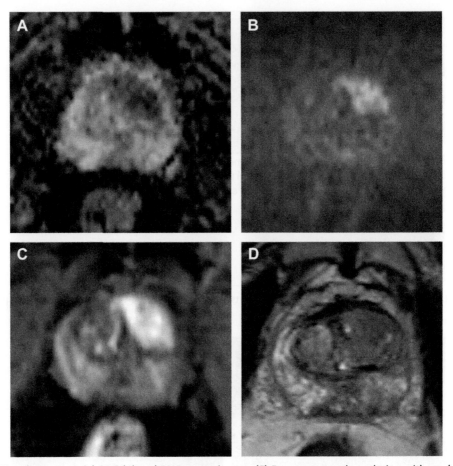

Fig. 10. TZ malignancy. Axial ADC (*A*) and DWI source images (*B*) Demonstrate a large lesion with marked diffusion restriction in the anterior left prostate. Post contrast T1WI (*C*) demonstrates relatively homogenous, intense "sheet like" enhancement in the left anterior prostate suspicious for csPCa. These suspicious DWI and DCE images are useful to identify areas of concern for characterization on T2WI. In this case, the T2WI (*D*) shows homogeneous intermediate intensity signal in the TZ measuring greater than 1.5 cm which is characteristic of csPCa. The final PI-RADS assessment is based on the T2WI for TZ lesions, making this is a PI-RADS 5 lesion. This lesion involves the hypointense AMS seen at the anterior aspect of the gland. Subsequent prostatectomy revealed corresponding Gleason 4 + 5 adenocarcinoma.

normal peripheral zone for an extended time and dissipates rapidly in malignant tissues. Therefore, tumor can often be identified as areas of sparing of increased T1 signal known as the "hemorrhage exclusion sign"[21] (Fig. 9). Thus, hemorrhage may actually aid tumor diagnosis and sizing in some cases. Hemorrhage can mimic enhancement on DCE images, and as such close scrutiny of precontrast T1WI data or subtraction images in areas of perceived enhancement should be employed to avoid this pitfall.[22]

Transition zone

Identifying and characterizing lesions in the TZ is more challenging than in the peripheral zone, as the background is variable and heterogeneous.

With experience, radiologists learn to recognize a characteristic "organized chaos" of the TZ consisting of round encapsulated BPH nodules of varying sizes with interspersed stromal tissue. Stromal BPH nodules can have markedly decreased T2 signal intensity, while glandular nodules have moderate to markedly increased T2 signal, though both patterns can exist in the same nodule. Malignancy in the TZ has a characteristically homogeneous intermediate signal intensity appearance on T2WI and should be described as such. The appearance of a "smudgy fingerprint" or "erased charcoal" are helpful descriptors of the characteristic T2WI appearance of malignancy (Fig. 10). BPH nodules can demonstrate abnormal diffusion signal, especially on the ADC map, where they frequently appear hypointense. Similarly, BPH nodules demonstrate highly variable enhancement patterns and can have extremely avid early enhancement. Due to these factors, the T2WI series is the dominant sequence that primarily assigns the PI-RADS v2.1 category, with DWI relegated to a tiebreaker function (see **Fig. 5**). Note that the DWI and DCE systems are identical for the TZ, though the dominant T2WI is different and more complicated than the PZ.

BPH is so frequently encountered that in PI-RADS v2.1, it is considered a normal finding. Therefore, regardless of other imaging features, when a BPH nodule or typical BPH stromal changes are confidently identified on T2WI, they are assessed as PI-RADS 1. An important and frequently misunderstood component of analyzing the TZ is deciding which nodules or lesions warrant further characterization and assessment, and which can be considered normal BPH. The objective is to identify and assess nodules or regions that have features known to be associated with malignancy and that differ from the background nodules on T2WI or DWI. Lesions on T2WI that have homogeneous intermediate signal intensity with obscured margins, lenticular shape, or invasive behavior should be scored regardless of other sequence characteristics. Additionally, DWI can be helpful in identifying suspicious regions, even though it is not the dominant sequence. If the majority of nodules do not demonstrate restricted diffusion, but one or a small number do have increased signal on high b-value images, these nodules warrant closer scrutiny and full PI-RADS assessment. Alternatively, if scattered areas of heterogeneous or nodular diffusion restriction are

a background feature of the examinee's BPH and the DWI signal in focal nodules does not differ from the background, these nodules do not necessarily need further assessment.

The characterization of lesions with nodule-like morphology in the TZ can be difficult, and PI-RADS v2.1 gives more detail than prior versions on how these should be assessed (**Fig. 11**). If they are round or oval and completely encapsulated by a distinct T2 dark rim on 2 planes, they should be characterized as PI-RADS 1 regardless of DWI or DCE characteristics. These typical nodules can have variable internal characteristics, including cystic change and heterogenous or homogenous signal intensity. If, however, the nodules are incompletely encapsulated or homogeneous and circumscribed without a distinct capsule they should be given a T2WI score of 2 (**Fig. 12**). Because atypical nodules can harbor malignancy, these nodules can then potentially be upgraded to a final assessment of 3 if they demonstrate clear diffusion restriction (ie, a DWI score 4 or 5) (**Fig. 13**). When nodules become more ill-defined with obscured margins, they fit into T2WI score 3 categorization, as well as other lesions with some suspicious features that do not fit into other categories. These PI-RADS 3 lesions are only upgraded to overall PI-RADS 4 when they restrict diffusion and have aggressive characteristics or size $\geq$ 1.5 cm (ie, DWI score 5).

The use of DCE images in the TZ has a limited role, though we advise that they still may contain pertinent, helpful information for identifying lesions. The positive or negative DCE assessment

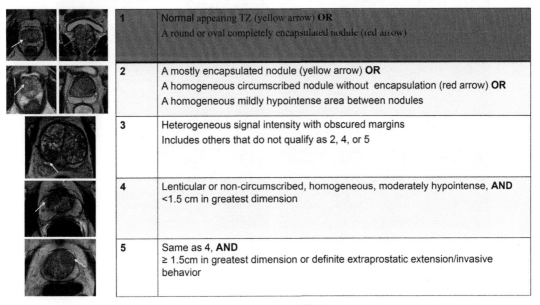

1	Normal appearing TZ (yellow arrow) **OR** A round or oval completely encapsulated nodule (red arrow)
2	A mostly encapsulated nodule (yellow arrow) **OR** A homogeneous circumscribed nodule without encapsulation (red arrow) **OR** A homogeneous mildly hypointense area between nodules
3	Heterogeneous signal intensity with obscured margins Includes others that do not qualify as 2, 4, or 5
4	Lenticular or non-circumscribed, homogeneous, moderately hypointense, **AND** <1.5 cm in greatest dimension
5	Same as 4, **AND** $\geq$ 1.5cm in greatest dimension or definite extraprostatic extension/invasive behavior

Fig. 11. PI-RADS v2.1 assessment in the transition zone using T2WI.

should still be performed in the TZ, though it will ultimately not play a role in the final PI-RADS assessment as DCE does not factor into the overall PI-RADS algorithm for the TZ. However, while both BPH nodules and significant malignancy can show avid enhancement, some enhancement patterns are more suspicious for csPCa, than others. BPH typically demonstrates a "popcorn-like" or swirled pattern. The homogeneous unencapsulated "sheet like" enhancement pattern has been suggested as a factor to consider in characterizing findings and has an association with significant malignancy[15] (see **Fig. 9**; **Fig. 14**). Similarly, confluent avid enhancement that crosses borders or extends to the capsule/AFS with obtuse angles of capsular abutment is a pattern suggesting significant prostate cancer. These patterns are not described in PI-RADS, but in practice, if they are seen, close scrutinization of the T2WI and DCE is necessary to determine if these regions warrant a higher PI-RADS assessment.

Central zone

The CZ analysis is a common pitfall for inexperienced prostate MRI interpretters.[23,24] Normally, the CZ can be seen as a cone of tissue at the base around the ejaculatory ducts, though it can be displaced and asymmetric secondary to BPH. It normally has hypointense signal on T2WI images and ADC maps and hyperintense signal on DWI.[25] Therefore, the normal CZ can be mistakenly interpreted as tumor in the PZ. While the normal CZ mimics prostate cancer, malignancy can also occur in the CZ, although most in most cases the cancer originates in the adjacent PZ. Due to unclear reasons, CZ tumors are, on average, more aggressive than tumors outside the CZ.[9,26] PI-RADS v2.1 provides more detail on CZ analysis than prior versions to help guide interpreters against this pitfall. The key is to realize that normal CZ tissue does not demonstrate early enhancement or substantially increased signal on high

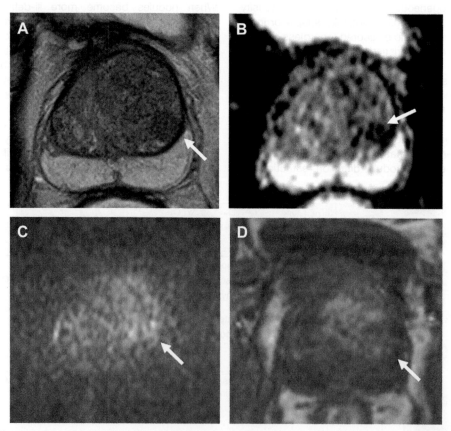

Fig. 12. Circumscribed BPH nodule. (*A*) Axial 2WI demonstrating a circumscribed T2 hypointense nodule without a capsule (*arrow*). This is assessed as PI-RADS 2 on T2WI. ADC map (*B*) demonstrates hypointense corresponding signal, though on high b value DWI images (*C*) signal is only mildly hyperintense resulting in a DWI assessment of PI-RADS 3. Post contrast images (*D*) show negative enhancement with signal similar to background. In PI-RADS v2.1, the assessment of this TZ nodule is based on the T2WI and it is not upgraded by DWI with PIRADS assessment less than 4, resulting in an overall assessment of PI-RADS 2. This was negative for malignancy on targeted biopsy.

b-value images. Therefore, lesions at the posterior base in the region where the CZ is located should only be assigned a score greater than PI-RADS 1 if an increased signal is seen on early DCE or high b-value images, especially when asymmetrically present (**Fig. 15**).

Anterior fibromuscular stroma

While it can be variable in thickness, the AFS is typically symmetric and identified at the anterior prostate as low signal on T2WI, DWI, and ADC maps with little or no early enhancement. The AFS does not contain glandular elements, and therefore PCa does not arise directly in the AFS. However, it can extend to the AFS from the TZ or PZ, and the characterization of this region is newly addressed in PI-RADS v2.1. AFS tumor is readily identified as areas of increased T2 signal relative to pelvic muscles, increased high b-value DWI signal, or early enhancement. When any of these features are identified, the lesion should be characterized by the zone of the prostate where the reader most suspects it arose (PZ or TZ). Identification of these anterior tumors is important, and when the AFS is involved, it should be discussed in the clinical report as they have an increased risk of extraprostatic extension.[27]

PROSTATE IMAGING AND DATA REPORTING SYSTEM ASSESSMENTS IN CASES WITHOUT ADEQUATE DIFFUSION-WEIGHTED IMAGING

At times, DWI will have artifact severe enough to render them uninterpretable for some or the entirety of the gland, most commonly from rectal gas or prosthetic hip implant artifacts. Many studies have clearly demonstrated that performance is best with DWI as a component of the protocol, and therefore when DWI has limitations, this should clearly be stated in the report, and it

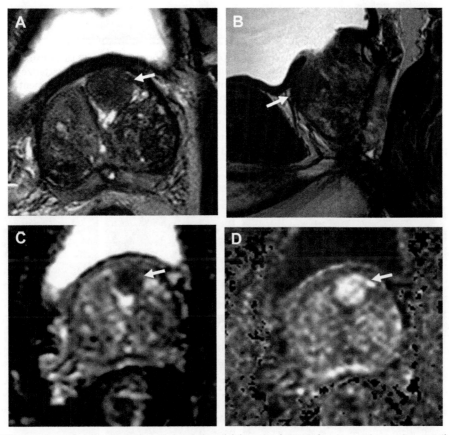

Fig. 13. *BPH nodule with DWI upgrading.* (*A*) Axial and (*B*) sagittal T2WI demonstrating a circumscribed T2 hypointense nodule without a complete capsule (*arrow*). The absence of the capsule is best seen posteriorly on the sagittal image. This is assessed as PI-RADS 2 on T2WI. ADC map (*C*) and calculated high b value DWI images (*D*) demonstrate marked diffusion restriction with size under 1.5 cm, resulting in a DWI assessment of PI-RADS 4. In PI-RADS v2.1, the assessment of this TZ nodule is based first on the T2WI assessment of 2, though it is upgraded to a final assessment of 3 based on the DWI.

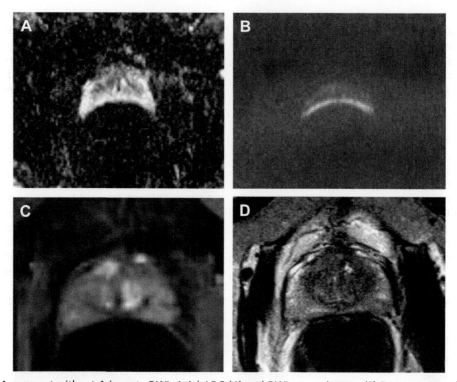

Fig. 14. Assessment without Adequate DWI. Axial ADC (*A*) and DWI source images (*B*) Demonstrate substantial architectural distortion from rectal gas significantly limiting the ability to detect or characterize lesions. Post contrast T1WI (*C*) demonstrates a small homogenous, intense "sheet like" focus of enhancement in the right anterior prostate TZ suspicious for csPCa. Note how this enhancement differs from the more characteristic heterogeneous enhancement in the remainder of the TZ. (*D*) T2WI demonstrates relatively homogeneous intermediate intensity signal at the site of enhancement measuring <1.5 cm. This lesion is characterized as PI-RADS 4 based on the T2WI appearance, though it may have been difficult to identify without the suspicious enhancement. Subsequent targeted biopsy revealed corresponding Gleason 3 + 4 adenocarcinoma.

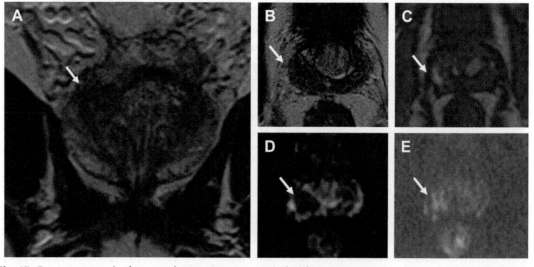

Fig. 15. Prostate cancer in the central zone. An asymmetrical T2 hypointense region (*arrows*) is identified at the peripheral zone on coronal (*A*) and axial (*B*) T2WI. The presence of enhancement on post contrast T1WI (*arrow, C*) raises concern for malignancy. The increased signal on high b value DWI (*D*) corresponding to area of decreased signal on ADC (*E*) also suggests a malignant lesion. This is characterized as PI-RADS 4 and biopsy demonstrated Gleason 4 + 5 adenocarcinoma.

will undoubtedly hinder diagnostic accuracy. However, as long as DCE images are obtained, PI-RADS assessments can still be performed using a modified algorithm with T2WI images representing the dominant sequence and DCE as a tiebreaker for PI-RADS 3 T2WI lesions (**Fig. 16**). If DCE is also not performed or is inadequate, the exam should not be used for cancer detection, though at times, staging may be possible with T2WI alone.

PROSTATE IMAGING AND DATA REPORTING SYSTEM WITHOUT DYNAMIC CONTRAST ENHANCED IMAGES

In cases where DCE is not performed or is inadequate due to contraindications or artifacts, the PI-RADS algorithm can still be applied. The only significant change involves DCE's role in potentially upgrading PI-RADS 3 lesions in the peripheral zone to PI-RADS 4 (see **Fig. 5**). In some centers, particularly in Europe, contrast is at times purposely not administered in a "biparametric" MRI protocol relying on T2WI and DWI. This remains a controversial topic, and complete discussion can be seen elsewhere.[28,29] Briefly, several studies at experienced centers have shown equivalent

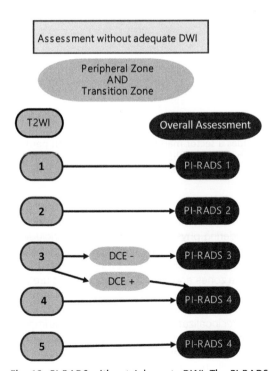

Fig. 16. PI-RADS without Adequate DWI. The PI-RADS schema for lesions where the DWI is inadequate or significantly hampered by artifact is later in discussion. Note that this applies to both the TZ and PZ, and T2WI becomes the dominant sequence for both.

results between biparametric and multiparametric protocols.[30] However, some studies still show small advantages to using DCE, and proponents point out the improved confidence, helpfulness in cases where diffusion is inadequate, and theoretical utility of contrast for inexperienced readers.[28] The PI-RADS committee continues to endorse contrast usage at this time, though it acknowledges that biparametric exams may be performed in some scenarios. The committee suggests they be limited to patients with the following: lower risk for csPCa; no prior biopsy; no prior biparametric MRI with continued suspicion of cancer; no prior prostate cancer interventions; not on active surveillance; no hip implants.

PROSTATE IMAGING AND DATA REPORTING SYSTEM VERSION 2.1 VALIDATION

Numerous studies have been performed validating PI-RADS v2, the immediate predecessor to the current version. These demonstrate on meta-analysis that the PI-RADS framework works as intended in characterizing risk in a stepwise fashion with pooled sensitivity of 89% and specificity of 73% for any cancer, surpassing PI-RADS v1.[31,32] However, some studies show inconsistent and, at times, poor inter-reader reproducibility of the system,[33] with only moderate agreement even among very experienced readers in one multicenter study.[34] Several studies show continued at least mild improvement in diagnostic accuracy with PI-RADS v2.1 over v2 on systematic review.[35] On meta-analysis done in 2021, the improvements in sensitivity and specificity were not significant, though limited data was available for this analyisis.[36] Like PI-RADS v2, PI-RADS v2.1 stratifies the risk of malignancy among the 5 categories as intended.[37]

Inter-reader reproducibility was a main target for improvement in PI-RADS v 2.1, particularly in the TZ. To that end, numerous vague statements in PI-RADS v2 have been clarified in v2.1, and the handling of BPH nodules is now more clearly delineated. Thus far, the results of preliminary studies on inter-reader reproducibility have been mixed, though overall show mildly improved inter-reader agreement.[35] One complicating feature is that in PI-RADS v.2, BPH changes were categorized at minimum to be PI-RADS 2, and therefore PI-RADS 1 was extremely rare. This is not ideal in a 5 category risk schema, and in PI-RADS 2.1 the changes to BPH assessment should yield many more PI-RADS 1 overall determinations, which has been observed in the literature.[38] However, this adjustment leads to more interobserver disagreement in overall PI-RADS assessment

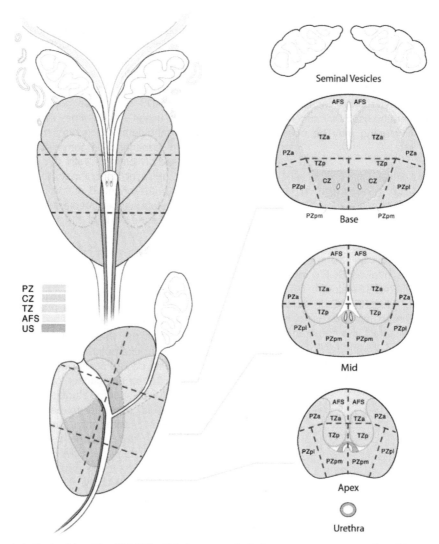

Fig. 17. *Prostate Sector Map.* The PI-RADS v 2.1 document includes a sector map reproduced here with permission. This map divides the prostate into 41 sectors which may help aid localization. Note how the peripheral zone is seen laterally and posteriorly at the base, though at the extreme apex it often extends to the anterior prostate as seen on the sagittal image.

attributable to this PI-RADS 1 vs. 2 distinction.[39] Overall, we believe the literature suggests modest improvements in both diagnostic accuracy and inter-reader reproducibility with the new criteria in PI-RADS v2.1. However, reader experience remains important, and we can expect continued changes to improve the criteria in future PI-RADS versions.

ADDITIONAL REPORTING COMPONENTS
Mapping lesions

PI-RADS v2.1 recommends that radiologists identify up to 4 lesions with assessments category ≥3. The method of localization is important, and we recommend communicating the optimal method with ordering physicians. PI-RADS does include a sector map to aid localization that was revised in version 2.1 to include 41 sectors covering the 3 prostate zones and the AFS, as well as the urethra and the seminal vesicles (**Fig. 17**). This map can be incorporated into reports as an aid in localization. Whatever localization method is chosen, it is important that the report also includes the index lesion that will guide treatment, which is defined as the lesion with the highest PI-RADS assessment. If there is more than one lesion with the same PI-RADS assessment, the index lesion is the lesion with the most aggressive features, or the largest lesion if there is no difference in aggressive features.

Staging

Staging any identified tumor is an important part of the PI-RADS interpretation process. Prostate MRI is generally considered the best way to characterize local T stage, and it has shown utility for staging superior to clinical staging alone in numerous studies.[40] When evaluating T stage, a key component involves differentiating T2 organ-confined disease versus T3a disease with extraprostatic extension (EPE) or T3b disease with seminal vesicle invasion (SVI). PI-RADS v2.1 gives some criteria for identifying known characteristics of extraprostatic disease, recommending the following key features: asymmetry of the neurovascular bundles, bulging contour, irregular or spiculated margin, obliteration of the rectoprostatic angle, over 1 cm of tumor contact with prostate capsule, capsular breach, bladder wall invasion. However, PI-RADS v2.1 does not provide additional guidance or weighting of these features, relies on radiologist discretion, and does not advocate for a specific reporting method. As such, there has been wide variability in accuracy and reproducibility, and existing systems have shown relatively low sensitivity for EPE.[40] More recently, Mehralivand and colleagues[41] developed a simple EPE grading system with more objective criteria to reduce variability inherent to subjective interpretations. In this system exams receive a grade of 0-3 as follows:

Grade 0- None of the following features.

Grade 1- Curvilinear contact length >1.5 cm OR capsular bulge/irregularity.

Grade 2- Contact length >1.5 cm AND capsular bulge/irregularity.

Grade 3- Frank breach of capsule OR invasion into adjacent structures.

This system generated an AUC of 0.77 for identifying EPE with sensitivity/specificity as follows: Grade ≥1: 75%/68%, Grade ≥2: 61%/81%, Grade 3: 30%/96%.[41] This system has since been validated to perform as well as or better than competing systems or subjective grading in several retrospective studies.[42–46] Additional prospective validation is needed, and features may need to be refined, though at present this appears an acceptable and potentially reproducible staging method.

In addition to EPE, identifying the involvement of critical surrounding structures is also important. SVI can be identified as focal or diffuse T2 intensity involving the normally thin-walled, fluid-filled structures. Increased enhancement and diffusion restriction can also be very helpful, and close scrutiny of coronal images to evaluate for direct extension from prostate base tumors is important.

For lesions at the apex, it is important to identify tumor abutting the external US, which is a round structure with signal isointense to skeletal muscle on T2WI. When tumor involves this structure, it carries higher risk of recurrence if unresected or incontinence if the sphincter is damaged at prostatectomy. Lastly, identifying tumor involving or adjacent to the neurovascular bundles is important as it may lead surgeons to alter their surgical approach and consider whether nerve-sparing surgery should be attempted. The neurovascular bundles are T2 hypointense small rounded structures near the posterior prostate capsule, most typically at the 5 and 7 o'clock positions.

Beyond local staging, bone metastases and lymph node metastases should be reported if clearly identified, though typically prostate MRI is not the primary mode of identifying metastatic disease.

Template

We highly recommend that a standard reporting template be used consistently throughout each radiology practice. Surveys show this is preferred by referring urologists, it improves reporting clarity,[47,48] and it may improve diagnostic performance.[49] There are example templates provided by the PI-RADS committee containing the most critical reporting elements. When reporting, we note that PI-RADS v2.1 does not specify how EPE be reported. We advocate that EPE be reported via the radiologist and urologist preferred method of verbal expression of probability using a standardized method to improve clarity (eg, extremely low, low, intermediate, high, very high risk of EPE).[47,50] This can be more easily incorporated into practice with a standard template using a pre-specified lexicon.

SUMMARY

All radiologists interpreting prostate MRI should have a firm knowledge of the principles of PI-RADS 2.1 and its use in practice. This article provides that basic framework and can serve as the foundation for prostate MRI interpretation in modern clinical practice.

CLINICS CARE POINTS

- PI-RADS v2.1 is the recommended standard of care in reporting prostate MRI for the detection, staging, and monitoring of prostate cancer that has not yet undergone treatment

- PI-RADS v2.1 makes small modifications and clarifications to PI-RADS v2, leaving the main framework intact
- PI-RADS application requires making assessments ranging from 1 to 5 on T2WI and DWI and binary assessments on DCE images
- These assessments are then used to generate an overall assessment that is based primarily on the DWI assessment in the peripheral zone and the T2WI assessment in the transition zone
- Lesion identification for further characterization involves finding foci that differ from background and have suspicious features on any sequence, not only the dominant sequence used for characterization.
- PI-RADS v2.1 clarifies AFS lesion assessments, which should be performed according to the zone where the cancer most likely arose
- Increased or asymmetric early enhancement or signal on high b-value DWI series is key to identifying cancer in the CZ

DISCLOSURE

Additional Disclosures not pertaining directly to article content: B. Spilseth: Francis Medical, consultant. AI Metrics, stockholder. Bot Image, stockholder. D. Margolis: Ad-hoc consulting, Promaxo, Inc; R. T Gupta: Consultant, Philips; S. Chang: Speaking honorarium, Bayer.

REFERENCES

1. Siddiqui MM, Rais-Bahrami S, Turkbey B, et al. Comparison of MR/ultrasound fusion–guided biopsy with ultrasound-guided biopsy for the diagnosis of prostate cancer. JAMA 2015;313(4):390.
2. Rosenkrantz AB, Verma S, Choyke P, et al. Prostate magnetic resonance imaging and magnetic resonance imaging targeted biopsy in patients with a prior negative biopsy: a consensus statement by AUA and SAR. J Urol 2016;196(6):1613–8.
3. Spilseth B, Ghai S, Patel NU, et al. A comparison of radiologists' and urologists' opinions regarding prostate MRI reporting: Results from a survey of specialty societies. Am J Roentgenol 2018;210(1):101–7.
4. Weinreb JC, Barentsz JO, Choyke PL, et al. PI-RADS Prostate Imaging - Reporting and Data System: 2015, Version 2. Eur Urol 2016;69(1):16–40.
5. Turkbey B, Rosenkrantz AB, Haider MA, et al. Prostate imaging reporting and data system version 2.1: 2019 update of prostate imaging reporting and data system version 2. Eur Urol 2019;76(3):340–51.
6. ACR American College of Radiology. PI-RADS v2 Prostate Imaging and Reporting and Data System: Version 2. Published online 2015. Available at: http://www.acr.org/Quality-Safety/Resources/PIRADS.
7. Hricak H, Dooms GC, McNeal JE, et al. MR imaging of the prostate gland: normal anatomy. AJR Am J Roentgenol 1987;148(1):51–8.
8. McNeal JE. The zonal anatomy of the prostate. Prostate 1981;2:35–49.
9. McNeal JE, Redwine EA, Freiha FS, et al. Zonal distribution of prostatic adenocarcinoma. Correlation with histologic pattern and direction of spread. Am J Surg Pathol 1988;12(12):897–906.
10. Cruz M, Tsuda K, Narumi Y, et al. Characterization of low-intensity lesions in the peripheral zone of prostate on pre-biopsy endorectal coil MR imaging. Eur Radiol 2002;12(2):357–65.
11. Pooli A, Johnson DC, Shirk J, et al. Predicting pathological tumor size in prostate cancer based on multiparametric prostate magnetic resonance imaging and preoperative findings. J Urol 2021;205(2):444–51.
12. Tan CH, Johnson V, Kundra V, et al. Diffusion-weighted MRI in the detection of prostate cancer: meta-analysis. Am J Roentgenol 2012;(October):822–9.
13. Wu LM, Xu JR, Ye YQ, et al. The clinical value of diffusion-weighted imaging in combination with T2-weighted imaging in diagnosing prostate carcinoma: a systematic review and meta-analysis. Am J Roentgenol 2012;199(1):103–10.
14. Greer MD, Shih JH, Lay N, et al. Validation of the dominant sequence paradigm and role of dynamic contrast-enhanced imaging in PI-RADS version 2. Radiology 2017;285(3):859–69.
15. Rosenkrantz AB, Babb JS, Taneja SS, et al. Proposed adjustments to PI-RADS version 2 decision rules: impact on prostate cancer detection. Radiology 2016;283(1):119–29.
16. Krishna S, McInnes M, Lim C, et al. Comparison of prostate imaging reporting and data system versions 1 and 2 for the detection of peripheral zone gleason score 3 + 4 = 7 cancers. Am J Roentgenol 2017;209(6):W365–73.
17. Berman RM, Brown AM, Chang SD, et al. DCE MRI of prostate cancer. Abdom Radiol 2016;41(5):844–53.
18. Hansford BG, Peng Y, Jiang Y, et al. Dynamic contrast-enhanced MR imaging curve-type analysis: Is it helpful in the differentiation of prostate cancer from healthy peripheral zone? Radiology 2015;275(2):448–57.
19. Tamada T, Sone T, Jo Y, et al. Prostate cancer: relationships between postbiopsy hemorrhage and tumor detectability at MR diagnosis. Radiology 2008;248(2):531–9.
20. Sarradin M, Lepiney C, Celhay O, et al. [Estimating minimum period of time to perform prostate MRI after prostate biopsy: Clinical and histological bleeding risk factors; from a prospective study]. Progrès en

Urol J l'Association française d'urologie la Société française d'urologie 2018;28(2):85–93, 2.

21. Barrett T, Vargas HA, Akin O, et al. Value of the hemorrhage exclusion sign on T1-weighted prostate MR images for the detection of prostate cancer. Radiology 2012;263(3):751–7.

22. Furlan A, Borhani AA, Westphalen AC. Multiparametric MR imaging of the prostate: interpretation including prostate imaging reporting and data system version 2. Radiol Clin North Am 2018;56(2):223–38.

23. Rosenkrantz AB, Taneja SS. Radiologist, be aware: ten pitfalls that confound the interpretation of multiparametric prostate MRI. Am J Roentgenol 2014; 202(1):109–20.

24. Thomas S, Oto A. Multiparametric MR imaging of the prostate: pitfalls in interpretation. Radiol Clin North Am 2018;56(2):277–87.

25. Gupta RT, Kauffman CR, Garcia-Reyes K, et al. Apparent diffusion coefficient values of the benign central zone of the prostate: Comparison with low- and high-grade prostate cancer. Am J Roentgenol 2015;205(2):331–6.

26. Vargas Ha, Akin O, Franiel T, et al. Normal central zone of the prostate and central zone involvement by prostate cancer: clinical and MR imaging implications. Radiology 2012;262(3):894–902.

27. Koppie TM, Bianco FJ, Kuroiwa K, et al. The clinical features of anterior prostate cancers. BJU Int 2006; 98(6):1167–71.

28. Kamsut S, Reid K, Tan N. Roundtable: arguments in support of using multi-parametric prostate MRI protocol. Abdom Radiol 2020;45(12):3990–6.

29. Scialpi M, Martorana E, Scialpi P, et al. Round table: arguments in supporting abbreviated or biparametric MRI of the prostate protocol. Abdom Radiol 2020; 45(12):3974–81.

30. Woo S, Suh CH, Kim SY, et al. Head-to-head comparison between biparametric and multiparametric MRI for the diagnosis of prostate cancer: A systematic review and meta-analysis. Am J Roentgenol 2018;211(5):W226–41.

31. Woo S, Suh CH, Kim SY, et al. Diagnostic performance of prostate imaging reporting and data system version 2 for detection of prostate cancer: a systematic review and diagnostic meta-analysis. Eur Urol 2017;72(2):177–88.

32. Zhang L, Tang M, Chen S, et al. A meta-analysis of use of prostate imaging reporting and data system version 2 (PI-RADS V2) with multiparametric MR imaging for the detection of prostate cancer. Eur Radiol 2017;27(12):5204–14.

33. Smith CP, Türkbey B. PI-RADS v2: Current standing and future outlook. Turkish J Urol 2018;44(3):189–94.

34. Rosenkrantz AB, Ginocchio LA, Cornfeld D, et al. Interobserver reproducibility of the PI-RADS version 2 lexicon: a multicenter study of six experienced prostate radiologists. Radiology 2016;000(0):152542.

35. Annamalai A, Fustok JN, Beltran-Perez J, et al. Interobserver agreement and accuracy in interpreting mpMRI of the prostate: a systematic review. Curr Urol Rep 2022;23(1):1–10.

36. Park KJ, Choi SH, Kim M hyun, et al. Performance of prostate imaging reporting and data system version 2.1 for diagnosis of prostate cancer: a systematic review and meta-analysis. J Magn Reson Imaging 2021;54(1):103–12.

37. Oerther B, Engel H, Bamberg F, et al. Cancer detection rates of the PI-RADSv2.1 assessment categories: systematic review and meta-analysis on lesion level and patient level. Prostate Cancer Prostatic Dis 2022;25(2):256–63.

38. Linhares Moreira AS, De Visschere P, Van Praet C, et al. How does PI-RADS v2.1 impact patient classification? A head-to-head comparison between PI-RADS v2.0 and v2.1. Acta radiol 2021;62(6):839–47.

39. Beetz NL, Haas M, Baur A, et al. Inter-Reader Variability Using PI-RADS v2 Versus PI-RADS v21: Most New Disagreement Stems from Scores 1 and 2. RoFo Fortschritte auf dem Gebiet der Rontgenstrahlen und der Bildgeb Verfahren 2021;194(8):852–61.

40. de Rooij M, Hamoen EHJ, Witjes JA, et al. Accuracy of Magnetic resonance imaging for local staging of prostate cancer: a diagnostic meta-analysis. Eur Urol 2016;70(2):233–45.

41. Mehralivand S, Shih JH, Harmon S, et al. A grading system for the assessment of risk of extraprostatic extension of prostate cancer at multiparametric MRI. Radiology 2019;290(3):709–19.

42. Park KJ, Kim MH, Kim JK. Extraprostatic tumor extension: comparison of preoperative multiparametric MRI criteria and histopathologic correlation after radical prostatectomy. Radiology 2020;296(1): 87–95.

43. Xiang JY, Huang XS, Xu JX, et al. MRI extraprostatic extension grade: accuracy and clinical incremental value in the assessment of extraprostatic cancer. BioMed Res Int 2022;2022. https://doi.org/10.1155/2022/3203965.

44. Reisæter LAR, Halvorsen OJ, Beisland C, et al. Assessing extraprostatic extension with multiparametric mri of the prostate: Mehralivand extraprostatic extension grade or extraprostatic extension likert scale? Radiol Imaging Cancer 2020;2(1). https://doi.org/10.1148/rycan.2019190071.

45. Xu L, Zhang G, Zhang X, et al. External validation of the extraprostatic extension grade on MRI and its incremental value to clinical models for assessing extraprostatic cancer. Front Oncol 2021;11(April):1–9.

46. Asfuroğlu U, Asfuroğlu BB, Özer H, et al. Which one is better for predicting extraprostatic extension on multiparametric MRI: ESUR score, Likert scale, tumor contact length, or EPE grade? Eur J Radiol 2022;149(October 2021). https://doi.org/10.1016/j.ejrad.2022.110228.

47. Spilseth B, Margolis DJ, Patel NU, et al. A prostate MRI reporting : results from a survey of specialty societies. Am J Roentgenol 2018;43(7):1807–12.

48. Magnetta MJ, Donovan AL, Jacobs BL, et al. Method to optimize prostate MRI. Am J Roentgenol 2018;210(January):108–12.

49. Shaish H, Feltus W, Steinman J, et al. Impact of a structured reporting template on adherence to prostate imaging reporting and data system version 2 and on the diagnostic performance of prostate MRI for clinically significant prostate cancer. J Am Coll Radiol 2018;15(5):749–54.

50. Wibmer A, Vargas HA, Sosa R, et al. Value of a standardized lexicon for reporting levels of diagnostic certainty in prostate MRI. Am J Roentgenol 2014;203(6):W651–7.

Contemporary Approach to Prostate Imaging and Data Reporting System Score 3 Lesions

Jorge Abreu-Gomez, MD[a],*, Christopher Lim, MD[b],
Masoom A. Haider, MD, FRCPC[c]

KEYWORDS

- Prostate cancer ● PI-RADS 3 ● mpMRI ● MR guided biopsy ● PSAD

KEY POINTS

- PI-RADS 3 lesions are equivocal for the presence of Clinically Significant Prostate Cancer (csPCa). Understanding the differences between PI-RADS version 2 and version 2.1 may allow for better identification and reporting of score 3 lesions.
- Ensuring optimal image quality and adequate radiologist training plays a key role in the number of reported PI-RADS 3 lesions. Increased number of equivocal lesions could undermine the confidence of MRI usefulness among referring physicians.
- A relatively low, but still significant number of csPCa ranging from 10% to 30.5% is identified in the PI-RADS 3 subgroup with variable results depending on disease prevalence, history of prior negative prostate biopsy or if the patient is under active surveillance. A PSA density (PSAD) $\geq$0.10 to 0.15 can aid in the selection of patients who may undergo biopsy.
- Fluidic and tissue based molecular markers have not been completely assessed in the PI-RADS 3 population. Larger studies are needed in this subset of patients to determine their benefits in terms of patient selection for biopsy.
- Texture features and convolutional networks are artificial intelligence tools have potential value in early studies in adding to the PI-RADS scoring system however further validation is needed.

INTRODUCTION

The Prostate Imaging Reporting and Data System (PI-RADS) initially released in 2012[1] with subsequent revisions in 2016 and 2019,[2,3] represents a score based system created in order to standardize the acquisition, interpretation and reporting of multiparametric MRI (mpMRI). Since its initial version, the system was designed to increase detection, localization and characterization of csPCa and at the same time, to reduce the diagnosis of clinically insignificant Prostate Cancer(ciPCa).[4] PI-RADS stratifies the overall level of suspicion using a 5-point scale ranging from very low likelihood (score 1) to very high likelihood (score 5). Overall score 3 corresponds to intermediate/equivocal likelihood for csPCa.[2,3]

[a] Joint Department of Medical Imaging, University Health Network, Mount Sinai Hospital and Women's College Hospital, University of Toronto, 610 University Avenue, Suite 3-920, Toronto, ON M5G 2M9, Canada; [b] Department of Medical Imaging, Sunnybrook Health Sciences Centre, University of Toronto, 2075 Bayview Avenue, Room AB 279, Toronto, ON M4N 3M5, Canada; [c] Lunenfeld-Tanenbaum Research Institute, Sinai Health System and the Joint Department of Medical Imaging, Sinai Health System, Princess Margaret Hospital, University of Toronto, 600 University Avenue, Toronto, ON, Canada M5G 1X5
* Corresponding author. Joint Department of Medical Imaging, University Health Network, Mount Sinai Hospital and Women's College Hospital, University of Toronto, 610 University Avenue, Suite 3-920, Toronto, ON M5G 2M9, Canada.
E-mail address: jorgeandres.abreugomez@uhn.ca

Radiol Clin N Am 62 (2024) 37–51
https://doi.org/10.1016/j.rcl.2023.06.008
0033-8389/24/© 2023 Elsevier Inc. All rights reserved.

The most recent PI-RADS version 2.1 (v2.1), was constructed to improve diagnostic accuracy and reduce interobserver variability.[3] One of the most important changes of the updated version consists in the increased weight of DWI features for the assessment of the transition zone (TZ)[5] and reclassification of the Benign Prostate Hyperplasia (BPH) nodules; as well as the introduction of the concept of "Atypical nodule," reserved for T2-weighted imaging (T2WI) score 2.[3]

In PI-RADS v2.1, T2WI remains as the dominant sequence for the assessment of the TZ. The definitions of scores 1 and 2 in the TZ were updated to normal appearing TZ or the presence of a "typical nodule" for score 1 and the presence of "atypical nodule" or a homogeneous, mildly hypointense area between nodules for score 2. Moreover, the role of DWI was highlighted with the possibility of upgrading T2WI score 2 or "atypical nodule" to overall score 3 based on the presence of restricted diffusion (DWI score $\geq$4). There were no changes in the definition of score 3 nor in the upgrading rule from overall score 3 to score 4 based on a DWI score of 5.[3] Thus, PI-RADS 2.1 may result in some TZ nodules being classified as 3 that would have been previously considered 2.

DWI remains as the dominant sequence for the assessment of the peripheral zone (PZ). The main changes consisted in the updated definition of score 2 as linear/wedge shaped area hypointense on ADC and/or hyperintense on high b-value DWI as well as the updated definition of score 3, now including a focal abnormality hypointense on ADC and/or hyperintense on high b-value DWI or a focal abnormality markedly hypointense on ADC or markedly hyperintense on high-b-value DWI, but not both. The definitions of scores 1, 4 and 5 remain unchanged.[3] Thus, the change in PZ scoring may result in some PZ PI-RADS 3 lesions being reclassified as 2.

APPROACH TO PI-RADS 3 LESIONS IN THE PERIPHERAL ZONE

DWI remains as the dominant sequence for assigning an overall score in the PZ according to PI-RADS v2.1. However, an update in the definition of score 3 has been performed and adequate understanding of this modification is required for optimal interpretation. Score 3 lesions should be focal in the first instance (discrete and different from the background). If we are dealing with a focal lesion, then our next question should be oriented to DWI characteristics. In this regard, 2 options can constitute a score 3. The first one, when the lesion is hypointense on ADC and/or hyperintense on high b-value DWI (Fig. 1) and the second,

when lesion is markedly hypointense on ADC or markedly hyperintense on high-b-value DWI, but not both. Fig. 2 illustrates a patient with a focal markedly hypointense lesion on ADC but not markedly hyperintense on high b-value DWI and Fig. 3 illustrates the opposite example, with a focal lesion markedly hyperintense on high b-value DWI bot not markedly hypointense on ADC.

In the PZ, DWI score 3 depends on dynamic contrast enhancement imaging (DCE) to upgrade the overall score from 3 to 4 if there is "positive," early enhancement (Fig. 4). On the other hand, if DCE is negative, the overall score remains as 3 (see Fig. 1). This "upgrading" rule did not have modifications from PI-RADS v2 to 2.1.[2,3]

The role of ADC quantification has not been formally addressed but is used by many in clinical practice outside of PI-RADS to help to avoid overcalling of PI-RADS 3 lesions when stable ADC measurement can be achieved on MRI local systems. The universal application of simple ADC thresholds in PI-RADS scoring remains hampered by intersite variations in equipment and protocols.

APPROACH TO PI-RADS 3 LESIONS IN THE TRANSITION ZONE

Assigning overall score 3 in a particular lesion requires adequate understanding of the score definition on the dominant sequence in the TZ (T2WI). For score 1, PI-RADS v2.1 introduced the concept of "typical nodule," defined as a round, completely encapsulated nodule with the capsule assessed at least in 2 planes (Fig. 5).[3] The newly described atypical nodules constitute one of the descriptors of score 2. These are defined as either almost but not fully encapsulated nodule or a homogeneous circumscribed nodule without encapsulation (Figs. 6 and 7). Of note, these nodules depend on DWI to assign an overall score, with a combined DWI score $\geq$4 resulting in an overall score 3 (Fig. 8) and a combined DWI score $\leq$4 resulting in an overall score 2 (Fig. 9). There has been some lack of clarity around the degree of brightness on high b value images and darkness on ADC maps that constitute sufficient restriction to push a T2 score 2 nodule to 3 and this may result in overcalling of TZ nodules as PI-RADS 3 and reduce the performance of PI-RADS v2.1 compared to v2.

T2WI score 3 has not been modified from PI-RADS v2, defined as a lesion demonstrating heterogeneous signal intensity with obscured margins. This also depends on DWI to assign an overall score. Thus, lesions presenting with a combined DWI score of 5 can be upgraded to score 4 (Fig. 10) and lesions with a combined DWI score $\leq$5 remaining as score 3 (Fig. 11).[3,5]

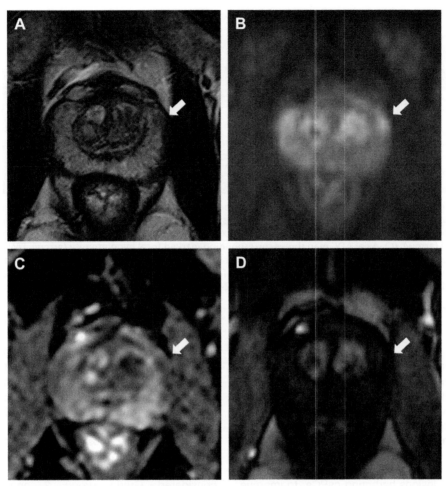

Fig. 1. Overall score 3 according to Prostate Imaging reporting and Data System v 2.1. 64-year-old man with history of elevated PSA to 5.6 ng/mL. (*A*), Axial T2WI shows a 7 mm slightly heterogeneous, predominantly hypointense focus in the left anterior mid PZ (*arrow*). T2WI score is 3. (*B*), Axial high b-value DWI shows corresponding focal hyperintensity (*arrow*). (*C*), Axial ADC map shows corresponding focal hypointensity (*arrow*). DWI score is 3. (*D*), Early DCE image shows no corresponding early enhancement (*arrow*). DCE is negative. DWI is the dominant sequence in determining overall score in the PZ. Since DCE is negative, overall score 3 was assigned. Targeted biopsy of lesion revealed PCa with ISUP grade group 1. DWI = Diffusion weighted image; ISUP= International Society of Urologic Pathology; PCa = prostate cancer; T2WI = T2-weighted image; PZ = Peripheral zone.

BIPARAMETRIC MAGNETIC RESONANCE IMAGING AND ITS INFLUENCE ON PI-RADS 3 LESIONS

The increment demand for the diagnostic workup of PCa with prostate MRI have led to increased waiting lists and concerns regarding difficult access to an optimal diagnostic MRI. Biparametric MRI (bpMRI) has been proposed as one of the possible solutions given the decreased exam length and the reduced costs avoiding the use of gadolinium.[6] The PI-RADS steering committee has addressed this need. Although it is estimated that in up to 80% of cases DCE has no effect on the overall PI-RADS score,[7,8] the lack of IV contrast can have an effect on reading performance, in particular for inexperienced readers[6,9] with consequent potential increase in number of indeterminate cases going for biopsies, even for expert readers. For example, in the multicenter 4M study, more indeterminate scores were assigned on bpMRI (8%-11%) when compared to mpMRI (6%) for 2 experienced readers.[10] Increased number of equivocal lesions could undermine the confidence of MRI utility among referring physicians and therefore, bpMRI should be considered in a risk based model mainly for low risk patients where there is a need to rule out csPCa.[6] The document states greater evidence is needed to define which patients would benefit

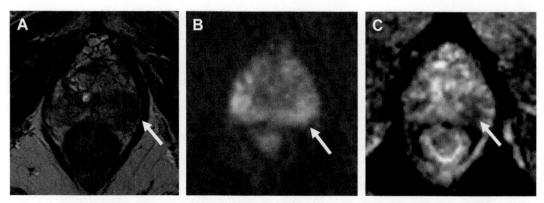

Fig. 2. Overall score 3 according to Prostate Imaging reporting and Data System v2.1. 58-year-old man with history of elevated PSA to 4.8 ng/mL. (A), Axial T2WI shows a 13 mm moderate hypointense focus centered in the left posterolateral mid PZ (arrow). T2WI score is 4. (B), Axial high b-value DWI shows no corresponding focal hyperintensity (arrow). (C), Axial ADC map shows corresponding marked focal hypointensity (arrow). DWI score is 3. DCE was negative (not shown). Targeted biopsy showed no malignancy. Follow up MRI demonstrated the complete resolution of the abnormality after treatment for prostatitis (not shown). DCE = dynamic contrast enhanced; DWI = Diffusion weighted image; T2WI = T2-weighted image; PZ = Peripheral zone.

from contrast administration and who can safely avoid it.

Although individual studies and systematic reviews support the use of bpMRI in the assessment of PCa,[11,12] to our knowledge, the impact of this approach has not been documented in the clinical practice. A study conducted by Belue and colleagues, addresses the status of bpMRI recognizing the PI-RADSv2.1 indications for the use of gadolinium as main considerations for the adoption of bpMRI. Gadolinium contrast injection is intended to provide better assessment PI-RADS 3 lesions harboring csPCa, to improve radiologist interpretation of MRIs with impaired diagnostic quality on T2w and DWI and assisting low experienced radiologists in prostate MR reporting.[3,13] According to their results, although several studies have been addressed the diagnostic yield of mpMRI versus bpMRI, most of the studies do not report the cancer grade group for each PI-RADS overall score, specifically for PI-RADS 3 where the "upgrade rule" from 3 to 4 is intended to increase the likelihood of csPCa, nor the overall quality of the examinations or the reporting radiologist expertise. Of the few studies that fulfilled most of the DCE indications, the utility of DCE varied according to the definition of csPCa being most useful on those which considered Grade group 2 and greater (≥Gleason score [GS] 3 + 4) and the PI-RADS score ≥3 as threshold for cancer significance. Of note, none of the studies included low

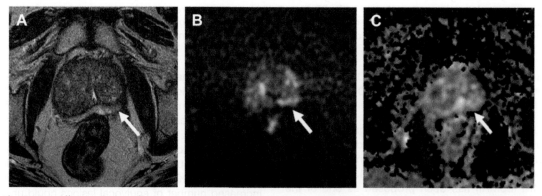

Fig. 3. Overall score 3 according to Prostate Imaging reporting and Data System v2.1. 68-year-old man with history of elevated PSA to 4.2 ng/mL. (A), Axial T2WI shows a 13 mm heterogeneous, mildly hypointense focus centered in the left posterior medial/lateral mid PZ (arrow). T2WI score is 3. (B), Axial high b-value DWI shows corresponding focal marked hyperintensity (arrow). (C), Axial ADC map shows no corresponding focal hypointensity (arrow). DWI score is 3. DCE was negative (not shown). Targeted biopsy showed no malignancy. DCE = dynamic contrast enhanced; DWI = Diffusion weighted image; T2WI = T2-weighted image; PZ = Peripheral zone.

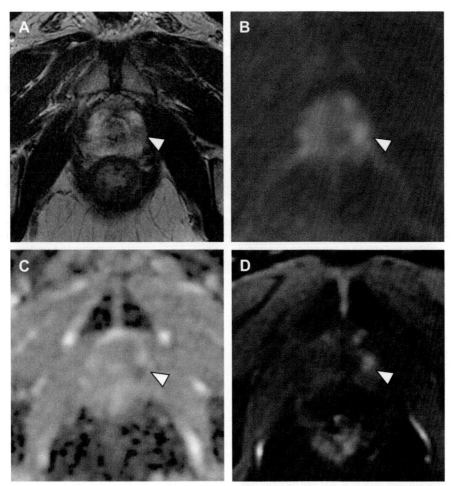

Fig. 4. Overall score 4 obtained using rule for upgrading from score 3 to score 4, according to Prostate Imaging reporting and Data System v2.1. 61-year-old man with history of elevated PSA to 8.2 ng/mL. (*A*), Axial T2WI shows a 7 mm circumscribed, moderate hypointense focus in the left anterior mid/apex PZ (*arrowhead*). T2WI score is 4. (*B*), Axial high b-value DWI shows corresponding focal hyperintensity (*arrowhead*). (*C*), Axial ADC map shows corresponding focal hypointensity (*arrowhead*). DWI score is 3. (*D*), Early DCE image shows corresponding early enhancement (*arrowhead*). DCE is positive. DWI is the dominant sequence in determining overall score in the PZ. However, score 3 on DWI is upgraded to overall score 4 if DCE is positive. Thus, overall score 4 was assigned. Targeted biopsy of lesion and prostatectomy specimen revealed PCa with ISUP grade group 3. DCE = dynamic contrast enhanced; DWI = Diffusion weighted image; ISUP= International Society of Urologic Pathology; PCa = prostate cancer; T2WI = T2-weighted image; PZ = Peripheral zone.

diagnostic quality examination which is a potential area of DCE strength and therefore, results should be interpreted with care because may not reflect the real life practice where the artifacts on DWI/T2w are encountered by the interpreting radiologist.[13]

Recently, Messina and colleagues, in a single center, prospective study assessed the diagnostic accuracy of the "upgrading rule" from PI-RADS score 3 to 4 based on early enhancement after contrast administration compared to true PI-RADS score 4 lesions based on high b-value/ADC. In their results, most of the cases of the upgraded PI-RADS 3 lesions were false positives, suggesting that use of

gadolinium has a detrimental effect on MRI accuracy for csPCa in PI-RADS 4 lesions.[14] In their cohort, however, all examinations were technically satisfactory and the potential role of DCE as safety net for quality impaired sequences was not assessed. These results are in contradiction with the study conducted by Druskin and colleagues, where PI-RADS 3 lesions were more likely to be csPCa if DCE was positive[15] and a retrospective study leaded by Taghipour and colleagues, using radical prostatectomy as gold standard. According to their results, a positive DCE increased the accuracy of detection of csPCa in 68.9% of lesions presenting with a DWI score of 3.[16]

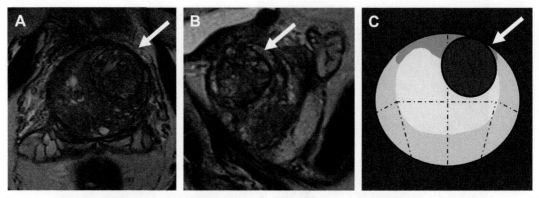

Fig. 5. Typical nodule, T2WI score 1 according to Prostate Imaging reporting and Data System v2.1. 73-year-old man with history of elevated PSA to 4.1 ng/mL. (*A*), Axial T2WI and (*B*), Sagittal T2WI show a round, circumscribed, completely encapsulated nodule in the left anterior base TZ (*arrows*). (*C*), Schematic diagram highlighting the complete capsule surrounding the nodule (*arrow*). A completely encapsulated nodule assessed at least in two planes is consistent with a typical nodule, score 1. T2WI = T2-weighted image; TZ = Transition zone.

PI-RADS 3 LESIONS AND CLINICALLY SIGNIFICANT PROSTATE CANCER

Detection rate of csPCa in PI-RADS 3 lesions varies greatly depending on several factors including disease prevalence among different patient population (biopsy naïve, previous negative biopsy or active surveillance), patient recruitment (prospective vs retrospective), definition of csPCa and the gold standard used for PCa confirmation (eg, MR in-bore biopsy, software fused MRI-US biopsy, cognitive MRI-US biopsy or radical prostatectomy).[17,18] Despite the effort of PI-RADS for reducing variability on Prostate MRI practice, it is still recognized differences in protocols among centers which will not be compliant with the quality standards proposed by PI-RADS system and will make the reporting radiologist uncertain of the findings.

Thus, a high quality MRI, compliant with PI-RADS 2.1 standards should provide the required information to reduce the number of equivocal/PI-RADS 3 lesions.[19] On the other hand, radiologist expertise on prostate mpMRI is considered another key factor in the number of reported PI-RADS 3 lesions with experienced radiologists reporting a smaller number of "equivocal" or "uncertain" cases versus less experienced readers.[18–20] Efforts in the formal quality assessment of the MR scanners/images/reporting and adequate training and continued the assessment of the interpreting radiologists are considered essential in prostate MRI practice with the aim to reduce the number of equivocal/PI-RADS 3 lesions.[19,21]

Management of patients with equivocal lesions on mpMRI and factors influencing biopsy decision process remain as an unmet need.[8] Shoots

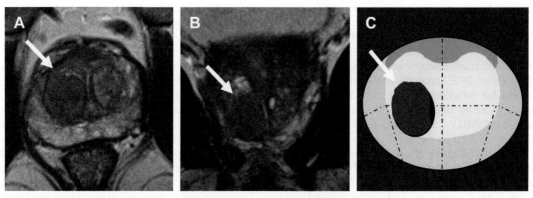

Fig. 6. Atypical nodule, T2WI score 2 according to Prostate Imaging reporting and Data System v2.1. 64-year-old man with history of elevated PSA to 5.0 ng/mL. (*A*), Axial T2WI and (*B*), Coronal T2WI show an almost but not fully encapsulated nodule predominantly occupying the right posterior mid TZ. The sites of capsule interruption are highlighted by the arrows in A and B. (*C*), Schematic representation of the incomplete capsule surrounding the nodule (*arrow*). T2WI = T2-weighted image; TZ = Transition zone.

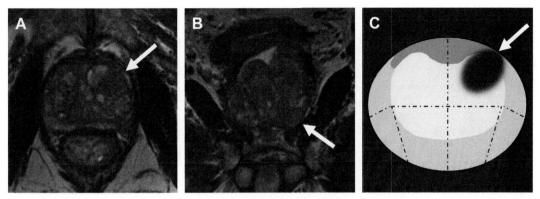

Fig. 7. Atypical nodule, T2WI score 2 according to Prostate Imaging reporting and Data System v2.1. 76-year-old man with history of elevated PSA to 4.6 ng/mL. (*A*), Axial T2WI and (*B*), Coronal T2WI show a homogeneous circumscribed nodule without encapsulation in the left anterior mid/apical TZ (*arrows*). (*C*), Schematic diagram highlighting the absence of capsule in the circumscribed nodule (*arrow*). T2WI = T2-weighted image; TZ = Transition zone.

and colleagues, showed cumulative data of 6 studies including 3 different patient populations: biopsy naïve, previous negative biopsy and active surveillance. His results demonstrated an overall csPCa rate of 21% for biopsy naïve patients, 16% for patients with prior negative biopsy and 17% for patients in active surveillance with an overall PCa detection rate of 39%, 30% and 47% respectively.[17] Maggi and colleagues, in a meta-analysis including 28 studies with 1759 PI-RADSv2 score 3 lesions, showed a reporting prevalence of 17.3% for equivocal PI-RADS 3 lesions. In their work, the detection rate of csPCa was further analyzed in biopsy naïve patients

and patients with negative prostate biopsy, yielding a rate of 21% and 17% respectively. The overall PCa rate was also determined, being 44% for biopsy naïve and 32% for the group of patients with prior negative biopsy.[8] Barkovich and colleagues in a systematic review including 13 studies, 2462 lesions in 1738 men of mixed population, showed a detection rate for CsPCa in PI-RADS 3 lesions of 11.5% with a total PCa detection rate of 25.5%. Of note, in their results, the majority of csPCa was consistent with International Society of Urologic Pathology (ISUP), grade group 2 with only 2.2% of the cases consistent with grade group $\geq$3.[22] **Table 1** summarizes

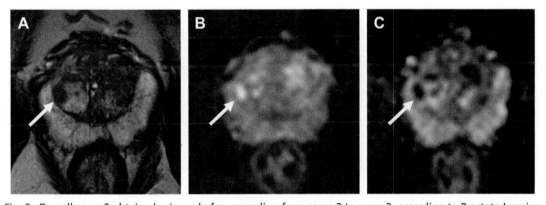

Fig. 8. Overall score 3 obtained using rule for upgrading from score 2 to score 3, according to Prostate Imaging reporting and Data System v2.1. 57-year-old man with history of elevated PSA to 5.7 ng/mL. (*A*), Axial T2WI shows a hypointense circumscribed "atypical" nodule without encapsulation in the right mid posterior TZ (*arrow*). T2WI score is 2. (*B*), Axial high b-value DWI shows corresponding marked hyperintensity (*arrow*). (*C*), Axial ADC map shows corresponding marked hypointensity (*arrow*). DWI score is 4. T2WI is the dominant sequence in determining overall score in the TZ. However, score 2 on T2WI is upgraded to overall score 3 if DWI score is $\geq$ 4. Thus, overall score 3 was assigned. Targeted biopsy of lesion revealed PCa with ISUP grade group 1. DWI = Diffusion weighted image; ISUP= International Society of Urologic Pathology; PCa = prostate cancer; T2WI = T2-weighted image; TZ = Transition zone.

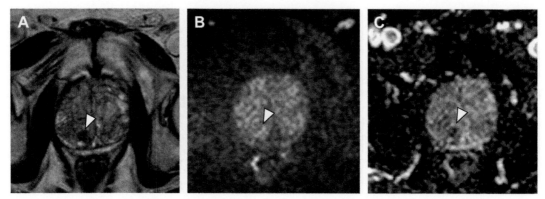

Fig. 9. Overall score 2 according to Prostate Imaging reporting and Data System v 2.1. 62-year-old man with history of elevated PSA to 5.7 ng/mL. (*A*), Axial T2WI shows a hypointense circumscribed "atypical" nodule without encapsulation in the right mid posterior TZ (*arrowhead*). T2WI score is 2. (*B*), Axial high b-value DWI shows no corresponding marked hyperintensity (*arrowhead*). (*C*), Axial ADC map shows corresponding hypointensity (*arrowhead*). DWI score is 3. T2WI is the dominant sequence in determining overall score in the TZ. Since DWI score is ≤ 4, overall score 2 was assigned. Targeted biopsy of lesion was not performed. DWI = Diffusion weighted image; T2WI = T2-weighted image; TZ = Transition zone.

the literature reporting the detection rate of PI-RADS v2 3 lesions for csPCa including the number of lesions for each study, the studied population, Magnet/coil specifications and country of origin.

WHAT TO DO WITH AN EQUIVOCAL OR PI-RADS 3 LESION?

Prevalence of equivocal results for csPCa is variable among practices ranging between 20% and 28% in large, prospective randomized studies.[35,36] Several factors can influence the assignment of a score 3 as stated above but at the radiologist level, is well known that moderately experienced readers are more likely to assign a score 3 to a given lesion than highly experienced readers.[20] There is no clear consensus on what would be the next step with a PI-RADS 3 lesion[37] with options including MRI follow up, targeted biopsy, systematic biopsy and/or saturation biopsy.

The PI-RADS steering committee recommends to follow the MRI-directed biopsy pathway (MRDB).[4,38,39] According to this recommendation,

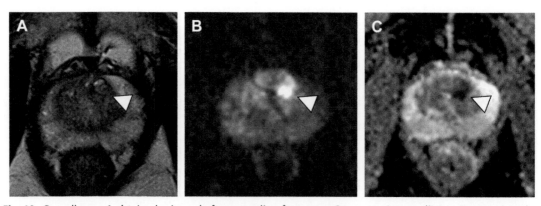

Fig. 10. Overall score 4 obtained using rule for upgrading from score 3 to score 4, according to Prostate Imaging reporting and Data System v2.1. 69-year-old man with history of elevated PSA to 7.8 ng/mL. (*A*), Axial T2WI shows a 15 mm, heterogeneous, predominantly hypointense lesion with obscured margins in the left mid anterior TZ (*arrowhead*). T2WI score is 3. (*B*), Axial high b-value DWI shows corresponding marked hyperintensity (*arrowhead*). (*C*), Axial ADC map shows corresponding marked hypointensity (*arrowhead*). DWI score is 5. T2WI is the dominant sequence in determining overall score in the TZ. However, score 3 on T2WI is upgraded to overall score 4 if DWI score is 5. Thus, overall score 4 was assigned. Targeted biopsy of lesion revealed PCa with ISUP grade group 2. DWI = Diffusion weighted image; ISUP= International Society of Urologic Pathology; PCa = prostate cancer; T2WI = T2-weighted image; TZ = Transition zone.

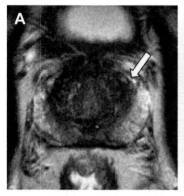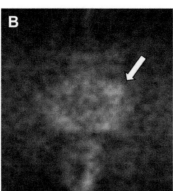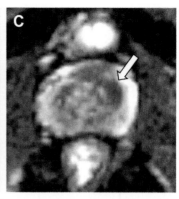

Fig. 11. Overall score 3 according to Prostate Imaging reporting and Data System v 2.1. 62-year-old man with history of elevated PSA to 5.3 ng/mL. (A), Axial T2WI shows a 16 mm, heterogeneous, predominantly hypointense lesion with obscured margins in the left anterior mid TZ (arrow). T2WI score is 3. (B), Axial high b-value DWI shows no corresponding marked hyperintensity (arrow). (C), Axial ADC map shows corresponding hypointensity (arrow). DWI score is 3. T2WI is the dominant sequence in determining overall score in the TZ. Since DWI score is < 5, overall score 3 was assigned. Targeted biopsy of lesion revealed PCa with ISUP grade group 2. DWI = Diffusion weighted image; ISUP= International Society of Urologic Pathology; PCa = prostate cancer; T2WI = T2-weighted image; TZ = Transition zone.

patients can be divided in 3 groups. In the first group, biopsy naïve patients, MRDB biopsy should be considered with or without systematic biopsy[40] with the alternative of avoiding biopsy in selected patients with no high-risk factors[40] ensuring a safety net monitoring. For the second group of patients with prior negative biopsy at persistent risk for PCa, MRDB can be considered alone as per European Association of Urology (EAU) guidelines[41] or MRDB targeted and systematic biopsy as per Society of Abdominal Radiology (SAR)/American Urologic Association (AUA) consensus statement.[42] Whole-prostate mapping biopsies is considered an alternative for this group of patients.[4] For the third group, patients with persistent risk with negative findings or nonexplanatory histology at MRDB without systematic biopsy cores, a systematic biopsy is recommended with or without MRDB. The options include a saturation or mapping biopsy.[4]

The EAU guidelines divide the patient population into 2 groups. For biopsy naïve patients with PI-RADS 3 lesions, combined targeted and systematic biopsy is recommended. For the second group of patients with prior negative biopsy, only a targeted biopsy from the equivocal lesion is recommended.[41]

ADDITIONAL CONSIDERATIONS AND FUTURE PERSPECTIVES
Clinical Parameters and Risk Modeling

Adaptive risk modeling that takes into account common clinical variables used in risk calculators such as the Prostate Cancer Prevention Trial (PCPT) risk calculator, PI-RADS score, PSA, prior results and fluidic or tissue based molecular markers to improve overall accuracy of CSPCa risk is a common an immediate goal in the urooncology community, A variety of clinical variables have been analyzed as potential aid in the biopsy decision of PI-RADS 3 lesions. A study conducted by Kim and colleagues, showed the age and location of tumor within the PZ as significant predictors for the detection of csPCa.[43] Martorana and colleagues proposed a 0.5 mL lesion volume as cutoff for discriminating fusion-targeted biopsy need in PI-RADS v2.1 score 3 lesions with a diagnostic accuracy of 73.2% and a negative predictive value of 96.5%. Multivariate analysis adding prostate volume and patient age improved diagnostic accuracy to 86.5%.[44]

PSAD has been shown to be related with the presence of csPca when a cut-off of 0.15 ng/mL^2 is used.[43] Felker and colleagues demonstrated that PSAD of 0.15 and greater had a statistically significant association with csPCa in PI-RADS 3 lesions among the transition zone ($P = .001$) and that in combination with an ADC value less than 1000 mm^2/s improves the detection of csPCa from 15% to 60% (AUC>0.9).[34] Optimal thresholds for PSAD have not been established, however a range of 0.1 to 0.15 for thresholds seems reasonable. Deniffel and colleagues looked at PI-RADS and PSAD models in a decision curve analysis compared to other proposed risk models incorporating MRI. With an acceptable modeled risk threshold of 10% for missing csPCa they showed that a strategy of avoiding biopsy in patients with PI-RADS 3 lesions and a PSAD less than 0.1 performed best avoiding biopsy in 63/1000 men and missing no cancers in the validation cohort.[45]

Table 1
Summary of the literature evidence assessing the detection rate of PI-RADS v2 category 3 lesions for Clinically Significant Prostate Cancer (csPCa)

Study	n	Population	Detection Rate for csPCa (%)	Magnet	Coil	Zone	Dates (Country)
Otti et al,[23] 2019	792	Biopsy naïve	30.5	1.5 T	Body array	PZ/TZ	Jul 2013 – Apr 2016 (UK)
Thai et al,[24] 2018	634	Not specified	11.1	3T	Endorectal/ Body array	TZ	Jan 2012 – Feb 2015 (USA)
Sheridan et al,[25] 2018	111	Not specified	17.1	3T	Body array	PZ/TZ	Jan 2015 – Jul 2016 (USA)
Mehralivand et al,[26] 2017	737	Not specified	12	3T	Endorectal/ Body array	PZ/TZ	May 2015 – May 2016 (USA)
Tan et al,[27] 2017	134	Biopsy naïve, prior negative biopsy and active surveillance	10	3T	Body array	PZ/TZ	May 2013 – Dec 2016 (USA)
Patel et al,[28] 2019	122	Not specified	24	3T	Endorectal/ Body array	PZ/TZ	Sept 2010- Jun 2013 (USA)
Curci et al,[29] 2018	286	Active surveillance	11	3T	Body array	PZ/TZ	Aug 2015 – Aug 2016 (USA)
Feng et al,[30] 2016	401	Not specified	5.1	3T	Body array	PZ/TZ	Jun 2013 – Jul 2015 (China)
Rosenkrantz et al,[31] 2017	343	Biopsy naïve, prior negative biopsy and active surveillance	11.4–27.1	3T	Body array	PZ/TZ	Sep 2013 – Feb 2015 (USA)
Zhao et al,[32] 2016	372	Not specified	26–35	3T	Body array	PZ/TZ	Nov 2010 – Dec 2013 (China)
Purysko et al,[33] 2017	170	Not specified	14–20	3T	Body array	PZ/TZ	Aug 2014 – Feb 2015 (USA)
Felker et al,[34] 2017	96	Not specified	15	3T	Body array	TZ	Apr 2014 – Apr 2016 (USA)

Molecular markers such as Prostate Cancer (PC)- specific biomarker prostate cancer gene 3 (PCA3) considered the most specific PC gene with increased diagnostic accuracy for PCa detection,[46] can aim in the selection of patients for biopsy. A study conducted by Kaufmann and colleagues, in 49 patients with equivocal, PI-RADS 3 lesions and previous negative biopsies demonstrated increase of diagnostic accuracy to 91.8% with the addition of PCA3 cutoff value of 35, suggesting the use of this cutoff to reduce the diagnostic uncertainty in this equivocal lesions and avoid potential unnecessary biopsies.[47]

To our knowledge, additional studies combining molecular markers and PI-RADS 3 lesions are lacking. However, other molecular markers such as the Prostatic health index (PHI), defined as a combination of relative concentrations of 3 different PSA forms: total PSA, free PSA, and [-2] proPSA, obtained using the mathematical formula: ([-2]proPSA/free PSA) $\times \sqrt{PSA}$) have been studied as an option to increase specificity before initial or repeat biopsy.[48] A study conducted by Gnanapragasam and colleagues, showed that the addition of PHI to mpMRI can avoid unnecessary repeat biopsies while preserving the detection of csPCa. In this study, adding PHI to mpMRI improved significant cancer prediction (AUC 0.75) compared to mpMRI + PSA alone (AUC 0.69). According to their results, at a threshold of $\geq$35, PHI + mpMRI demonstrated an NPV of 0.97 for excluding significant tumors. Tosoian and colleagues found 0 patients with a PI-RADS score 3 and PHI less than 27 harboring csPCa, suggesting a potential threshold of 27 for the identification of csPCa. In their cohort, the incorporation of PHI reduced the rate of unnecessary biopsies without changing the frequency of detection of csPCa.[49]

Serum biomarker 4K score test is based on a 4-kallikrein panel including kallikrein-related peptidase 2 (hK2), total PSA, intact and free PSA in combination with patient age, digital rectal examination and biopsy history.[48] Initial retrospective studies analyzing 4K score with PI-RADS $\geq$3 have shown that using a threshold of 4Kscore $\geq$7.5% in combination with MR findings, the percentage of missed csPCa is about 0.7% with 2.45% of unnecessary biopsies avoided. However, further addition of PSAD $\geq$ 0.15 to the model would led to only missing 2.2% of csPCa while avoiding 11.5% biopsies.[50] A study conducted by Wagaskar and colleagues, showed that a combination of both, the 4K score test greater than 7% and mpMRI scores $\geq$3 reduces the number of biopsies without compromising the detection of csPCa and can aid in reducing the detection of non-csPCa.[51]

ARTIFICIAL INTELLIGENCE (AI) IN PI-RADS 3 LESIONS

Machine Learning (ML), a subfield of AI, refers to the creation of algorithms that analyzes datasets and learns from human experts to predict outcomes.[52] Algorithms are usually supervised (where the ground-truth is formed directly by human experts) or unsupervised (algorithm development is independent of human experts), trained on large datasets.[52,53] There has been extensive work evaluating ML of radiomic features, which include texture, shape and size.[54] The most studied radiomic feature in prostate MRI is texture analysis, a mathematical method assessing the spatial heterogeneity by analyzing the distribution and relationship of voxel gray-scale levels[55] and has shown to be promising at detecting prostate cancers and can provide information on tumor grade.[56,57] There has been extensive work evaluating ML of radiomic features of PI-RADS 3 lesions demonstrating mixed results. For example, Hou and colleagues found radiomic machine learning models combining T2W, DWI and ADC maps could help csPCa in PI-RADS 3 lesions at a single center.[58] Similarly, in a single center study, Hectors and colleagues found ML of T2W radiomic features could improve the diagnosis of csPCs in PI-RADS 3 lesions.[59] However, these results were not generalizable in the multicenter study by Lim and colleagues, which found radiomic ML of T2W and ADC features achieved only moderate accuracy in PI-RADS category 3 lesions.[60] Although there is interest in radiomics to provide non-invasive tumor assessment, there appear to be significant limitations often related to lack of standardization, which limits the applicability of results, requiring more robust multicenter standardized study before it can be used in clinical practice.

A subset of ML known as deep convolutional neural networks (CNN), shows promise in medical imaging.[52] CNN is the creation of an algorithm when imaging data is transformed into multiple hidden layers that mimics the human brain neural network. CNN has been demonstrated to aid with prostate cancer lesion detection[61,62] and tumor aggressiveness.[53,63,64] However, the results are less robust when applied to indeterminate PI-RADS 3 lesions. For example, Sanford and colleagues developed an AI algorithm assigning a PI-RADS score on segmented lesion with moderate agreement with expert radiologist and similar cancer detection rates.[62] However, the AI algorithm performed worse for lower PI-RADS 3 and 4 lesions compared to PI-RADS 5 lesions.[62] Winkel and colleagues developed a deep learning system assessing the accuracy and efficiency of bi-parametric prostate MRI with similar accuracy between the algorithm and expert radiologist for PI-RADS $\geq$4 lesions; however, the algorithm was worse compared to radiologist when incorporating PI-RADS 3 lesions.[61] Similarly, Shelb and colleagues, developed a type of CNN algorithm at evaluating T2W and DWI images which performed similar to PI-RADS assessment, particularly for PI-RADS $\geq$4 lesions but the algorithm was again less robust when also evaluating PI-RADS 3 lesions.[65] There are many challenges for the use of AI in prostate imaging with issues of particular importance for indeterminate PI-RADS 3 lesions. For example, there is higher inter-reader variability in assigning PI-RADS 3 lesion which varies between expert and non-expert centers.[61,66] Because of the heterogeneous PI-RADS 3 classification of lesions, the result of AI algorithms in indeterminate lesions have inherent noise, affecting diagnostic accuracy and applicability.[61] The prevalence of csPCs in PI-RADS 3 lesions is relatively low, ranging from approximately 13% to 27%[67] and the datasets used are relatively small, which leads to the risk of overfitting of the algorithm. Deep learning has great potential when trained on large datasets; however, in the setting of PI-RADS 3 lesion, most studies are composed of small single institution incorporating only hundreds of patients at best.[68] Another issue of importance is the formulation of an appropriate reference standard for the evaluation of PI-RADS 3 lesions.[52] Possible reference standards include systematic biopsy, targeted biopsy (cognitive fusion, software fusion or MRI-in-bore) and surgical radical prostatectomy specimens. As the majority of PI-RADS 3 lesions are not cancer, surgical radical prostatectomy (which could be considered the ideal ground truth giving information on all prostate lesions) cannot solely be used as the majority of men with PI-RADS 3 lesions will not undergo surgery and a significant proportion of cases will be omitted from analysis. Similarly, targeted biopsy has limitations if a lesion is not accurately sampled or is not detected on MRI and excluded from analysis. Therefore, an ideal algorithm should be trained and tested on men using a combination of radical prostatectomy, targeted biopsy and systematic biopsy (to identify men without cancer) as the ground truth and be verified with men both with and without cancer.[52] AI in the assessment of PI-RADS category 3 lesions is a rapidly evolving field with immense interest and impact for improving management decisions. In the future, large multi-institutional datasets will need to be developed to allow for robust algorithm develop and to ensure generalizability of results to all men.

SUMMARY

PI-RADSv2.1 brought important modifications for the assessment of category 3 lesions in both the peripheral and transition zone. The impact of these changes has been small. The PI-RADS 3 category can be problematic and combination with PSAD is the most likely approach to aid in clinical decision making. This is being supplemented in practice with commercially available fluidic makers but further evidence in prospective trials of the utilis of these approaches to improve the accuracy of PI-RADS alone in the detection of csPCa is still needed. Continued efforts are in place to ensure widespread standardisation and quality assurance of mpMRI as well as adequate training and certification of reporting radiologists. Clear steps in the management of PI-RADS 3 lesions remains an unmet need and several initial studies have been raised the potential utility of serum biomarkers for the selection of patients who may undergo biopsy and decrease the number of unnecessary biopsies while maintaining a high yield for csPCa detection. Artificial intelligence, as developing tool in Radiology has also been studied in the setting of equivocal lesions on mpMRI. However, further prospective studies are also required for machine learning to determine the benefit in both reducing the number of reported PI-RADS 3 lesions as well as the refinement of imaging biomarkers useful for the selection of patients for biopsy.

CLINICS CARE POINTS

- PI-RADS 3 lesions are equivocal for csPCa. The number of reported equivocal lesions mainly depends on MRI quality and radiologist training/expertise.

- PI-RADS v2.1 incorporates updated definitions for overall score 3 lesions which are key in the correct identification and reporting.

- Given the increased demand for prostate MRI, biparametric MRI can be considered as an alternative for low-risk patients where there is a need to rule out csPCa acknowledging this technique may increase the number of indeterminate cases going for biopsies.

DISCLOSURE

No relevant disclosures regarding the educational content of this article.

REFERENCES

1. Barentsz JO, Richenberg J, Clements R, et al. ESUR prostate MR guidelines 2012. Eur Radiol 2012;22(4): 746–57.

2. Weinreb JC, Barentsz JO, Choyke PL, et al. PI-RADS Prostate Imaging - Reporting and Data System: 2015, Version 2. Eur Urol 2016;69(1):16–40.

3. Turkbey B, Rosenkrantz AB, Haider MA, et al. Prostate Imaging Reporting and Data System Version 2.1: 2019 Update of Prostate Imaging Reporting and Data System Version 2. Eur Urol 2019; 76(3):340–51. Available at: https://linkinghub. elsevier.com/retrieve/pii/S0302283819301800.

4. Padhani AR, Barentsz J, Villeirs G, et al. PI-RADS Steering Committee: The PI-RADS Multiparametric MRI and MRI-directed Biopsy Pathway. Radiology 2019;292(2):464–74.

5. Barrett T, Rajesh A, Rosenkrantz AB, et al. PI-RADS version 2.1: one small step for prostate MRI. Clin Radiol 2019;74(11):841–52.

6. Schoots IG, Barentsz JO, Bittencourt LK, et al. PI-RADS Committee Position on MRI Without Contrast Medium in Biopsy-Naive Men With Suspected Prostate Cancer: Narrative Review. AJR Am J Roentgenol 2021;216(1):3–19.

7. Zawaideh JP, Sala E, Shaida N, et al. Diagnostic accuracy of biparametric versus multiparametric prostate MRI: assessment of contrast benefit in clinical practice. Eur Radiol 2020;30(7):4039–49.

8. Maggi M, Panebianco V, Mosca A, et al. Prostate Imaging Reporting and Data System 3 Category Cases at Multiparametric Magnetic Resonance for Prostate Cancer: A Systematic Review and Meta-analysis. Eur Urol Focus 2020;6(3):463–78.

9. Gatti M, Faletti R, Calleris G, et al. Prostate cancer detection with biparametric magnetic resonance imaging (bpMRI) by readers with different experience: performance and comparison with multiparametric (mpMRI). Abdom Radiol (New York) 2019;44(5):1883–93.

10. van der Leest M, Israël B, Cornel EB, et al. High Diagnostic Performance of Short Magnetic Resonance Imaging Protocols for Prostate Cancer Detection in Biopsy-naïve Men: The Next Step in Magnetic Resonance Imaging Accessibility. Eur Urol 2019; 76(5):574–81.

11. Pecoraro M, Messina E, Bicchetti M, et al. The future direction of imaging in prostate cancer: MRI with or without contrast injection. Andrology 2021;9(5): 1429–43.

12. Tamada T, Kido A, Yamamoto A, et al. Comparison of Biparametric and Multiparametric MRI for Clinically Significant Prostate Cancer Detection With PI-RADS Version 2.1. J Magn Reson Imaging 2021;53(1):283–91.

13. Belue MJ, Yilmaz EC, Daryanani A, et al. Current Status of Biparametric MRI in Prostate Cancer Diagnosis: Literature Analysis. Life 2022;12(6).

14. Messina E, Pecoraro M, Laschena L, et al. Low cancer yield in PI-RADS 3 upgraded to 4 by dynamic contrast-enhanced MRI: is it time to reconsider scoring categorization? Eur Radiol 2023. https:// doi.org/10.1007/s00330-023-09605-0.

15. Druskin SC, Ward R, Purysko AS, et al. Dynamic Contrast Enhanced Magnetic Resonance Imaging Improves Classification of Prostate Lesions: A Study of Pathological Outcomes on Targeted Prostate Biopsy. J Urol 2017;198(6):1301–8.

16. Taghipour M, Ziaei A, Alessandrino F, et al. Investigating the role of DCE-MRI, over T2 and DWI, in accurate PI-RADS v2 assessment of clinically significant peripheral zone prostate lesions as defined at radical prostatectomy. Abdom Radiol (New York) 2019;44(4):1520–7.

17. Schoots IG. MRI in early prostate cancer detection: how to manage indeterminate or equivocal PI-RADS 3 lesions? Transl Androl Urol 2018;7(1): 70–82.

18. Moldovan PC, Van den Broeck T, Sylvester R, et al. What Is the Negative Predictive Value of Multiparametric Magnetic Resonance Imaging in Excluding Prostate Cancer at Biopsy? A Systematic Review and Meta-analysis from the European Association of Urology Prostate Cancer Guidelines Panel. Eur Urol 2017;72(2):250–66.

19. Barentsz JO, van der Leest MMG, Israël B. Reply to Jochen Walz. Let's Keep It at One Step at a Time: Why Biparametric Magnetic Resonance Imaging Is Not the Priority Today. Eur Urol 2019;76:582–3. How to Implement High-quality, High-volume Prostate Magnetic Resonance Imaging: Gd Contrast Can Help. Vol. 76, European urology. Switzerland; 2019. p. 584–583.

20. Greer MD, Brown AM, Shih JH, et al. Accuracy and agreement of PI-RADSv2 for prostate cancer mpMRI: A multireader study. J Magn Reson Imaging 2017;45(2):579–85.

21. Abreu-Gomez J, Shabana W, McInnes MDF, et al. Regional Standardization of Prostate Multiparametric MRI Performance and Reporting: Is There a Role for a Director of Prostate Imaging? AJR Am J Roentgenol 2019;213(4):844–50.

22. Barkovich EJ, Shankar PR, Westphalen AC. A Systematic Review of the Existing Prostate Imaging Reporting and Data System Version 2 (PI-RADSv2) Literature and Subset Meta-Analysis of PI-RADSv2 Categories Stratified by Gleason Scores. AJR Am J Roentgenol 2019;212(4): 847–54.

23. Otti VC, Miller C, Powell RJ, et al. The diagnostic accuracy of multiparametric magnetic resonance imaging before biopsy in the detection of prostate cancer. BJU Int 2019;123(1):82–90.

24. Thai JN, Narayanan HA, George AK, et al. Validation of PI-RADS Version 2 in Transition Zone Lesions for

the Detection of Prostate Cancer. Radiology 2018; 288(2):485–91.

25. Sheridan AD, Nath SK, Syed JS, et al. Risk of Clinically Significant Prostate Cancer Associated With Prostate Imaging Reporting and Data System Category 3 (Equivocal) Lesions Identified on Multiparametric Prostate MRI. AJR Am J Roentgenol 2018; 210(2):347–57.

26. Mehralivand S, Bednarova S, Shih JH, et al. Prospective Evaluation of PI-RADS™ Version 2 Using the International Society of Urological Pathology Prostate Cancer Grade Group System. J Urol 2017;198(3):583–90.

27. Tan N, Lin W-C, Khoshnoodi P, et al. In-Bore 3-T MR-guided Transrectal Targeted Prostate Biopsy: Prostate Imaging Reporting and Data System Version 2-based Diagnostic Performance for Detection of Prostate Cancer. Radiology 2017;283(1):130–9.

28. Patel NU, Lind KE, Garg K, et al. Assessment of PI-RADS v2 categories ≥ 3 for diagnosis of clinically significant prostate cancer. Abdom Radiol (New York) 2019;44(2):705–12.

29. Curci NE, Lane BR, Shankar PR, et al. Integration and Diagnostic Accuracy of 3T Nonendorectal coil Prostate Magnetic Resonance Imaging in the Context of Active Surveillance. Urology 2018;116: 137–43.

30. Feng Z-Y, Wang L, Min X-D, et al. Prostate Cancer Detection with Multiparametric Magnetic Resonance Imaging: Prostate Imaging Reporting and Data System Version 1 versus Version 2. Chin Med J (Engl) 2016;129(20):2451–9.

31. Rosenkrantz AB, Babb JS, Taneja SS, et al. Proposed Adjustments to PI-RADS Version 2 Decision Rules: Impact on Prostate Cancer Detection. Radiology 2017;283(1):119–29.

32. Zhao C, Gao G, Fang D, et al. The efficiency of multiparametric magnetic resonance imaging (mpMRI) using PI-RADS Version 2 in the diagnosis of clinically significant prostate cancer. Clin Imaging 2016;40(5): 885–8.

33. Purysko AS, Bittencourt LK, Bullen JA, et al. Accuracy and Interobserver Agreement for Prostate Imaging Reporting and Data System, Version 2, for the Characterization of Lesions Identified on Multiparametric MRI of the Prostate. AJR Am J Roentgenol 2017;209(2):339–49.

34. Felker ER, Raman SS, Margolis DJ, et al. Risk Stratification Among Men With Prostate Imaging Reporting and Data System version 2 Category 3 Transition Zone Lesions: Is Biopsy Always Necessary? AJR Am J Roentgenol 2017;209(6):1272–7.

35. Ahmed HU, El-Shater Bosaily A, Brown LC, et al. Diagnostic accuracy of multi-parametric MRI and TRUS biopsy in prostate cancer (PROMIS): a paired validating confirmatory study. Lancet [Internet] 2017;389(10071):815–22.

36. Kasivisvanathan V, Rannikko AS, Borghi M, et al. MRI-Targeted or Standard Biopsy for Prostate-Cancer Diagnosis. N Engl J Med 2018;378(19): 1767–77.

37. Gomez Rivas J, Giganti F, Alvarez-Maestro M, et al. Prostate Indeterminate Lesions on Magnetic Resonance Imaging-Biopsy Versus Surveillance: A Literature Review. Eur Urol Focus 2019;5(5): 799–806.

38. Padhani AR, Weinreb J, Rosenkrantz AB, et al. Prostate Imaging-Reporting and Data System Steering Committee: PI-RADS v2 Status Update and Future Directions. Eur Urol 2019;75(3):385–96.

39. Drost F-JH, Osses DF, Nieboer D, et al. Prostate MRI, with or without MRI-targeted biopsy, and systematic biopsy for detecting prostate cancer. Cochrane Database Syst Rev 2019;4(4):CD012663.

40. National Institute for Health and Care Excellence (NICE). Prostate cancer: diagnosis and management (update). Internet. 2019. Available at: https://www.nice.org.uk/guidance/ng131. Accessed April 15, 2023.

41. EAU Guidelines. March 10-13, Milan, Italy. Edn. https://uroweb.org/eau-guidelines/citing-usage-republication.

42. Rosenkrantz AB, Verma S, Choyke P, et al. Prostate Magnetic Resonance Imaging and Magnetic Resonance Imaging Targeted Biopsy in Patients with a Prior Negative Biopsy: A Consensus Statement by AUA and SAR. J Urol 2016;196(6):1613–8.

43. Kim TJ, Lee MS, Hwang S II, et al. Outcomes of magnetic resonance imaging fusion-targeted biopsy of prostate imaging reporting and data system 3 lesions. World J Urol 2019;37(8):1581–6.

44. Martorana E, Aisa MC, Grisanti R, et al. Lesion Volume in a Bi- or Multivariate Prediction Model for the Management of PI-RADS v2.1 Score 3 Category Lesions. Turkish J Urol 2022;48(4):268–77.

45. Deniffel D, Healy GM, Dong X, et al. Avoiding Unnecessary Biopsy: MRI-based Risk Models versus a PI-RADS and PSA Density Strategy for Clinically Significant Prostate Cancer. Radiology 2021;300(2):369–79.

46. Busetto GM, De Berardinis E, Sciarra A, et al. Prostate cancer gene 3 and multiparametric magnetic resonance can reduce unnecessary biopsies: decision curve analysis to evaluate predictive models. Urology 2013;82(6):1355–60.

47. Kaufmann S, Bedke J, Gatidis S, et al. Prostate cancer gene 3 (PCA3) is of additional predictive value in patients with PI-RADS grade III (intermediate) lesions in the MR-guided re-biopsy setting for prostate cancer. World J Urol 2016;34(4):509–15.

48. Rivas JG, Alvarez-Maestro M, Czarniecki M, et al. Negative Biopsies With Rising Prostate-Specific Antigen. What To Do? EMJ Urol 2017;5(1):76–82.

49. Tosoian JJ, Druskin SC, Andreas D, et al. Use of the Prostate Health Index for detection of prostate

cancer: results from a large academic practice. Prostate Cancer Prostatic Dis 2017;20(2):228–33.

50. Baskin AS, de la Calle C, Fasulo V, et al. Mp26-11 Clinical Utility of 4Kscore When Combined With Psa, Trus and Mpmri for the Detection of High-Grade Prostate Cancer. J Urol 2021; 206(Supplement 3):466–7.

51. Gross J, Vetter J, Andriole G, et al. Mp26-13 Evaluating the four-kallikrein panel and mpmri in predicting prostate biopsy outcomes. J Urol 2021; 206(Supplement 3):467–8.

52. Turkbey B, Haider MA. Artificial Intelligence for Automated Cancer Detection on Prostate MRI: Opportunities and Ongoing Challenges, From the AJR Special Series on AI Applications. AJR Am J Roentgenol 2022;219(2):188–94.

53. Cuocolo R, Cipullo MB, Stanzione A, et al. Machine learning applications in prostate cancer magnetic resonance imaging. Eur Radiol Exp 2019;3(1):35.

54. Varghese BA, Cen SY, Hwang DH, et al. Texture Analysis of Imaging: What Radiologists Need to Know. AJR Am J Roentgenol 2019;212(3):520–8.

55. Schieda N, Lim CS, Zabihollahy F, et al. Quantitative Prostate MRI. J Magn Reson Imaging 2021;53(6): 1632–45.

56. Rozenberg R, Thornhill RE, Flood TA, et al. Whole-Tumor Quantitative Apparent Diffusion Coefficient Histogram and Texture Analysis to Predict Gleason Score Upgrading in Intermediate-Risk 3 + 4 = 7 Prostate Cancer. AJR Am J Roentgenol 2016; 206(4):775–82.

57. Wibmer A, Hricak H, Gondo T, et al. Haralick texture analysis of prostate MRI: utility for differentiating non-cancerous prostate from prostate cancer and differentiating prostate cancers with different Gleason scores. Eur Radiol 2015;25(10):2840–50.

58. Hou Y, Bao M-L, Wu C-J, et al. A radiomics machine learning-based redefining score robustly identifies clinically significant prostate cancer in equivocal PI-RADS score 3 lesions. Abdom Radiol (New York) 2020;45(12):4223–34.

59. Hectors SJ, Chen C, Chen J, et al. Magnetic Resonance Imaging Radiomics-Based Machine Learning Prediction of Clinically Significant Prostate Cancer in Equivocal PI-RADS 3 Lesions. J Magn Reson Imaging 2021;54(5):1466–73.

60. Lim CS, Abreu-Gomez J, Thornhill R, et al. Utility of machine learning of apparent diffusion coefficient (ADC) and T2-weighted (T2W) radiomic features in PI-RADS version 2.1 category 3 lesions to predict prostate cancer diagnosis. Abdom Radiol (New York) 2021;46(12):5647–58.

61. Winkel DJ, Tong A, Lou B, et al. A Novel Deep Learning Based Computer-Aided Diagnosis System Improves the Accuracy and Efficiency of Radiologists in Reading Biparametric Magnetic Resonance Images of the Prostate: Results of a Multireader, Multicase Study. Invest Radiol 2021;56(10):605–13.

62. Sanford T, Harmon SA, Turkbey EB, et al. Deep-Learning-Based Artificial Intelligence for PI-RADS Classification to Assist Multiparametric Prostate MRI Interpretation: A Development Study. J Magn Reson Imaging 2020;52(5):1499–507.

63. Le MH, Chen J, Wang L, et al. Automated diagnosis of prostate cancer in multi-parametric MRI based on multimodal convolutional neural networks. Phys Med Biol 2017;62(16):6497–514.

64. Belue MJ, Turkbey B. Tasks for artificial intelligence in prostate MRI. Eur Radiol Exp 2022;6(1):33.

65. Schelb P, Kohl S, Radtke JP, et al. Classification of Cancer at Prostate MRI: Deep Learning versus Clinical PI-RADS Assessment. Radiology 2019;293(3): 607–17.

66. Greer MD, Shih JH, Barrett T, et al. All over the map: An interobserver agreement study of tumor location based on the PI-RADSv2 sector map. J Magn Reson Imaging 2018;48(2):482–90.

67. Oerther B, Engel H, Bamberg F, et al. Cancer detection rates of the PI-RADSv2.1 assessment categories: systematic review and meta-analysis on lesion level and patient level. Prostate Cancer Prostatic Dis 2022;25(2):256–63.

68. Cuocolo R, Cipullo MB, Stanzione A, et al. Machine learning for the identification of clinically significant prostate cancer on MRI: a meta-analysis. Eur Radiol 2020;30(12):6877–87.

Pitfalls in Prostate MR Imaging Interpretation

Devaki Shilpa Sudha Surasi, MD, CMQ[a,*], Praneeth Kalva, BS[b], Ken-Pin Hwang, PhD[c], Tharakeswara Kumar Bathala, MD, MS[a]

KEYWORDS

- Prostate MR imaging • Multiparametric MR imaging • Prostate cancer • Pitfalls in interpretation

KEY POINTS

- Normal anatomic structures such as the normal central zone, anterior fibromuscular stroma, periprostatic venous plexus, neurovascular structures, and thick surgical capsule can potentially be misinterpreted as prostate cancer.
- Benign lesions which can mimic prostate cancer include prostatitis, benign prostatic hyperplasia nodules, focal prostate atrophy, and prostate calcifications.
- Postprocedural and posttreatment changes can persist for several weeks, and a good understanding of these pitfalls is essential for accurate interpretation of multiparametric prostate MR imaging.

INTRODUCTION

Prostate cancer is the most frequently diagnosed non-cutaneous cancer and the second leading cause of cancer-related death in men.[1] Over the past 2 decades, evidence has been collected supporting the use of prostate MR imaging in the screening and diagnosis of prostate cancer, along with traditional diagnostic tools such as digital rectal examination, serum prostate-specific antigen (PSA) levels, and transrectal prostate biopsy.[2] Prostate MR imaging is now routinely used in the screening, diagnosis, staging, imaging guidance, and therapy for prostate cancer.[2] The introduction of Prostate Imaging-Reporting and Data System (PI-RADS) has made it possible to standardize imaging interpretation and reporting for prostate MR imaging.[3] Although the existence of a standardized protocol significantly helps the radiologist in the interpretation and reporting of prostate imaging, prostate MR imaging is not free of diagnostic pitfalls, because many benign conditions or even normal anatomic structures may mimic prostate carcinoma.[4] In addition, the appearance of each

prostate gland on MR imaging is nearly unique due to variations in men's levels of benign prostatic hyperplasia (BPH) and changes brought on by prostatitis or prior treatments.[5] It is critical to be aware of these limitations, as false-positive and false-negative MR imaging results can lead to over- or undertreatment, respectively.[6] For this reason, it is essential to have a thorough understanding of the anatomy of the prostate gland as well as the typical and atypical imaging appearance of prostate cancer and the conditions that can mimic it.[7]

The objective of this review is to examine specific challenges associated with prostate MR imaging interpretation, including benign conditions, normal anatomic structures, and postprocedural changes that may interfere with accurate diagnosis of prostate cancer. In addition, this review aims to propose potential approaches to mitigate common errors.

Normal Central Zone

The ejaculatory ducts are encircled by a layer of tissue known as the central zone (CZ), which

[a] Division of Diagnostic Imaging, The University of Texas MD Anderson Cancer Center, 1400 Pressler, Unit 1483, Houston, TX 77030, USA; [b] University of Texas Southwestern Medical School, 5323 Harry Hines Blvd, Dallas, TX 75390, USA; [c] Division of Diagnostic Imaging, The University of Texas MD Anderson Cancer Center, 1400 Pressler, Unit 1472, Houston, TX 77030, USA
* Corresponding author. 1400 Pressler, Unit 1483 Houston, TX 77030.
E-mail address: dssurasi@mdanderson.org

Radiol Clin N Am 62 (2024) 53–67
https://doi.org/10.1016/j.rcl.2023.07.001

extends from the base to the middle third of the prostate.[8,9] In 80% to 90% of patients, the CZ can be seen as a ring of tissue between the peripheral and transition zones (TZs) on MR imaging.[7] The CZ displays a hypointense signal on T2-weighted imaging with symmetric components that look like Mickey Mouse ears or a heart in the coronal plane.[10] In addition, it exhibits restricted diffusion, which may be seen as both low and high signal intensities on apparent diffusion coefficient (ADC) maps and diffusion-weighted images (DWIs), respectively.[10] On dynamic contrast-enhanced (DCE) images, the CZs symmetric distribution around the ejaculatory ducts and the absence of early arterial enhancement aid to distinguish it from prostate cancer (Fig. 1). However, CZ asymmetries can occasionally develop as a result of nearby BPH nodules, which may be a source of misinterpretation. Owing to its low T2 signal intensity and ADC values, the CZ may be misinterpreted for prostate cancer, especially when asymmetric. To prevent a false-positive interpretation of the CZ as a suspicious lesion, it is essential to have a thorough knowledge of the anatomy of the posterior prostate base.

The PI-RADS v2.1 score system lacks defined criteria for CZ lesions.[11] However, it is advised to use the criteria for the zone from which the malignancy involving the CZ seems to have originated because CZ involvement is more likely to begin from the peripheral zone (PZ) or TZ.[11]

Tumors in the CZ have been linked to higher grades and stages of the disease compared with tumors without CZ involvement; therefore, it is crucial to correctly identify prostate cancer cases that involve the CZ. Although less than 5% of prostate cancers develop in the CZ, these tumors are more aggressive, have higher Gleason scores, are more likely to invade the seminal vesicles, have extracapsular extension, and are more likely to experience biochemical recurrence after prostatectomy.[12]

Anterior Fibromuscular Stroma

The anterior fibromuscular stroma (AFMS) is a structure interlacing with muscle fibers of the urinary sphincter, levator ani, and detrusor muscles. It is located in the anterior portion of the prostate and made up of connective tissue, smooth muscle, and some skeletal muscle. It does not contain glandular tissue and does not give rise to prostate cancer.[13] On T2-weighted, high-b-value DW MR images and ADC maps, the AFMS often manifests as low signal intensity, which can occasionally conceal or mimic prostate cancer (Fig. 2). Owing to its fibrous and muscular structure, it exhibits a type 1 (progressive) enhancement curve on DCE-MR imaging. Cancers that affect the AFMS usually begin in the tissues that are nearby TZ or PZ.[14] The AFMS varies in thickness, being thinner in people with more BPH. Because of its hypointense appearance on T2-weighted images and ADC maps, the AFMS can be misinterpreted for malignancy. Asymmetry of the AFMS brought on by adjacent BPH nodules can also resemble malignancy. However, there are two crucial distinctions on DCE and DWI that can assist in distinguishing AFMS from malignancy. First, unlike cancer, the AFMS does not exhibit a hyperintense signal on DWI. Second, prostate cancer often has early vascular enhancement, whereas the AFMS exhibits delayed mild enhancement on DCE imaging.[14]

In an analysis of radical prostatectomy specimens, 20% of all prostate cancers are pure anterior tumors. The rate of extracapsular extension is typically higher in these anterior malignancies.[15]

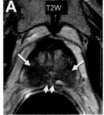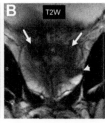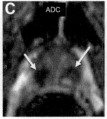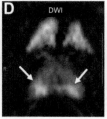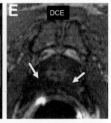

Fig. 1. Central zone mimicking prostate cancer. (A) Axial and (B) Coronal T2-weighted images show symmetric foci with hypointense signal at the base of the prostate (white arrows) corresponding to the central zone. The ejaculatory ducts (white arrowheads, A) can be seen at the same level in the axial plane (C) The central zone with mild hypointense signal on an apparent diffusion coefficient map (white arrows) and (D) hyperintense signal on a high-b-value (1400 s/mm²) diffusion-weighted image (white arrows). (E) The central zone demonstrates no early enhancement on a dynamic contrast-enhanced T1-weighted image (white arrows). Also noted is biopsy-proven prostate cancer (3 + 4) in the left mid-peripheral zone which abuts the left central zone superiorly and gives the appearance of involvement of the left central zone, best seen on (B) coronal T2-weighted image (white arrowhead).

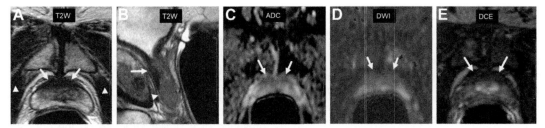

Fig. 2. Anterior fibromuscular stroma mimicking transition zone lesion. (*A*) Axial and (*B*) sagittal T2-weighted images show a thick anterior fibromuscular stroma with hypointense signal (*white arrows*) that is similar to the signal of the obturator muscle (*white triangle, A*). (*C*) The anterior fibromuscular stroma has mild hypointense signal on an apparent diffusion coefficient map (*arrows*) and (*D*) on a high-b-value (1400 s/mm^2) image (*arrows*). (*E*) The anterior fibromuscular stroma demonstrates no early enhancement on a dynamic contrast-enhanced T1-weighted image (*arrows*). Inferiorly, (*B*) prostate cancer abutting the anterior fibromuscular stroma. (*B*) The Sagittal T2-weighted image also shows a lesion with intermediate/low signal intensity in the anterior aspect of the transition zone (*arrowhead*) abutting the anterior fibromuscular stroma (*white arrow*). Unlike the anterior fibromuscular stroma, the lesion (not shown) in the transition zone had a hyperintense signal on a high-b-value (1400 s/mm^2) diffusion-weighted image with corresponding hypointense signal on an apparent diffusion coefficient map. On dynamic contrast-enhanced T1-weighted image, the lesion showed early arterial enhancement, which helps to distinguish it from the anterior fibromuscular stroma. MR imaging-US fusion biopsy of the lesion showed prostate cancer with a Gleason score of 4 + 3.

They can be distinguished from other prostate abnormalities because they show early enhancement pattern on DCE imaging and are hyperintense on high-b-value DWI.[14]

Periprostatic Venous Plexus

The prostatic venous plexus, situated primarily along the lateral aspect of the gland, serves as the route for venous drainage. It connects with the dorsal venous plexus (Santorini) and the hemorrhoidal venous plexus located at the back, ultimately draining into the internal iliac vein.[16] On MR imaging, the venous plexus appears as tubular structures outside the prostatic capsule (Fig. 3). However, as individuals age, these structures become less prominent.[17] Prominent veins within the venous plexus exhibit variable signal intensity on T2-weighted MR and ADC images. These veins can display low signal intensity due to flow phenomenon, and in certain cases, they may be incorrectly identified as lesions within the prostate, especially in areas where the prostatic pseudocapsule is thin.[18] Often happens at the apex of the prostate where the pseudocapsule is sparse, and there is a combination of limited glandular tissue and intermingled periprostatic supporting tissue. More commonly, the venous plexus demonstrates high signal on T2-weighted MR images, making it difficult to distinguish from the glandular tissue. This can result in inappropriate inclusion of the venous plexus in the prostate contour, which may result in inaccurate calculation of gland volume and segmentation of the gland for MR/ultrasound (US) fusion biopsy. Because the veins directly drain the prostate, they display strong enhancement on DCE MR imaging. Identifying these veins involves tracing their linear morphology across multiple slices and planes.[19]

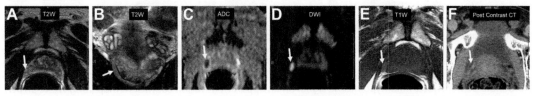

Fig. 3. Right periprostatic vein mimicking peripheral zone lesion. (*A*) Axial and (*B*) coronal T2-weighted images show a tubular structure with intermediate signal intensity in the right posterolateral periprostatic fat (*white arrow*), which represents a periprostatic vein coursing along the prostatic capsule. (*C*) This area has hypointense signal on apparent diffusion coefficient map (*white arrow*) and (*D*) hyperintense signal on high-b-value (1400 s/mm^2) image (*white arrow*). (*E*) The periprostatic vein demonstrates enhancement on dynamic contrast-enhanced T1-weighted image (*white arrow*). (*F*) Axial post-contrast computed tomography (CT) image shows enhancing periprostatic vein (*white arrow*).

Neurovascular Structures

The cavernous neural plexus, located near the prostate, gives rise to nerve branches that supply the corpora cavernosa, playing a crucial role in sexual function.[20,21] Surgeons aim to preserve these nerves during prostatectomy to optimize functional recovery.[22] However, if there is suspicion of tumor spread beyond the capsule, a wider excision may be performed, which could involve the partial or complete removal of these nerves.[22] This neural plexus is closely associated with arteries, veins, and smaller nerve branches that penetrate the prostatic capsule and provide innervation to the prostate itself. Together, they form the neurovascular bundle (NVB).[22] Traditionally, the NVB has been seen as a distinct structure running along the posterolateral margin of the prostate, covered by the lateral pelvic fascia, at around the 5 and 7 o'clock positions (**Fig. 4**).[20] Few anatomic studies challenge this view, suggesting that in approximately half of cases, there is no well-defined bundle formation, and the nerve trunks are sparsely distributed along both the anterior and posterior lateral aspects of the prostate.[13,22,23]

The proximity of NVB to the PZ presents a clinical challenge when assessing focal lesions in this area.[7] On axial slices, the NVB appears as a distinct rounded structure when viewed head-on. These structures exhibit decreased T2 signal intensity and appear as signal voids on the ADC map.[7] In some cases, the NVB may seem to be located within the PZ on the ADC map due to anatomic distortion of the prostate. These characteristics have led to instances where the NVB was mistakenly considered suspicious for a mass lesion in the PZ, similar to the pitfalls caused by the periprostatic venous plexus. To correctly identify the NVB, one should look for their typical location along the posterolateral margin of the PZ, their rounded contour when viewed head-on in individual axial slices, the tubular morphology when traced across consecutive slices, and the potential presence of a similar structure on the opposite side.[10] T2-weighted images, with their higher spatial resolution, are generally helpful in confirming that a potential lesion identified on DWI or DCE-MR imaging represents the normal NVB.[7] Furthermore, the expected delayed venous enhancement of the NVB due to its association with small venous structures.

Prostatitis

Prostatitis is a condition characterized by inflammation of the prostate gland, which can cause lower urinary tract symptoms and elevated levels of PSA.[24–26] It is a common reason for men to seek medical attention and can sometimes lead to unnecessary biopsies. Prostatitis has a bimodal age distribution, affecting men in the 20 to 40 age group as well as those more than 70 years. It can be classified into different types and subtypes, with the two main groups being bacterial prostatitis and granulomatous prostatitis. Acute bacterial prostatitis is commonly caused by infections such as *Escherichia coli* or *Staphylococcus*, and it presents with local and systemic symptoms. If not treated properly, acute bacterial prostatitis can progress to chronic prostatitis.[27] Inflammation in the PZ can lead to a paradoxic shortening of

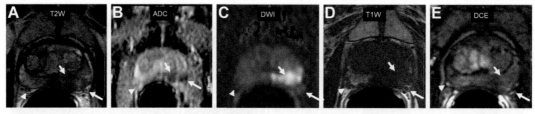

Fig. 4. Neurovascular bundle mimicking the appearance of prostate cancer and extraprostatic extension. (*A*) Axial T2-weighted image shows a PI-RADS 5 lesion in the left peripheral zone (*short white arrow*) corresponding to a biopsy-proven 4 + 3 Gleason score prostate cancer. The neurovascular bundle structures are located in the recto-prostatic angle at the 5 o'clock and 7 o'clock positions (*long white arrow and arrowhead*). The prostate cancer abuts the neurovascular bundle on the left. (*B*) Separate from the tumor (*short white arrow*) , the left neurovascular bundle demonstrates mild hypointense signal on an apparent diffusion coefficient map (*long white arrow*). The neurovascular bundle structures are located in the recto-prostatic angle at the 5 o'clock and 7 o'clock positions (*long white arrow and arrowhead*). and (*C*) mild hyperintense signal on a high-b-value (1400 s/mm²) diffusion-weighted image mimicking extraprostatic extension (*long white arrow*). The neurovascular bundle structures are located in the recto-prostatic angle at the 5 o'clock and 7 o'clock positions (*long white arrow and arrowhead*). (*D*) On the axial T1 and (*E*) dynamic contrast-enhanced T1-weighted images, the neurovascular bundles can be recognized as tubular-shaped enhancing structures (*arrowhead and long white arrow*). PI-RADS 5 lesion in the left peripheral zone (*short white arrow*).

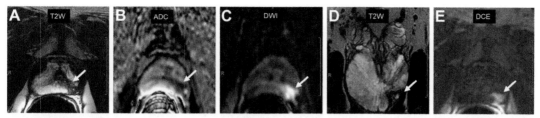

Fig. 5. Prostatitis. (*A*) Axial and (*D*) coronal T2-weighted images show wedge-shaped foci of hypointense signal in the left peripheral zone at the level of the apex (*white arrow*). (*B*) The peripheral zone has areas of markedly hypointense signal on apparent diffusion coefficient map (*white arrow*) and (*C*) markedly hyperintense signal on a high-b-value (1400 s/mm^2) diffusion-weighted image (*white arrow*). (*E*) The peripheral zone demonstrates diffuse early enhancement on a dynamic contrast-enhanced T1-weighted image (*white arrow*). MR imaging -US fusion biopsy revealed acute and chronic inflammation with areas of atrophy.

T2 and restricted diffusion, which can resemble cancer.

On multiparametric MR imaging (mpMR imaging), focal prostatitis typically appears as a nodular or linear area of reduced signal intensity on T2-weighted images and shows restricted diffusion in DWI sequences (**Fig. 5**). It also exhibits positive enhancement on DCE sequences.[28] These characteristics are similar to those of prostate cancer, especially considering their common glandular localization in the PZ of the prostate. Differentiating prostatitis from prostate cancer on MR imaging can be challenging, as both conditions can cause signal abnormalities on various sequences. The morphology of the PZ lesion can provide some clues, with well-defined and nodular lesions being more suspicious for cancer, whereas inflammatory lesions tend to be less mass-like, exhibiting ill-defined or linear margins.[7,28] Prostatitis can also have a lobar distribution or involve the PZ diffusely. In addition, the presence of inflammatory infiltration in the periprostatic tissue, increased reactive locoregional lymph nodes, and elevated PSA levels can further complicate the distinction between prostatitis and clinically significant prostate cancer. In cases where the distinction is not possible, repeat MR imaging may be considered to assess changes in the lesion and guide subsequent management decisions.[10,19,29] There is however no consensus in the literature on the optimum time to repeat the MR imaging, because inflammatory changes can persist long after the infectious process has been cleared.

Granulomatous Prostatitis

A nodular form of chronic prostatitis known as granulomatous prostatitis (GP) can be idiopathic or linked to several other disorders, including infections and systemic diseases including sarcoidosis and vasculitis, tuberculous prostatitis, or surgical procedures such as transurethral resection of the prostate. Bacillus Calmette–Guerin intravesical instillation used to treat bladder cancer can also cause it.[30] The incidence of GP in prostate biopsies varies between 0.36% and 2%. In addition to high PSA values, GP might appear with a firm palpable nodule or a hard and fixed lesion on digital rectal examination. On mpMR imaging, GP is characterized by low signal intensity on T2-weighted images, low ADC values, and moderate enhancement on DCE images.[19,31,32] These characteristics, however, can overlap with those of prostate cancer, thereby misinterpreting the lesion on mpMR imaging. It can be difficult to distinguish between prostate cancer and this condition because it can affect various regions of the prostate gland and appear with MR imaging findings similar to prostate cancer. Certain MR imaging findings can help with GP diagnosis in the acute or early phases. Abscesses and regions of caseous necrosis show central hyperintense signal on T2-weighted images and rim enhancement on DCE T1-weighted imaging (**Fig. 6**), which are not often seen in prostate cancer.[10,31,32] However, in the later phases of GP, needle biopsy and histopathology may be required to rule out tumor. When evaluating for GP, it is always important to look at the patient's history for any predisposing conditions. Patients diagnosed with tuberculous prostatitis may require follow-up MR imaging after antituberculosis treatment to confirm interval resolution.[33–35]

Benign Prostatic Hyperplasia

BPH is a widely prevalent condition that affects men predominantly over the age of 50 years. It is characterized by the growth of the TZ of the prostate, which is located all around the prostatic urethra. Depending on the glandular and stromal components and cystic alterations present, BPH nodules have variable MR imaging signal properties.[36,37] Typical BPH nodules demonstrate

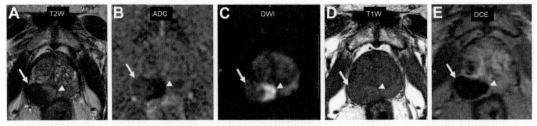

Fig. 6. Granulomatous prostatitis secondary to intravesical Bacillus Calmette–Guerin therapy for bladder cancer mimicking prostate tumor. (*A*) Axial T2-weighted image shows a focal lesion with a hypointense signal (*white arrow*) and a crescent-shaped intermediate signal (*arrowhead*) in the right peripheral zone. (*B*) The lesion (*white arrow*) demonstrates a crescent-shaped hypointense signal (*arrowhead*) on apparent diffusion coefficient map and (*C*) hyperintense signal on a high-b-value (1400 s/mm2) diffusion-weighted image (*arrowhead*). Pre contrast T1W (*D*) and post contrast DCE image (*E*) shows the lesion (*white arrow*) with no demonstrable enhancement. However the lesion demonstrates diffuse peripheral enhancement (*arrowhead*). Biopsy revealed granulomatous prostatitis with central caseous necrosis.

hypointense rim or capsule on T2-weighted images.[11] It can be difficult to differentiate between BPH nodules and prostate cancer when the capsule is absent or insufficient, particularly if the nodules exhibit homogenous hypointense signal on T2-weighted imaging and restricted diffusion.[38,39] The TZ assessment criteria were changed in PI-RADS v2.1 to reflect the challenges in differentiating between BPH nodules and prostate cancer.[11] Atypical BPH nodules, which are either partially encapsulated nodules or homogenous hypointense nodules without a capsule, may be upgraded to PI-RADS 3 if they have markedly restricted diffusion (**Fig. 7**).[11] Similar to BPH nodules in the TZ, BPH nodules can also be found in the PZ (**Fig. 8**); their diagnosis depends on their

position close to the TZ and the existence of encapsulation. It is important to remember nevertheless that prostate tumors with pseudocapsules have been documented and may be related to high-grade and high-stage disease.[40,41] It is essential to distinguish between stromal BPH nodules and TZ malignancies based on the shape, borders, and invasion patterns of the nodule on T2-weighted imaging. Lower ADC values correlate with a higher likelihood of a malignant nodule; hence, quantitative evaluation of signal intensity in the ADC map can also be useful.[42] The diagnosis often requires a second MR imaging or targeted biopsy due to the difficulty in reliably differentiating between stromal BPH nodules and TZ malignancies. Because TZ tumors are

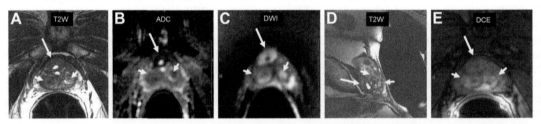

Fig. 7. Benign prostatic hypertrophy (BPH). (*A*) Axial and (*D*) sagittal T2-weighted images show an enlarged transition zone (*short white arrows*) containing mixed areas of high, intermediate, and low signal intensity related to BPH nodules. (*B*) The BPH nodules have variable signal intensity on apparent diffusion coefficient map (*short white arrows*) and (*C*) on a high-b-value (1400 s/mm2) diffusion-weighted image (*short white arrows*), and (*E*) variable levels of enhancement on a dynamic contrast-enhanced T1-weighted image (*short white arrows*). In the absence of focal abnormalities that are different from the background of BPH, the presence of clinically significant prostate cancer is highly unlikely. However, an oval-shaped nodule in the anterior gland may represent atypical stromal hyperplasia nodule mimicking prostate cancer. (*A*) Axial and (*D*) sagittal T2-weighted image shows an encapsulated nodule (*long white arrow*) with homogenous intermediate signal intensity with cystic changes in the anterior transition zone that is different from the background. (*B*) The nodule has hypointense signal on apparent diffusion coefficient map (*long white arrow*), (*C*) hyperintense signal on a high-b-value (1400 s/mm2) diffusion-weighted image (*long white arrow*), and (*E*) early arterial enhancement on a dynamic contrast-enhanced T1-weighted image (*long white arrow*). Based on the appearance of the nodule on T2-weighted imaging, the nodule was characterized as PI-RADS 3. MR imaging-US fusion biopsy of the nodule revealed stromal hyperplasia and prostate cancer with Gleason score of 4 + 3.

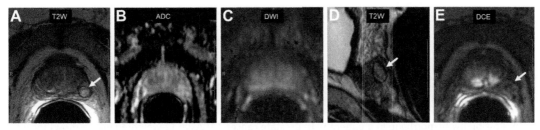

Fig. 8. Extruded benign prostatic hyperplasia (BPH) nodule. (*A*) Axial and (*B*) coronal T2-weighted images show an encapsulated nodule in the left peripheral zone (*white arrow*). (*C*) The nodule is poorly visualized on apparent diffusion coefficient map and (*D*) high-b-value (1400 s/mm²) diffusion-weighted image. (*E*) On dynamic contrast-enhanced T1-weighted image, the nodule demonstrates mild and delayed enhancement (*white arrow*).

commonly missed using conventional biopsy techniques, MR imaging is essential in the detection of these malignancies, especially when the tumor is located in the anterior TZ. Overall, to distinguish between BPH nodules versus prostate cancer, ensure appropriate management decisions, and prevent needless intrusive procedures, a thorough review of clinical data, imaging features, and careful interpretation is required.[42,43]

Thick Surgical Capsule

The surgical capsule is a fibromuscular structure between the PZ and TZ of the prostate. It serves as an anatomic landmark for surgical procedures targeting the TZ.[44,45] During embryonic development, the periurethral septum gives rise to the surgical capsule, which is made up of fibrous and muscular tissue. When BPH is present in the TZ, this structure, which is loose and poorly defined in younger men, proliferates and thickens. It eventually gathers into the surgical capsule, a crescentic band encircling the hypertrophied TZ.[44,45] This capsule causes intravesical protrusion and bladder outlet blockage and presses inward on the expanded TZ.

The surgical capsule is a vital landmark for establishing the limit of the treatment volume during transurethral enucleation of the TZ to treat symptomatic BPH. On MR imaging, the surgical capsule shows as a thin crescentic band around the TZ that has less T2 signal strength.[46] Individual patients may have varying conspicuity and asymmetry. Similar to the CZ, the surgical capsule has a lower ADC.[10,19] However, when coupled with T2-weighted imaging, its usual position and form can aid in differentiating it from focal tumor lesions on the ADC map.[46,47] On DCE sequence, the surgical capsule does not show rapid contrast enhancement, in contrast to malignant tumors (**Fig. 9**). To prevent being mistaken for a focal tumor lesion, it is essential to be aware of its normal architecture and signal characteristics on various sequences.[46,47]

Post-Biopsy Hemorrhage

Intraprostatic hemorrhage occurs after a prostate biopsy procedure due to the failure of blood clotting caused by the anticoagulant properties of citrate produced by the normal prostate gland.[48] The

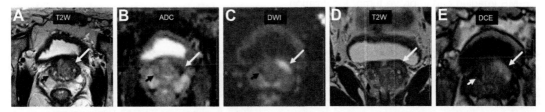

Fig. 9. Thick surgical capsule. (*A*) Axial and (*D*) coronal T2-weighted images show asymmetric thickening of surgical capsule that separates peripheral and transition zones (*short black arrow*). (*B*) The thick surgical capsule has hypointense signal intensity on apparent diffusion coefficient map (*short black arrow*), (*C*) on high-b-value (1400 s/mm²) diffusion-weighted image (*short black arrow*), and (*E*) delayed enhancement on dynamic contrast-enhanced T1-weighted image (*short white arrow*). Surgical capsule on left side at this level shows more asymmetric curvilinear hypointense signal which extends into the adjacent transition zone (*long white arrow*) on (*A*) axial T2-weighted image, (*B*) hypointense signal intensity on apparent diffusion coefficient map (*long white arrow*), (*C*) hyperintense signal on high-b-value (1400 s/mm²) diffusion-weighted image (*long white arrow*), and (*E*) early arterial enhancement on a dynamic contrast-enhanced T1-weighted image (*long white arrow*). Based on the appearance on T2-weighted imaging, the lesion was characterized as PI-RADS 5. MR imaging-US fusion biopsy of the lesion revealed prostate cancer with a Gleason score of 4 + 3.

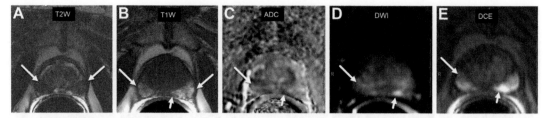

Fig. 10. Post-biopsy hemorrhage in a patient with prostate cancer. (*A*) Axial T2-weighted image shows focal hypointense signal in bilateral peripheral zone (*long arrows*). (*B*) On T1-weighted image, the same area demonstrates a hyperintense signal compatible with post-biopsy hemorrhage (*long arrows*), except for a focal area with a hypointense signal (*short white arrow*). (*C*) The area spared from hemorrhage on the T1-weighted image has a focal hypointense signal on an apparent diffusion coefficient map (*short white arrow*) and (*D*) hyperintense signal on a high-b-value (1400 s/mm2) diffusion-weighted image (*short white arrow*). (*E*) The lesion demonstrates early arterial enhancement on dynamic contrast-enhanced T1-weighted image (*short white arrow*). The focal area spared from hemorrhage showed prostate cancer with Gleason score 3 + 4 in the radical prostatectomy specimen. No focal signal abnormality is noted in the right posteriolateral peripheral zone (*long white arrow*) on ADC (C), DWI (D) and post contrast T1W image (*E*).

hemorrhage can remain in the gland for weeks or even months after the biopsy.[49,50] Reliable tumor localization can be challenging on MR imaging in the presence of post-biopsy hemorrhage. On MR imaging, post-biopsy hemorrhage appears as focal, diffuse, or striated high signal on T1-weighted images, low signal intensity on T2-weighted images, and ADC maps (**Fig. 10**).[49,50] Sometimes, it may cause a mildly high signal on DWI and mimic tumor or obscuring tumor areas. In contrast with benign prostate tissue, prostate cancer is poor in citrate and therefore not affected by post-biopsy hemorrhage. This results in the "hemorrhage exclusion sign, in which benign tissue affected by hemorrhage demonstrate hyperintense signal on T1-weighted images, while cancer has low signal intensity."[49,50] Prostate cancer typically has lower homogenous T2 signal and ADC values than hemorrhagic benign PZs. Using functional sequences such as DWI and DCE-MR imaging can improve tumor localization

in the setting of post-biopsy hemorrhage. Subtraction images and careful assessment of T1-weighted images can also aid in evaluating the distribution of hemorrhage and facilitate tumor identification.[49,50]

Most mpMR imaging studies are carried out before prostate biopsies, lowering the likelihood of this error. However, if an MR imaging is performed later, it is advisable to wait at least 6 to 8 weeks post-biopsy, especially for lesion localization purposes.[49,50] Waiting for the resolution of hemorrhage can lead to patient anxiety and potential delays in treatment. Thus, delays should be balanced with the need for timely diagnosis and treatment.[51] This delay can be avoided for staging purposes as post-biopsy hemorrhage is less likely to obscure extraprostatic extension.

Prostate Calcification

Prostate calcification is another frequent finding in prostate MR imaging, representing a potential

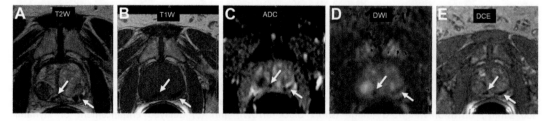

Fig. 11. Focal calcification at the interface of peripheral and transition zone. (*A*) Axial T2-weighted image shows bilateral foci of hypointense signal at the interface of peripheral and transition zone (*white arrows*). (*B*) On axial T1-weighted image, the same areas demonstrate foci of hypointense signal (*white arrows*). (*C*) These areas demonstrate hypointense signal on apparent diffusion coefficient map (*white arrows*) and (*D*) on high-b-value (1400 s/mm²) diffusion-weighted image (*white arrows*). (*E*) On dynamic contrast-enhanced T1-weighted image, no enhancement was noted corresponding to the abnormal areas of hypointense signal (*white arrows*). Computed tomography scan confirmed the presence of calcification at these locations (not shown).

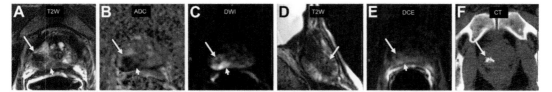

Fig. 12. Focal calcification in the peripheral zone. (A) Axial and (D) sagittal T2-weighted images show foci of hypointense signal in the right peripheral zone (*long white arrows*). (B) These areas demonstrate hypointense signal on apparent diffusion coefficient map (*long white arrow*) and (C) on high-b-value (1400 s/mm^2) diffusion-weighted image (*long white arrow*). (E) On dynamic contrast-enhanced T1-weighted image, no enhancement was noted corresponding to the abnormal areas of hypointense signal (*long white arrow*). (F) Computed tomography scan confirms the presence of calcification at these locations (*long white arrow*). (A) Axial T2-weighted image shows a focal hypointense signal in the right posteromedial peripheral zone (*short white arrow*). (B) This area demonstrates marked hypointense signal on apparent diffusion coefficient map (*short white arrow*) and (C) markedly hyperintense signal on high-b-value (1400 s/mm^2) diffusion-weighted image (*short white arrow*). (E) The lesion demonstrates early enhancement on a dynamic contrast-enhanced T1-weighted image (*short white arrow*). MR imaging-US Fusion biopsy revealed prostate cancer with Gleason score 4 + 4.

diagnostic pitfall. They are commonly found at the junction between the TZ and PZ of the prostate, often in the context of BPH (**Fig. 11**).[19] These calcifications can be associated with various other disease processes, such as infection and metabolic abnormalities. They are believed to develop from the calcification of corpora amylacea, which are presumed to be precursors to calcified "stones."[52] Although corpora amylacea can be present within areas of prostatic adenocarcinoma, their incidence is generally low and more commonly associated with low-Gleason grade cancers.[53] Prostate calcifications exhibit characteristic imaging features on MR imaging. Prostatic calcifications typically appear hypointense on T2-weighted and ADC images, low signal intensity on DWI, and lack of enhancement on DCE-MR imaging.[5] The differentiation of these calcifications from prostate cancer is crucial, and correlation with CT imaging can be helpful in confirming focal calcifications (**Fig. 12**).[10] Recognizing prostate calcifications is also important in the context of

energy ablation treatments, because they can interfere with energy ablation treatments such as high-intensity focused ultrasound (HIFU).

Focal Prostate Atrophy

Focal prostate atrophy (FPA) is a frequently encountered histologic diagnosis, observed in 73% of biopsy specimens.[54,55] Proliferative inflammatory atrophy (PIA) is the most prevalent subtype.[54,55] It can be caused by a variety of factors, including inflammation, radiation therapy, androgenic therapy, and recurrent ischemic insult. It has not been demonstrated to be linked to prostate cancer. However, in men who have a persistent suspicion of prostate cancer, finding PIA in negative biopsies correlates with a decreased frequency of detecting prostate cancer.[56] Focal atrophy is characterized by a significant reduction in the prostate gland's volume and can have a cuneiform or geographic distribution. On histology and MR imaging, FPA can look like prostate cancer,

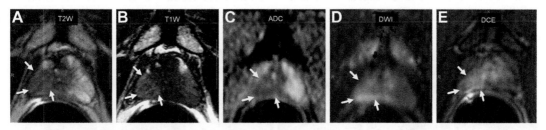

Fig. 13. Focal prostate atrophy in the right side of the peripheral zone mimicking prostate cancer. (A) Axial T2-weighted image shows a linear hypointense signal in the right peripheral zone at the level of apex (*arrows*). (B) On axial T1-weighted image, the same area demonstrates mild hyperintense signal (*arrows*). (C) This area has mild hypointense signal on apparent diffusion coefficient map (*arrows*) and (D) mild hyperintense signal on high-b-value (1400 s/mm^2) diffusion-weighted image (*arrows*). (E) The lesion demonstrates early arterial enhancement on dynamic contrast-enhanced T1-weighted image (*arrows*). MR imaging-US Fusion biopsy revealed focal atrophy and chronic prostatitis.

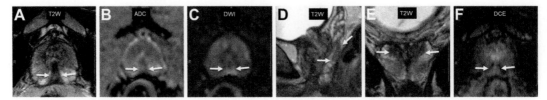

Fig. 14. Pseudolesion in the midline peripheral zone. (*A*) Axial and (*D*) sagittal T2-weighted images show a linear and wedge-shaped hypointense signal in the posterior midline peripheral zone at the level of base and mid gland (*arrows*). (*E*) On coronal T2-weighted image, the same area shows a tear-drop-shaped signal abnormality due to the presence of compressed central zone (*arrows*). (*B*) This area has mild hypointense signal on an apparent diffusion coefficient map (*arrows*) and (*C*) mild hyperintense signal on a high-b-value (1400 s/mm^2) diffusion-weighted image (*arrows*). (*F*) The lesion demonstrates delayed enhancement on dynamic contrast-enhanced T1-weighted image (*arrows*). This area was stable on follow-up MR imaging after 2.5 years.

potentially leading to overdiagnosis.[55] The findings suggest that a notable correlation exists between the degree of atrophy and the rise in levels of total or free serum PSA, which may be attributed to impaired epithelial cells in atrophic acini.[57]

On prostate MR imaging, focal atrophy appears as a hypointense area on T2-weighted images with moderate diffusion restriction and moderate enhancement on DCE imaging (**Fig. 13**).[5] When compared with prostate cancer, the degree to which diffusion restriction and tissue enhancement are present is typically less pronounced.[46]

Pseudolesion in the Midline Posterior Peripheral Zone

Pseudolesion in the midline posterior PZ on prostate MR imaging refers to a low T2 signal intensity focus that can resemble prostate cancer due to diffusion restriction.[5,29] This phenomenon is believed to be caused by the fusion of the prostatic capsule and fascia in this specific region.[13,58] The fusion occurs near the base of the prostate at the junction of the two lobes, where the posterior prostatic fascia and seminal vesicles fascia (Denonvillier fascia) merge with the capsule.[13,58] As a result, the prostatic capsule thickens smoothly, leading to a low T2 signal intensity focus

on imaging. Differentiating this pseudolesion from prostate cancer is based on several key MR imaging clues. These clues include its midline location, concave contour, and the lack of rapid enhancement with washout (**Fig. 14**).[5,29] In contrast, prostate cancer typically demonstrates different imaging characteristics, such as a peripheral location, convex contour, and early enhancement on DCE.[5,29]

Posttreatment Changes

Posttreatment changes on prostate MR imaging are important confounding factors for the detection of recurrent prostate cancer and to guide treatment decisions. Radiation therapy, radical prostatectomy, prostate-sparing focused therapy, androgen deprivation therapy (ADT), and other types of treatments can all result in certain imaging abnormalities on MR imaging.[59] These changes should be interpreted in the context of the treatment received, clinical setting, and PSA levels.[59]

After treatment, there are common mimics that should be identified, such as granulation tissue and hemorrhage, which show early enhancement on DCE but appear benign on DWI. Recurrent tumors, on the other hand, show early enhancement

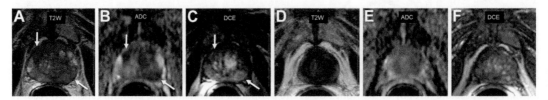

Fig. 15. Posttreatment recurrence after antiandrogen therapy (ADT). (*A*) Axial T2-weighted image demonstrates focal hypointense lesions in bilateral peripheral zone (*arrows*) with corresponding restricted diffusion (*B*) and early enhancement (*C*) suggestive of prostate cancer. Imaging was repeated after 7 months of ADT. (*D*) Axial T2-weighted image demonstrates diffuse low signal in the peripheral zone with poor distinction of the zonal anatomy. (*E*) On apparent diffusion coefficient map and (*F*) dynamic contrast-enhanced T1-weighted images, no focal signal abnormality is identified.

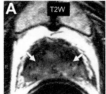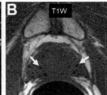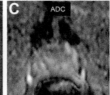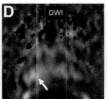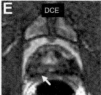

Fig. 16. Posttreatment recurrence after low-dose rate brachytherapy. (*A*) Axial T2-weighted image demonstrates low signal in the peripheral zone with multiple brachytherapy seeds throughout the gland (*arrows*). There is poor distinction of the zonal anatomy. (*B*) On axial T1-weighted image, brachytherapy seeds are better visualized. (*C*) Apparent diffusion coefficient map and (*D*) high-b-value (1400 s/mm^2) diffusion-weighted images demonstrate poor image quality with diffuse susceptibility artifact due to brachytherapy seeds, which limits evaluation. However, there is mild focal hyperintense signal on a high-b-value (1400 s/mm^2) diffusion-weighted image (*arrow*) (*D*). (*E*) This area corresponds to a focal area of early arterial enhancement on a dynamic contrast-enhanced T1-weighted image (*arrow*). An MR imaging-US fusion biopsy of the lesion revealed prostate cancer Gleason score 3 + 4 in the background of radiotherapy changes.

and are more hypointense on T2W images than posttreatment changes. The presence of metallic clips from surgery makes DCE MR imaging more reliable than DWI for evaluating recurrence. Early arterial enhancement on DCE MR imaging is highly suggestive of recurrence,[60] but all these changes should be correlated with the clinical setting, type of treatment received, and PSA levels.

Both benign and malignant tissues in the prostate may change after ADT, radiation therapy, and other energy ablation procedures. Owing to fibrotic tissues, these changes may lead to the loss of zonal anatomy and deformation of the gland's morphology (**Fig. 15**).[51] It may be difficult to discern between cancer and normal tissues when looking at T2-weighted images because of diffuse low signal intensity. In addition, the evaluation of DWI and ADC maps might be compromised by artifacts from brachytherapy seeds and radiation fiducial markers (**Fig. 16**).[61] In this situation, DCE MR imaging is often helpful

in detecting residual or recurrent tumors, especially when areas show early arterial enhancement.[61] It is crucial to remember that benign prostatic enlargement can exhibit hypervascularity as well, which could provide false-positive results on DCE imaging. Targeted biopsy may be required to confirm suspicious lesions in the prostate, especially when only local recurrence is present.[62,63]

Alternative treatments for prostate cancer include focal therapies such as cryotherapy, HIFU, and photodynamic therapy. These therapies may result in periprostatic fibrosis and scarring, loss of zonal differentiation, thickness of the prostatic capsule, and other changes that can be seen on an MR imaging.[59,63] After targeted treatments, enhancing soft tissue lesions should be considered as a sign of recurrence (**Fig. 17**), but it can be difficult to differentiate a viable tumor from reactive enhancing prostatic tissue, especially at the edges of the treated area.[59,63]

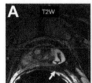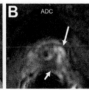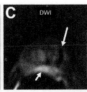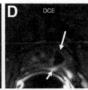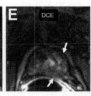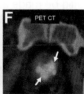

Fig. 17. Prostate cancer recurrence after left hemigland cryoablation. (*A*) Axial T2-weighted image shows a focal hyperintense area in the left hemigland related to necrotic cavity from previous cryoablation without evidence of restricted diffusion lond (*white arrow*) (*B, C*) or enhancement (*D*). However, focal hypointense lesion (*short white arrow*) in the left posteromedial peripheral zone on (*A*) axial T2-weighted image with corresponding hypointense signal (*B*) on apparent diffusion coefficient map (*short white arrow*) and hyperintense signal (*B*) on a high-b-value (1400 s/mm2) diffusion-weighted image (*short white arrow*) is suspicious for recurrent tumor. (*D*) This area demonstrates early arterial enhancement (*short white arrow*) on dynamic contrast-enhanced T1-weighted image. (*E*) Area of heterogeneous early enhancement superior to the ablation cavity at the level of the base on dynamic contrast-enhanced T1-weighted image with corresponding prostate specific membrane antigen (PSMA) activity on (*F*) PSMA PET/CT. An MR imaging-US fusion biopsy of the lesion revealed recurrent prostate cancer with Gleason score 4 + 3.

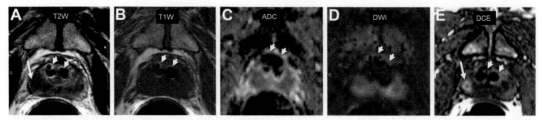

Fig. 18. Prostatic urethra implant compromising image quality. (*A*) Axial T2-weighted and (*B*) axial T1-weighted images show focal susceptibility artifacts in the transition zone of the prostate related to prostatic urethra implants (*short white arrows*). (*C*) The implants cause susceptibility artifacts that obscure a significant portion of the transition zone on apparent diffusion coefficient map (*short white arrows*) and (*D*) on high-b-value (1400 s/mm²) diffusion-weighted image (*short white arrows*). (*E*) On dynamic contrast-enhanced T1-weighted image, the implants show no enhancement (*short white arrows*). There is a focal hypointense lesion (*long white arrow*) in the right peripheral zone on (*A*) axial T2-weighted image with corresponding early arterial enhancement (*long white arrow*) on a dynamic contrast-enhanced T1-weighted image (*E*). This lesion is poorly visualized (*C*) on apparent diffusion coefficient map or (*B*) on high-b-value (1400 s/mm²) diffusion-weighted image due to poor image quality.

Changes After Prostatic Implants or Periprostatic Injection of Biodegradable Substances

The prostatic urethral lift is a minimally invasive treatment for BPH that can be performed on an ambulatory basis with the use of local anesthesia.[64] The procedure involves the utilization of permanent implants to retract the prostatic tissue and facilitate the opening of the prostatic urethra.[64] Based on nonclinical evaluations, these implants are MR-conditional, allowing patients to endure MR imaging scans immediately after the procedure.[65] However, they create artifacts that may obscure certain areas of the prostate gland, particularly on DWI (**Fig. 18**).[51] These artifacts are commonly observed in the TZ where the implants are situated.[51] These implants can be confused with fiducial markers used in radiotherapy. Although the implants can be imaged safely, individuals considering this treatment should be made aware of the potential impact on the quality of prostate MR imaging images.[51]

Rectal spacing with SpaceOAR (Augmenix, Inc, Waltham, MA, USA) or Barrigel (Palette Life Sciences, Inc) improved rectal dosimetry and reduced acute grade 2 or higher GI toxicity following radiotherapy.[66,67] SpaceOAR is a synthetic hydrogel composed of polyethylene glycol and Barrigel is a nonanimal origin stabilized sodium hyaluronate. These gel formulations are injected between posterior surface of prostate and rectum to establish a gap between the prostate and the rectum. Its purpose is to reduce the harmful effects of radiation on the rectum and minimize the impact on a patient's quality of life following prostate cancer radiation therapy.[68] The gel displays a bright signal on T2-weighted MR imaging images and should be positioned within the anterior perirectal fat, specifically between the anterior wall of the rectum and the posterior margin of the prostate (**Fig. 19**).[69] However, this intense signal can be misleading, resembling the appearance of an abscess or mucinous tumors originating from either the rectum or prostate.[51]

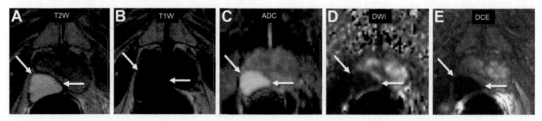

Fig. 19. Patient with prostate cancer following the placement of hydrogel before initiation of radiotherapy. (*A*) Axial T2-weighted and (*C*) apparent diffusion coefficient map images show the hydrogel located between the prostate and rectum with hyperintense signal. The hydrogel has hypointense signal on (*B*) axial T1-weighted and (*D*) high-b-value (1400 s/mm²) diffusion-weighted images (*arrows*). (*E*) The hydrogel demonstrates no enhancement on dynamic contrast-enhanced T1-weighted image (*arrows*).

SUMMARY

mpMR imaging has proven to be a valuable tool in diagnosing and staging prostate cancer, often surpassing traditional methods such as transrectal ultrasound-guided biopsy. Standardized protocols such as PI-RADS v2.1 aid radiologist in evaluating prostate mpMR imaging, taking into account zonal anatomy and the main sequences used for cancer detection. Radiologists must thoroughly study prostate imaging in different planes and sequences while being knowledgeable about the pitfalls discussed to prevent misinterpretation of images. The use of additional sequences, such as DWI, can assist in cases of uncertainty on T2-weighted imaging. Incorporating DWI/ADC maps and DCE can significantly improve the sensitivity for detecting tumors. This review emphasizes the importance of recognizing various factors that can complicate the interpretation of prostate MR imaging. Both normal anatomic structures and pathologic conditions can mimic the appearance of prostate cancer on MR imaging, highlighting the need for awareness to minimize interpretation errors and reconcile discrepancies between biopsy and MR imaging findings. Given these challenges, an MR imaging-guided biopsy should be considered for patients with an equivocal MR imaging who have clinical suspicion of prostate cancer.

CLINICS CARE POINTS

- Multiparametric MRI of the prostate is a commonly used modality of choice for the screening, diagnosis, staging, imaging guidance and treatment of prostate cancer, however, it is not free from interpretive challenges.

- DCE and DWI sequences can be helpful in the evaluation of anterior fibromuscular stroma can be misinterpreted for malignancy owing to the hypointense appearance on T2-weighted images and ADC maps.

- Stromal BPH nodules and TZ malignancies can be differentiated based on the shape, borders and invasion patterns of the nodule on T2-weighted imaging.

DISCLOSURE

D.S. Sudha Surasi reports research support from Blue Earth Diagnostics for an investigator-initiated trial. The other authors have no conflicts to report.

REFERENCES

1. Siegel RL, Miller KD, Wagle NS, et al. Cancer statistics, 2023. CA. A Cancer Journal for Clinicians 2023; 73(1):17–48.
2. Network. NCC. Prostate Cancer V.1.2023. 2023; Available at: https://www.nccn.org/guidelines/guidelines-process/transparency-process-and-recommendations/GetFileFromFileManagerGuid?FileManagerGuidId=48c2a3b5-a7c2-4222-9f48-59921011b4a7. Accessed June 6, 2023.
3. Purysko AS, Baroni RH, Giganti F, et al. PI-RADS version 2.1: A critical review, from the AJR special series on radiology reporting and data systems. Am J Roentgenol 2021;216(1):20–32.
4. Panebianco V, Giganti F, Kitzing YX, et al. An update of pitfalls in prostate mpMRI: a practical approach through the lens of PI-RADS v. 2 guidelines. Insights into Imaging 2018;9(1):87–101.
5. Thomas S, Oto A. Multiparametric MR imaging of the prostate: pitfalls in interpretation. Radiol Clin 2018; 56(2):277–87.
6. Quon JS, Moosavi B, Khanna M, et al. False positive and false negative diagnoses of prostate cancer at multi-parametric prostate MRI in active surveillance. Insights Imaging 2015;6(4):449–63.
7. Rosenkrantz AB, Taneja SS. Radiologist, be aware: ten pitfalls that confound the interpretation of multiparametric prostate MRI. Am J Roentgenol 2013; 202(1):109–20.
8. McNeal JE. Regional morphology and pathology of the prostate. Am J Clin Pathol 1968;49(3):347–57.
9. Surasi DSS, Chapin B, Tang C, et al. Imaging and management of prostate cancer. Semin Ultrasound CT MR 2020;41(2):207–21.
10. Panebianco V, Barchetti F, Barentsz J, et al. Pitfalls in interpreting mp-MRI of the prostate: a pictorial review with pathologic correlation. Insights into Imaging 2015;6(6):611–30.
11. Turkbey B, Rosenkrantz AB, Haider MA, et al. Prostate imaging reporting and data system version 2.1: 2019 update of prostate imaging reporting and data system version 2. Eur Urol 2019;76(3): 340–51.
12. Vargas HA, Akin O, Franiel T, et al. Normal central zone of the prostate and central zone involvement by prostate cancer: clinical and MR imaging implications. Radiology 2012;262(3):894–902.
13. Kiyoshima K, Yokomizo A, Yoshida T, et al. Anatomical features of periprostatic tissue and its surroundings: a histological analysis of 79 radical retropubic prostatectomy specimens. Jpn J Clin Oncol 2004; 34(8):463–8.
14. Ward E, Baad M, Peng Y, et al. Multi-parametric MR imaging of the anterior fibromuscular stroma and its differentiation from prostate cancer. Abdominal Radiology 2017;42(3):926–34.

15. Koppie TM, Bianco FJ Jr, Kuroiwa K, et al. The clinical features of anterior prostate cancers. BJU Int 2006;98(6):1167–71.

16. Cristini C, Pierro GBD, Leonardo C, et al. Safe digital isolation of the Santorini plexus during radical retropubic prostatectomy. BMC Urol 2013;13.

17. Allen KS, Kressel HY, Arger PH, et al. Age-related changes of the prostate: evaluation by MR imaging. Am J Roentgenol 1989;152(1):77–81.

18. Poon PY, Bronskill MJ, Poon CS, et al. Identification of the periprostatic venous plexus by MR imaging. J Comput Assist Tomogr 1991;15(2):265–8.

19. Eusebi L, Carpagnano FA, Sortino G, et al. Prostate multiparametric MRI: common pitfalls in primary diagnosis and how to avoid them. Current Radiology Reports 2021;9(3).

20. Nunes LW, Schiebler MS, Rauschning W, et al. The normal prostate and periprostatic structures: correlation between MR images made with an endorectal coil and cadaveric microtome sections. Am J Roentgenol 1995;164(4):923–7.

21. Tempany CMC, Rahmouni AD, Epstein JI, et al. Invasion of the neurovascular bundle by prostate cancer: evaluation with MR imaging. Radiology 1991; 181(1):107–12.

22. Lee SE, Hong SK, Han JH, et al. Significance of neurovascular bundle formation observed on preoperative magnetic resonance imaging regarding postoperative erectile function after nerve-sparing radical retropubic prostatectomy. Urology 2007;69(3):510–4.

23. Panebianco V, Salciccia S, Cattarino S, et al. Use of Multiparametric MR with neurovascular bundle evaluation to optimize the oncological and functional management of patients considered for nerve-sparing radical prostatectomy. J Sex Med 2012; 9(8):2157–66.

24. Coker TJ, Dierfeldt DM. Acute bacterial prostatitis: diagnosis and management. Am Fam Physician 2016;93(2):114–20.

25. Gill BC, Shoskes DA. Bacterial prostatitis. Curr Opin Infect Dis 2016;29(1):86–91.

26. Ramakrishnan K, Salinas RC. Prostatitis: acute and chronic. Prim Care Clin Off Pract 2010;37(3):547–63.

27. Holt JD, Garrett WA, McCurry TK, et al. Common questions about chronic prostatitis. Am Fam Physician 2016;93(4):290–6.

28. Meier-Schroers M, Kukuk G, Wolter K, et al. Differentiation of prostatitis and prostate cancer using the prostate imaging - reporting and data system (PI-RADS). Eur J Radiol 2016;85(7):1304–11.

29. Yu J, Fulcher AS, Turner MA, et al. Prostate cancer and its mimics at multiparametric prostate MRI. Br J Radiol 2014;87(1037):20130659.

30. Shukla P, Gulwani HV, Kaur S. Granulomatous prostatitis: clinical and histomorphologic survey of the disease in a tertiary care hospital. Prostate International 2017;5(1):29–34.

31. Lee SM, Wolfe K, Acher P, et al. Multiparametric MRI appearances of primary granulomatous prostatitis. Br J Radiol 2019;92(1098):20180075.

32. Rais-Bahrami S, Nix JW, Turkbey B, et al. Clinical and multiparametric MRI signatures of granulomatous prostatitis. Abdominal Radiology 2017;42(7): 1956–62.

33. Bertelli E, Zantonelli G, Cinelli A, et al. Granulomatous prostatitis, the great mimicker of prostate cancer: can multiparametric MRI features help in this challenging differential diagnosis? Diagnostics 2022;12(10):2302.

34. Bour L, Schull A, Delongchamps NB, et al. Multiparametric MRI features of granulomatous prostatitis and tubercular prostate abscess. Diagn Interv Imaging 2013;94(1):84–90.

35. Kawada H, Kanematsu M, Goshima S, et al. Multiphase contrast-enhanced magnetic resonance imaging features of Bacillus Calmette–Guérin-induced granulomatous prostatitis in five patients. Korean J Radiol 2015;16(2):342–8.

36. Chatterjee A, Gallan AJ, He D, et al. Revisiting quantitative multi-parametric MRI of benign prostatic hyperplasia and its differentiation from transition zone cancer. Abdominal Radiology 2019;44(6): 2233–43.

37. Guneyli S, Ward E, Thomas S, et al. Magnetic resonance imaging of benign prostatic hyperplasia. Diagn Interventional Radiol 2016;22(3):215–9.

38. Hoeks CMA, Hambrock T, Yakar D, et al. Transition zone prostate cancer: Detection and localization with 3-T multiparametric MR imaging. Radiology 2013;266(1):207–17.

39. Shannon BA, McNeal JE, Cohen RJ. Transition zone carcinoma of the prostate gland: A common indolent tumour type that occasionally manifests aggressive behaviour. Pathology 2003;35(6):467–71.

40. Bonde AA, Korngold EK, Foster BR, et al. Prostate cancer with a pseudocapsule at MR imaging: A marker of high grade and stage disease? Clin Imag 2016;40(3): 365–9.

41. Ranasinghe WKB, Troncoso P, Surasi DS, et al. Defining diagnostic criteria for prostatic ductal adenocarcinoma at multiparametric MRI. Radiology 2022;303(1):110–8.

42. Oto A, Kayhan A, Jiang Y, et al. Prostate cancer: differentiation of central gland cancer from benign prostatic hyperplasia by using diffusion-weighted and dynamic contrast-enhanced MR imaging. Radiology 2010;257(3):715–23.

43. Tang J, Yang JC, Zhang Y, et al. Does benign prostatic hyperplasia originate from the peripheral zone of the prostate? A preliminary study. BJU Int 2007; 100(5):1091–6.

44. Kahokehr AA, Gilling PJ. Which laser works best for benign prostatic hyperplasia? Curr Urol Rep 2013; 14(6):614–9.

45. Semple JE. Surgical capsule of the benign enlargement of the prostate its development and action. Br Med J 1963;1(5346):1640–3.

46. Kitzing YX, Prando A, Varol C, et al. Benign conditions that mimic prostate carcinoma: MR imaging features with histopathologic correlation. Radiographics 2016;36(1):162–75.

47. Chatterjee A, Thomas S, Oto A. Prostate MR: pitfalls and benign lesions. Abdominal Radiology 2020; 45(7):2154–64.

48. White S, Hricak H, Forstner R, et al. Prostate cancer: effect of postbiopsy hemorrhage on interpretation of MR images. Radiology 1995;195(2):385–90.

49. Barrett T, Vargas HA, Akin O, et al. Value of the hemorrhage exclusion sign on T1-weighted prostate MR images for the detection of prostate cancer. Radiology 2012;263(3):751–7.

50. Rosenkrantz AB, Mussi TC, Hindman N, et al. Impact of delay after biopsy and post-biopsy haemorrhage on prostate cancer tumour detection using multi-parametric MRI: a multi-reader study. Clin Radiol 2012;67(12):e83–90.

51. Purysko AS, Childes BJ, Ward RD, et al. Pitfalls in prostate MRI interpretation: a pictorial review. Semin Roentgenol 2021;56(4):391–405.

52. Sfanos KS, Wilson BA, De Marzo AM, et al. Acute inflammatory proteins constitute the organic matrix of prostatic corpora amylacea and calculi in men with prostate cancer. Proc Natl Acad Sci U S A 2009;106(9):3443–8.

53. Christian JD, Lamm TC, Morrow JF, et al. Corpora amylacea in adenocarcinoma of the prostate: Incidence and histology within needle core biopsies. Mod Pathol 2005;18(1):36–9.

54. Benedetti I, Bettin A, Reyes N. Inflammation and focal atrophy in prostate needle biopsy cores and association to prostatic adenocarcinoma. Ann Diagn Pathol 2016;24:55–61.

55. Freitas DM, Andriole GL Jr, Castro-Santamaria R, et al. Extent of Baseline Prostate Atrophy Is Associated With Lower Incidence of Low- and High-grade Prostate Cancer on Repeat Biopsy. Urology 2017; 103:161–6.

56. Servian P, Celma A, Planas J, et al. Clinical significance of proliferative inflammatory atrophy in negative prostatic biopsies. Prostate 2016;76(16): 1501–6.

57. Billis A, Meirelles LR, Magna LA, et al. Extent of prostatic atrophy in needle biopsies and serum PSA levels: is there an association? Urology 2007; 69(5):927–30.

58. Walz J, Epstein JI, Ganzer R, et al. A critical analysis of the current knowledge of surgical anatomy of the prostate related to optimisation of cancer control and preservation of continence and erection in candidates for radical prostatectomy: an update. Eur Urol 2016;70(2):301–11.

59. Patel P, Oto A. Magnetic resonance imaging of the prostate, including pre- and postinterventions. Semin Intervent Radiol 2016;33(3):186–95.

60. Panebianco V, Villeirs G, Weinreb JC, et al. Prostate magnetic resonance imaging for local recurrence reporting (PI-RR): international consensus -based guidelines on multiparametric magnetic resonance imaging for prostate cancer recurrence after radiation therapy and radical prostatectomy. Eur Urol Oncol 2021;4(6):868–76.

61. Gaur S, Turkbey B. Prostate MR imaging for post-treatment evaluation and recurrence. Urol Clin North Am 2018;45(3):467–79.

62. Mertan FV, Greer MD, Borofsky S, et al. Multiparametric magnetic resonance imaging of recurrent prostate cancer. Top Magn Reson Imaging 2016; 25(3):139–47.

63. Potretzke TA, Froemming AT, Gupta RT. Post-treatment prostate MRI. Abdominal Radiology 2020; 45(7):2184–97.

64. Magistro G, Weinhold P, Stief CG, et al. The new kids on the block: prostatic urethral lift (Urolift) and convective water vapor energy ablation (Rezūm). Curr Opin Urol 2018;28(3):294–300.

65. A Straightforward Minimally Invasive Treatment. 2023; Available at: https://www.urolift.com/physicians/procedure-device. Accessed May 25, 2023.

66. Dempsey PJ, Power JW, Yates A, et al. Creation of a protective space between the rectum and prostate prior to prostate radiotherapy using a hydrogel spacer. Clin Radiol 2022;77(3):e195–200.

67. Mariados NF, Orio PF III, Schiffman Z, et al. Hyaluronic acid spacer for hypofractionated prostate radiation therapy: a randomized clinical trial. JAMA Oncol 2023;9(4):511–8.

68. Montoya J, Gross E, Karsh L. How i do it: hydrogel spacer placement in men scheduled to undergo prostate radiotherapy. Can J Urol 2018;25(2): 9288–93.

69. Sheridan AD, Nath SK, Huber S, et al. Role of MRI in the use of an absorbable hydrogel spacer in men undergoing radiation therapy for prostate cancer: what the radiologist needs to know. Am J Roentgenol 2017;209(4):797–9. Pitfalls in Prostate MRI Interpretation.

Active Surveillance for Prostate Cancer
Expanding the Role of MR Imaging and the Use of PRECISE Criteria

Cameron Englman, MD[a,b], Tristan Barrett, MD, FRCR[c,d],
Caroline M. Moore, MD, FRCS[b,e], Francesco Giganti, MD, PhD[a,b],*

KEYWORDS

- Prostate cancer • Active surveillance • mpMRI • MRI • PRECISE • Biopsy

KEY POINTS

- AS enrollment criteria and protocols differ between institutions and guidelines.
- Multiparametric MR imaging during AS improves the accuracy of prostate biopsies, assists in the selection of eligible patients, and can be used to monitor cancer progression.
- The PRECISE recommendations standardize reporting of serial MR imaging scans during AS.
- We include a clinical primer to help clinicians navigate the PRECISE case report form.
- There is increasing evidence to support MR imaging-led AS programs and the need for an individualized risk-stratified approach to AS.
- Important limitations to mpMRI and the PRECISE recommendations exist that should be addressed in future updates.

Active surveillance (AS) is a conservative management approach increasingly used for patients with low- and intermediate-risk prostate cancer (PCa).[1] It is an alternative to active treatment, where patients are closely followed up to identify if and when cancer progression occurs, avoiding unnecessary treatment for clinically localized disease and identifying progression to trigger deferred procedures without losing the window of curability. AS differs from watchful waiting, which is a less-aggressive system of PCa monitoring that does not involve frequent testing or biopsies for patients who do not want or cannot have treatment therapies, and is now the preferred management option for low-risk disease.[1,2]

Multiparametric magnetic resonance imaging (mpMRI) of the prostate can detect clinically significant cancer and has emerged as a noninvasive method to monitor AS patients for PCa progression.[3,4] The Prostate Cancer Radiological Estimation of Change in Sequential Evaluation (PRECISE) recommendations[5] were published in 2016 to standardize reporting of serial mpMRIs during AS and have been applied in different MR imaging-led AS cohorts.[6–11]

The aim of this article is four-fold: (1) discuss current AS protocols; (2) look at the expanding role of mpMRI in AS protocols; (3) describe the PRECISE criteria, providing a clinical primer to help report using these recommendations; and (4) synthesize

[a] Department of Radiology, University College London Hospital NHS Foundation Trust, 3rd Floor, Charles Bell House, 43-45 Foley Street, London, W1W7TY, UK; [b] Division of Surgery & Interventional Science, University College London, 3rd Floor, Charles Bell House, 43-45 Foley Street, London, W1W7TY, UK; [c] Department of Radiology, University of Cambridge, Box 218, Addenbrooke's Hospital, Hills Road, Cambridge, CB2 0QQ, UK; [d] Department of Radiology, Cambridge University Hospitals NHS Foundation Trust, Box 218, Addenbrooke's Hospital, Hills Road, Cambridge, CB2 0QQ, UK; [e] Department of Urology, University College London Hospital NHS Foundation Trust, 3rd Floor, Charles Bell House, 43-45 Foley Street, London, W1W7TY, UK
* Corresponding author. Division of Surgery & Interventional Science, University College London, 3rd Floor, Charles Bell House, 43-45 Foley Street, London, W1W 7TS.
E-mail address: f.giganti@ucl.ac.uk

Radiol Clin N Am 62 (2024) 69–92
https://doi.org/10.1016/j.rcl.2023.06.009

the literature on MR imaging-led AS cohorts, examining the current limitations and offering suggestions on future directions for research.

ACTIVE SURVEILLANCE

From 1990 to 2010, more than 90% of patients diagnosed with low-risk PCa by prostate-specific antigen (PSA) and biopsy were treated radically according to a study on 11,892 patients from 36 sites across the United States.[12] Yet, definitive treatments such as radical prostatectomy (RP) and radiotherapy have significant morbidity and serious side effects including urinary and sexual function problems.[13]

AS was first described explicitly in a 2002 report for a trial on 250 low-risk PCa patients of expectant management with periodic biopsies and treatment only for those reclassified as of high risk.[14,15] Following substantial evidence on the indolent nature of low-grade PCa and favorable outcomes with conservative management, there has been increasing consensus about the value and benefits of AS. This approach has now become widely adopted internationally, with the percentage of low-risk PCa patients managed conservatively increasing from about 10% in 2000 to over 90% in a few regions.[16–18]

Randomized controlled trials comparing definitive therapy to conservative management have found similar long-term survival rates.[19,20] In the PIVOT trial,[19] 731 men with localized PCa were randomly assigned to either RP or observation, and after 19.5 years of follow-up (median = 12.7 years), RP did not significantly reduce overall or cancer-specific mortality compared with the observation arm. Furthermore, the ProtecT trial,[13] a large, randomized UK study that compared RP, radiotherapy, and "active monitoring" for localized PCa, recently reported its 15-year follow-up results and demonstrated no significant difference in overall or cancer-specific survival between the three cohorts. It should be noted that the conservative arm in both trials lacked the rigorous follow-up of modern AS protocols with no imaging or mandated biopsies and that both had a degree of cross-over between treatment arms.

Currently, there is significant intercenter heterogeneity in AS enrollment criteria and protocols (**Table 1**). While AS is largely accepted for low-risk PCa, this is not the case for intermediate-risk patients. Results from large, prospective studies that included patients with intermediate-risk PCa have been positive,[21–23] and the DETECTIVE study[24] demonstrated good outcomes for patients with favorable Grade Group (GG) 2 disease (PSA <

10 ng/ml, stage $\leq$ T2, and few positive cores on biopsy). The UK National Institute for Health and Care Excellence (NICE) guidelines[1] were the first to support AS for GG2 patients in 2015, and now others support this approach for "selected" intermediate-risk patients.[25,26] Protocols usually include monitoring PSA kinetics, digital rectal examinations, magnetic resonance (MR) imaging, and biopsies. Prostate biopsies, which are commonly used to assess changes in cancer grade, can be transrectal ultrasound scan-guided or transperineal and may be a random systematic biopsy (usually 12 cores) and/or targeted at specific lesions found on MR imaging. Protocol-based biopsies can be performed at different prespecified time points throughout AS, whereas confirmatory biopsies, if carried out, are usually performed within 12 months from diagnosis or AS inclusion.

However, biopsies are also a major barrier to the uptake, adherence, and tolerability of AS, with the PRIAS study[27] demonstrating lower compliance rates when protocol-based biopsies are used. These concerns must be weighed against the risk of delays in detecting PCa progression and missing the window of opportunity for curative treatment. Currently, there is no accepted consensus on the recommended frequency or timing of biopsies.

MR IMAGING IN AS

Multiparametric MR imaging consists of a combination of anatomic and functional sequences (**Fig. 1**) and has played an expanding role in AS. Increasing availability, improved image quality, growing expertise in the interpretation of scans, and more data on MR imaging accuracy and limitations are all influencing its use.[15] Indeed, 90% of academic centers in the United States and 72% of health care services in the United Kingdom now perform MR imaging of the prostate, with an additional 24% offering biparametric MR imaging (ie, without the injection of intravenous contrast)[30,31] although the rates of prebiopsy MR imaging for patients on AS range from 1.9% to 28.2% in studies on US populations.[32–34] MR imaging has several roles in AS and can assist with the selection of eligible patients, directing prostate biopsies, and monitoring for cancer progression.

Good-quality image acquisition is a prerequisite for the repeated use of MR imaging during AS. The Prostate Imaging-Reporting and Data System (PI-RADS)[35] guidelines indicate that both 1.5- and 3-T magnets can provide adequate and reliable scans when acquisition parameters are optimized. The same acquisition protocol would ideally be used for baseline and follow-up scans, but this is not

Table 1
Active surveillance enrollment criteria and protocols used at different institutes or recommended in guidelines

| Groups | Enrollment Criteria | | | Prostate Biopsy | | | | | | |
	Gleason Score	PSA Level (ng/mL)	Clinical Stage	DRE	PSA	Imaging	Confirmatory	Repeat	Initiation of at	Terminating as
Institutions										
Royal Marsden Hospital[23]	≤3 + 4	≤15	≤T2a	3 monthly (year 1), 4 monthly (year 2), then 6 monthly	3 monthly (year 1), 4 monthly (year 2), then 6 monthly	mpMRI at baseline and every 2 y	At 24 mo	Every 2 y	GS ≥ 4 + 3, positive cores >50% of total cores, PSAV >1 ng/ml per year	N/A
UCL[7]	≤3 + 4	≤20	≤T2b	N/A	Every 3–6 mo	mpMRI at 12 mo then based on imaging and clinical features	N/A	Based on imaging and clinical factors	GS ≥ 4 + 3	N/A
UoT[22]	≤3 + 4	≤15	≤T2b	N/A	Every 3 mo (up to 2 y) then 6 mo	Not routinely recommended	At 12 mo	Every 2 y	Pathology upgrade	N/A
UCSF[28]	≤3 + 3	≤10	≤T2	Every 3 mo	Every 6 mo	TRUS at 6 mo	At 9 mo	Every 1–2 y	GS > 6, positive cores > 2, PSADT < 3 y	N/A
Guidelines										
AUA[26]	≤3 + 3, ≤3 + 4	10–20, ≤10	≤T2a	Unspecified[a]	Unspecified[a]	mpMRI if magnet ≥ 1.5 T and reviewed by an experienced radiologist	Within 24 mo	Unspecified[a]	Clinical upstaging or upgrading at subsequent bx	N/A
EAU[2]	≤3 + 3	≤10	≤T2a	Every 12 mo	Every 6 mo	Before confirmatory bx	Timing not specified[b]	Not routinely recommended[c]	Decision based on a change in the bx results or T-stage progression	N/A

(continued on next page)

Table 1
(continued)

Groups	Enrollment Criteria			Prostate Biopsy					Initiation of at	Terminating as
	Gleason Score	PSA Level (ng/mL)	Clinical Stage	DRE	PSA	Imaging	Confirmatory	Repeat		
CCO[29]	≤3 + 3	≤10	≤T2a	Every 12 mo	Every 3–6 mo	Indicated when clinical findings discordant with the pathologic findings	Within 6–12 mo	Every 3–5 y	Gleason score ≥ 7 (if Gleason pattern 4 > 10% total cancer) or significant increase in cancer volume	Turning 80-year-old (end serial bx)
NICE[1]	≤3 + 3 ≤3 + 4	<10 10–20	≤T2a ≤T2b	Every 12 mo	Every 3–6 mo	Offer to mpMRI-naive patients at 12–18 mo	Not recommended[d]	Not routinely performed[c]	Evidence of disease progression – not specified	N/A
NCCN[25]	≤3 + 4	<10	<T2a	Every ≥ 12 mo	Every ≥ 6 mo	As an optional confirmatory tool at enrollment, repeating every ≥ 12 mo	Within 6 mo[e]	Every ≥ 12 mo	Gleason pattern 4 or 5 at bx or an > number of cores involved or in core length involvement	<10-y life expectancy (end serial bx)

AS, active surveillance; AT, active treatment; AUA, American Urologic Association; bx, biopsy; CCO, Cancer Care Ontario; DRE, digital rectal examination; EAU, European Association of Urology; mo, months; mpMRI, multiparametric magnetic resonance imaging; N/A, not available; NICE, National Institute for Health and Care Excellence; NCCN, National Comprehensive Cancer Network; N/A, not available; PSA, prostate-specific antigen; PSADT, PSA doubling time; TRUS, transrectal ultrasound; UCL, University College London; UCSF, University of California, San Francisco; UoT, University of Toronto.

a Although serial testing is recommended, no specific time interval is provided.

b No need for confirmatory biopsy if the primary biopsy was a targeted biopsy.

c Should be performed if progression is suspected (based on PSA, DRE, or mpMRI).

d All men diagnosed with PCa should have had a mpMRI-guided biopsy performed prior to the diagnosis; if not, a mpMRI should be offered, and a targeted biopsy performed if the results are discordant with the initial biopsy findings.

e Not obligatory, should be performed if the initial biopsy was less than 10 cores or assessment discordant.

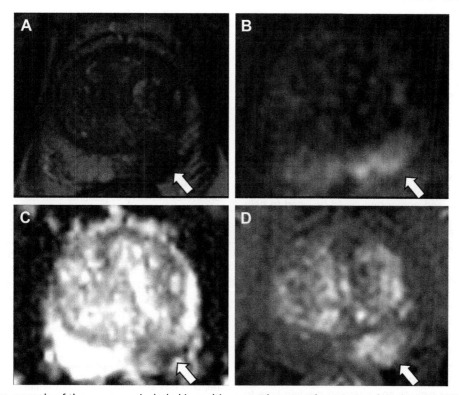

Fig. 1. An example of the sequences included in multiparametric magnetic resonance imaging. A 1.5 T scan of a 74-year-old patient with 10 mm GS 4 + 3 on biopsy and a lesion (*arrow*) in the left peripheral zone between 4 and 6 o'clock. The following sequences should be included in mpMRI: (*A*) T2-weighted image (T2-WI), to look at the anatomy of the prostate; (*B, C*) diffusion-weighted image (DWI) including a sequence of multiple *b* values, a dedicated high *b* value sequence (shown in B), and an apparent diffusion coefficient (ADC) map (shown in C) to examine the cellularity of the lesion; (*D*) a dynamic contrast-enhanced (DCE) sequence, which requires the injection of an intravenous contrast medium, to assess the vascularity of a lesion. Prostate cancer usually appears hypointense on T2-WI (*A*), hyperintense on the high *b* value sequence (*B*), and hypointense on the ADC map (*C*) and demonstrates early wash-in (*D*) and early wash-out on DCE sequences.

always practical for patients on AS for significant periods since protocols and technology evolve over time.

Adequate reporting expertise and consistency are also extremely important. Traditionally, PCa lesions have been measured using a 1-5 Likert scale, which was highly influenced by reporter expertise and implied subjective assessment of the whole prostate gland. However, the PI-RADS scoring system was introduced in 2012 to standardize MR imaging reporting,[36] and this was followed by the PRECISE recommendations in 2016 for reporting serial MR imaging during AS.[5] The importance of reporting scan quality has been further emphasized by the introduction of the Prostate Imaging Quality System (PI-QUAL) scoring system in 2020.[37]

Selection of AS Patients at Baseline

MR imaging can improve risk stratification and patient selection for AS. Turkbey and colleagues[38]

compared MR imaging with current clinicopathological criteria such as Cancer of the Prostate Risk Assessment (CAPRA), Einstein, and D'Amico to retrospectively determine AS eligibility for 133 patients undergoing RP. They found MR imaging was the most accurate method (sensitivity = 93%, positive predictive value = 57%, overall accuracy = 92%, $P < .005$), and when used in combination, the sensitivity and accuracy of each clinic-pathological criterion improved. Moreover, correlations between pathology results from template-mapped biopsies with the gland sampled every 5 mm, which is considered the gold standard for PCa detection, and RP specimens show that MR imaging has a good sensitivity ($\sim$90%) for the detection and localization of GG $\geq$ 2 cancers.[39,40] A 2019 meta-analysis comparing MR imaging with template-mapped biopsies in biopsy-naive and repeat-biopsy settings demonstrated that MR imaging had a pooled sensitivity and specificity of 91% and 37% for GG $\geq$ 2 cancers and 95% and

35% for GG $\geq$ 3 cancers, indicating its clinical potential for ruling out a high-grade disease.[40] Hence, the use of MR imaging before the first biopsy has become widespread to aid prognostic assessment.[4,41]

MR Imaging Before Confirmatory Biopsy

MR imaging-targeting can also improve reclassification on confirmatory biopsies and identify AS patients who had PCa undersampled at the initial biopsy. A study demonstrated that an MR imaging-based nomogram could be used to help exclude patients from AS.[42] Another study on the use of MR imaging-targeted confirmatory biopsy reclassified 59% of patients initially selected for AS by systematic biopsy.[43] A meta-analysis of MR imaging confirmatory biopsies on 1028 patients found the pooled sensitivity, specificity, positive likelihood ratio, and negative likelihood ratio were 69%, 78%, 3.1, and 0.4, respectively.[44] A study to determine the prognostic implications of confirmatory biopsy results found that no cancer on targeted biopsy was associated with a reduced risk of GG progression (hazard ratio = 0.41, $P < .01$), as well as an increased median time to progression (74.3 vs 44.6 months, $P < .01$).[45] In the ASIST trial,[46] patients with a recent diagnosis of GG1 who were referred for confirmatory biopsy were randomized to either MR imaging or non-MR imaging arms. Although initial results found no difference in the upgrading rates between the two groups,[46] which was attributed to the learning curve for MR imaging-targeted biopsies with higher volume centers performing better, after 2 years of follow-up, MR imaging before confirmatory biopsy resulted in 50% fewer AS failures (19% vs 35%, $P = .017$) and less progression to higher-grade cancer (10% vs 23%, $P = .048$).[47] Finally, a systematic review on the added value of MR imaging and MR imaging-targeted biopsies to confirmatory biopsies during AS found that 27% had cancer upgrading (to Gleason score $\geq 3 + 4$) using a combined approach of MR imaging-targeted and systematic, MR imaging-targeted and standard confirmatory biopsies alone would have missed cancer upgrading in 10% and 7% of cases, respectively, and 35% of MR imaging-positive patients were upgraded compared with only 12% of MR imaging-negative patients.[48]

MR Imaging for AS Monitoring

While correctly identifying AS candidates is essential, monitoring for PCa progression is equally as important. Growth of a lesion, change in lesion parameters, or the development of new lesions can be equated with true pathologic progression, which raises the possibility of MR imaging-led AS with triggers for biopsies based solely on imaging findings. This approach may limit the number of biopsies required, if a stable MR imaging scan can reduce the need for time-based biopsies and improve AS compliance; however, this remains controversial. Fujihara and colleagues[49] demonstrated if surveillance biopsy was triggered based only on MR imaging progression, 63% of initially scheduled biopsies would be postponed. Although this approach missed histologic progression (GG2) in 12% of patients with no radiological progression, no high-grade (GG $\geq$ 3) cancers were missed. The MRIAS trial[50] followed up AS patients for 3 years with annual MR imaging, 6-month PSA, and exit biopsy at 3 years. Protocol-driven biopsies were performed for predefined targets, such as a new persistent lesion or rising PSA kinetics, and most patients (71%) avoided biopsy before 3 years, the progression rate was relatively low (21%), and the incidence of high-risk cancer missed by MR imaging was only 1%. In the United Kingdom, two major London hospitals, University College London Hospital (UCLH) and Guy's Hospital, use MR imaging for AS, but while Guy's uses protocol-based biopsies, UCLH does not, and the dropout rate for a stable disease is greater than 20% and less than 1%, respectively.[51,52]

THE PRECISE RECOMMENDATIONS

A 2015 systematic review found no consistency across reporting of serial MR imaging scans during AS, which prevented meaningful analysis and comparison of the data between studies.[53] This inspired the European School of Oncology Task Force to meet and discuss 394 statements on the topic, which resulted in the publication of the PRECISE recommendations.[5] Key recommendations included the adoption of a case report form (Fig. 2) and reporting of a PRECISE score (Fig. 3), as well as a checklist for investigators working on MR imaging-led AS cohorts.

The PRECISE score is a 1-5 scale that has been shown to be reproducible with agreement levels comparable to other scoring systems such as PI-RADS v.2.[54] It is intended to lead to the identification of AS patients who progress (ie, PRECISE score 4-5) in a timely manner and thereby prompt rebiopsy or treatment, as well as the avoidance of repeat biopsy and lower surveillance intensity in case of radiological stability (ie, PRECISE score 1-3), thereby reducing the burden of surveillance on the individual patient and the broader health care system. A retrospective analysis of 80 patients on AS,[54] where two expert radiologists assessed scans from two different cohorts

PRECISE Case report form for men having MRI on active surveillance

Reporting radiologist		Date of scan		Date of report	
PSA		PSA date		PSA density	
Prostate volume on T2-weighted imaging		Magnet strength		Coil used	
Likelihood of clinically significant disease (1–5)*		PI-RADS 2 score (maximal)		TNM stage	
Likelihood of extraprostatic extension (T3a) (1–5)*		Likelihood of seminal vesicle invasion (T3b) (1–5)*			

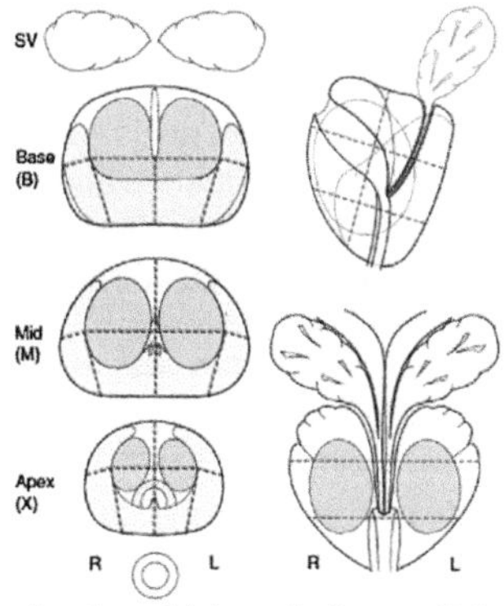

Lesion	Appeared since last scan?	Not visible	D1	D2	D3	Volume (D1 x D2 x D3 x 0.52)	Volume by planimetry	Likelihood of clinically significant disease (1–5)*	PI-RADS-2 score
1									
2									
3									

	Sequence where lesion best seen	Volume where lesion best seen	Volume on T2-weighted imaging
Lesion 1			
Lesion 2			
Lesion 3			

Draw and number each lesion on the diagram, with the most significant lesion being number 1.

*Likert score of 1–5 for likelihood where 1= Very low likelihood; 2= Low likelihood 3 = Intermediate/equivocal; 4 = High likelihood ; 5 = Very high likelihood

	Date of previous MRI	Likelihood of change from previous MRI (1–5 score)	Parameter which has changed eg volume on T2W-I, visibility on DWI, Likert score or PI-RADS score, T3a or T3b disease
Lesion 1			
Lesion2			
Lesion 3			

Fig. 2. Case report form for reporting of magnetic resonance imaging at baseline and during follow-up in patients on active surveillance. MRI, magnetic resonance imaging; PI-RADS, Prostate Imaging Reporting and Data System; PRECISE, Prostate Cancer Radiological Estimation of Change in Sequential Evaluation; PSA, prostate-specific antigen; T2-WI, T2-weighted image. (*Reprinted with permission from* Moore and colleagues[5])

independently, found high interobserver reproducibility, with agreement per patient and per scan for each PRECISE score of 79% and 81%, respectively. However, further work is needed to confirm these results with multiple readers of differing experience, in a variety of health care settings and incorporating different MR systems and vendors.

PRECISE CLINICAL PRIMER

We provide a practical guide on reporting MR imaging using the PRECISE case report form and a primer to familiarize radiologists with the PRECISE scoring system. We present a variety of cases and images to demonstrate the difference between scores. We divide the case report form into three sections corresponding to the boxes on the page and discuss each step that should be followed.

Clinical Details and Overall Likelihood of Clinically Significant PCa

1. The first box requires the necessary clinical and patient details including the scan and report date, the name of the reporting radiologist,

Likert	Assessment of likelihood of radiologic progression	Example
1	Resolution of previous features suspicious on MRI	Previously enhancing area no longer enhances
2	Reduction in volume and/or conspicuity of previous features suspicious on MRI	Reduction in size of previously seen lesion that remains suspicious for clinically significant disease
3	Stable MRI appearance: no new focal/diffuse lesions	Either no suspicious features or all lesions stable in size and appearance
4	Significant increase in size and/or conspicuity of features suspicious for prostate cancer	Lesion becomes visible on diffusion-weighted imaging; significant increase in size of previously seen lesion
5	Definitive radiologic stage progression	Appearance of extracapsular extension, seminal vesicle involvement, lymph node involvement, or bone metastasis

MRI = magnetic resonance imaging.

Fig. 3. Breakdown of the PRECISE scoring system as shown in the original recommendations. (*Reprinted with permission from* Moore and colleagues[5])

and the date and result of the most recent serum PSA level.

2. The prostate volume on T2-weighted imaging should be measured either by planimetry (ie, using manual slice-by-slice segmentation of the prostate or with automated segmentation algorithms)[55] or using the ellipsoid formula (ie, [anteroposterior × transverse × longitudinal diameter] × [$\pi/6$]), with PSA density subsequently derived as PSA (ng/ml)/prostate volume (cc).

3. Record details about the MR scanner including the magnet field strength (either 1.5- or 3-T) and the coils used (eg, with/without an endorectal coil).

4. A rating of the *overall* likelihood of clinically significant disease is required using a Likert scale (where 1 = very low likelihood and 5 = very high likelihood), the *maximal* PI-RADS score for any lesion seen on the scan, as well as the Tumor, Node and Metastasis staging including 1 to 5 Likert scores for the likelihood of extraprostatic extension (T3a) and seminal vesicle invasion (T3b).

Description of the Current Lesion/s

1. The reporter is then required to comment on the three most conspicuous lesions, with the most significant "index" lesion being number one. For each lesion, they are required to note whether they appeared since the last scan, if they remain visible, and their volumes. Assessment of the likelihood of clinically significant PCa should be performed using the PI-RADS score and a more subjective Likert scale. PI-RADS recommends the use of the dominant sequence for reading prostate lesions (ie, diffusion-weighted imaging for the peripheral zone and T2-weighted imaging for the transition zone).[35] Likert uses similar interpretation principles to PI-RADS but is less didactic in the use of a dominant sequence and is more experience-based.[56] This section also includes a figure where the reporter can draw and number each lesion.

2. In accordance with PI-RADS recommendations, lesion size should be measured on the apparent diffusion coefficient (ADC) map for lesions within the peripheral zone and on T2-weighted imaging for transition zone lesions.[35] However, if lesion measurement is difficult or compromised on these sequences, the measurement should be made on the sequence that best depicts the lesion. Lesion volume can be determined using one of four different techniques (**Fig. 4**). Planimetry or the ellipsoid formula are considered the most accurate, but single plane or biaxial measurements may

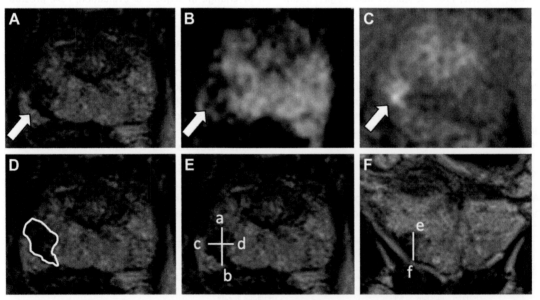

Fig. 4. The various methods for measuring lesion size on multiparametric magnetic resonance imaging. A 1.5 T scan of a 56-year-old patient with 5 mm GS 3 + 3 in the right peripheral zone on targeted biopsy. The lesion between 7 and 9 o'clock (*arrow*) is clearly visible on (*A*) T2-WI, (*B*) ADC map, and (*C*) DCE sequences. (*D*) The lesion volume on planimetry is obtained by contouring the lesion slice by slice on the axial image, while the volume using the ellipsoid formula is obtained using the three diameters from the (*E*) axial and (*F*) coronal acquisition according to the formula: (ab × cd × ef) × ($\pi/6$). The size of a lesion can also be measured using a single maximum diameter or by the biaxial measurement of maximum diameters (ie, estimated square area), as per the original case report form shown in **Fig. 2**.

also be used when the quality of sequences is compromised by artifacts or when lesions are very small and only seen on one or two slices. It is recommended that the volume of the lesion is recorded using the same method for serial studies, as this will prevent errors from inconsistent measurements and, ideally, radiologists should be blinded to the previous lesion measurements at this point.

PRECISE Scores

1. This section requires reporters to review previous MR imaging scans and therefore is not reported for the baseline study. The date of the last MR imaging is recorded, a PRECISE score for the likelihood of radiological change compared to prior imaging should be provided, and a comment included on any parameters which have changed. Images should be compared to both the previous imaging and baseline study when determining the PRECISE score, with the recommended parameters for assessing any change being lesion size, conspicuity (ie, visibility), change in the PI-RADS score (indicating upgrade of existing lesions or new lesions), and any features of extraprostatic disease (including extracapsular extension, seminal vesicle invasion, nodal involvement, and metastasis). The final PRECISE score reflects either resolution (PRECISE 1, Fig. 5) or reduction (PRECISE 2, Fig. 6) of features suspicious for tumor such as conspicuity or size of the lesion compared to previous

scans, overall radiological stability (PRECISE 3, Fig. 7), or radiological progression in lesion size/conspicuity (PRECISE 4, Fig. 8) or stage progression (PRECISE 5, Fig. 9).

SYNTHESIS OF AVAILABLE EVIDENCE ON MR IMAGING-LED AS

Two recent systematic reviews have synthesized the literature on MR imaging-led AS.[57,58] The first study included 15 studies with 2240 patients and provided pooled diagnostic estimates of serial MR imaging for PCa progression during AS.[57] The PRECISE recommendations were used in six studies (Table 2), and nine used institution-specific definitions. The pooled sensitivity, specificity, and accuracy of serial MR imaging for progression were 59%, 75%, and 73%, respectively. The positive predictive value ranged from 37% to 50% with a negative predictive value of MR imaging for progression ranging from 81% to 88%. There was also a nonsignificant trend toward improved performance of the cohorts using the PRECISE recommendations. In the second analysis, only seven studies (including 800 patients) were assessed.[58] The pooled sensitivity and specificity of MR imaging for disease progression were 61% and 78%, respectively. These studies concluded that serial MR imaging alone is not enough to reliably exclude PCa progression and suggest that blood markers and clinical factors must also be used to determine the timing of follow-up biopsies.

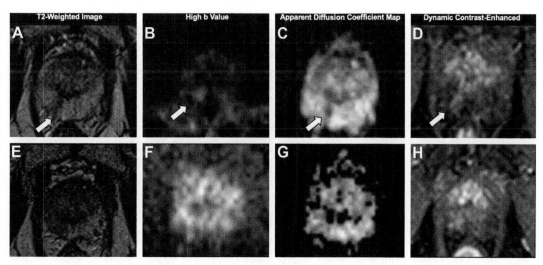

Fig. 5. Case of resolution in suspicious features for prostate cancer on magnetic resonance imaging (PRECISE 1). (A–D) A 1.5 T MR scan of a 69-year-old patient showing a wedge-shaped focus (arrow) in the right peripheral zone (Likert 3/5). The patient had only 1 mm Gleason 3 + 3 disease at targeted biopsy. A subsequent 1.5 T scan (E–H) demonstrates no focal lesions (Likert 2/5). The PRECISE score was 1 (ie, resolution of previous features suspicious on magnetic resonance imaging).

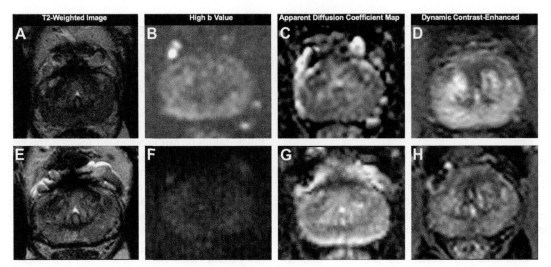

Fig. 6. A case of reduction in suspicious features for prostate cancer on magnetic resonance imaging (PRECISE 2). (*A-D*) A 1.5 T MR scan of a 61-year-old patient showing a diffuse patchy T2 signal associated with mildly restricted diffusion and diffuse enhancement (Likert 3/5). Systematic biopsy showed 3.5 mm Gleason 3 + 4 disease in the left peripheral zone at mid-gland. (*E-H*) A subsequent 3T scan demonstrates improvement of the diffuse changes with no focal lesions (Likert 2/5). The PRECISE score was 2 (ie, reduction in conspicuity of previous features suspicious on MRI).

At least another three MR imaging-led AS cohort studies have been published since these systematic reviews. Chu and colleagues[59] showed that both consistently visible and increasingly suspicious lesions on imaging were associated with GG ≥ 2 detection and definitive treatment in 125 patients. Castillo and colleagues[60] reported on 90 patients who underwent serial imaging and observed radiological progression in 29% of

patients with a suspicious baseline scan (PI-RADS = 3) and 25% with a nonsuspicious baseline scan (PI-RADS ≤ 2). In addition, Thankapannair and colleagues[61] investigated a tailored risk-monitoring strategy and enrolled 156 patients into a prospective stratified three-tier follow-up program based on Cambridge Prognostic Group, PSA density, and MR imaging Likert score at entry. Rates of pathologic progression, AS dropout, and

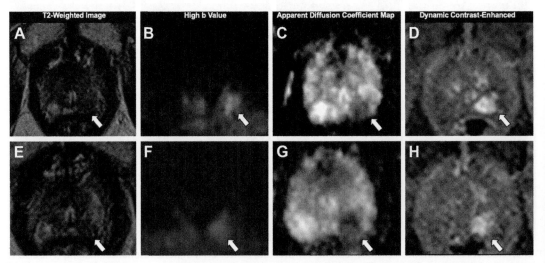

Fig. 7. A case of a stable lesion on serial magnetic resonance imaging (PRECISE 3). (*A–D*) A 1.5 T MR scan of a 73-year-old patient showing a focal lesion (*arrow*) within the left mid-apical peripheral zone (Likert 4/5). Targeted biopsy showed 8 mm Gleason 3 + 4 disease, and the patient opted for AS. A subsequent 1.5 T scan (*E–H*) shows a stable lesion (Likert 4/5). The PRECISE score was 3 (ie, stable MR features over time).

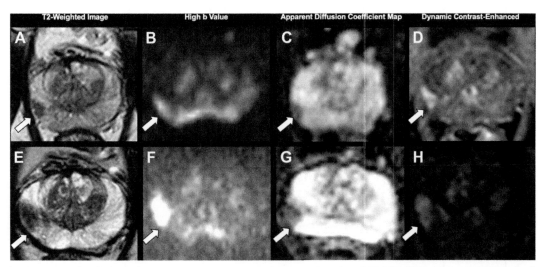

Fig. 8. A case of radiological progression on magnetic resonance imaging (PRECISE 4). (*A–D*) A 1.5 T MR scan of a 64-year-old patient showing a 6 mm wedge-shaped lesion in the right peripheral zone (Likert 4/5). Targeted biopsy revealed 3 mm Gleason 3 + 4 disease, and the patient opted for AS. (*E–H*) A subsequent 3T scan demonstrates increased size and conspicuity of the lesion (Likert 5/5) but no measurable extraprostatic extension. The PRECISE score was 4 (ie, MR features suggesting disease progression). A targeted biopsy revealed 3.5 mm Gleason 4 + 3 disease, and the patient was treated with high-intensity focal ultrasound.

patient choice for treatment were assessed. Overall, 86.5% of patients remained on AS or converted to watchful waiting by the end of the evaluation period, and modeling suggested a potential 22% reduction in the need for outpatient appointments and 42% less MR imaging use than the current NICE guidelines. They concluded that the early outcomes of their study supported a risk-stratified follow-up intensity, but the study is limited by a short follow-up period, a relatively small cohort, and only a single center's experience.

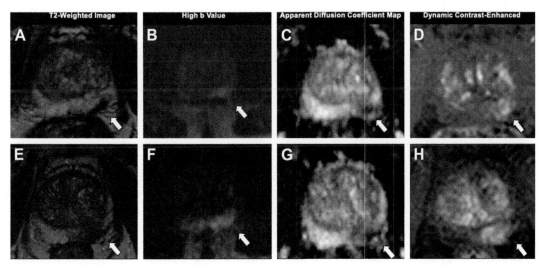

Fig. 9. A case of definitive-stage progression on magnetic resonance imaging (PRECISE 5). (*A-D*) A 1.5 T MR scan of a 70-year-old patient on AS for Gleason 3 + 4 disease showing a suspicious lesion (*arrow*) in the left peripheral zone in the mid-gland at 5 o'clock (Likert 4/5). A subsequent 1.5 T scan (*E-H*) demonstrates progression in both the size and conspicuity of the tumor (Likert 5/5), as well as early macroscopic extracapsular disease extension. The PRECISE score was 5 (ie, MR features suggesting definitive stage progression). A radical prostatectomy was performed, and histology demonstrated Gleason 4 + 3 disease (pT3a).

Table 2
Published cohort studies that report according to the PRECISE recommendations

Study, Year	Country	Study Period	Cohort (n)	AS Eligibility Criteria	Age (yr), Median (IQR)	PSA (ng/mL), Median (IQR)	PSAD (ng/mm³), Median (IQR)	GG1 (%)	GG2 (%)	FU (mo), Median (IQR)	MRI Modality	Reporting Criteria	No. of MRI Reporters	MRI Interval	FU Bx	Definition of Progression	Sensitivity, Specificity, PPV, NPV	Key Messages
Caglic et al,[8] 2020	UK	2011–2018	295	≤3 + 4	66 (61–69)	5.6 (5–7.9)	0.10 (0.07–0.16)	84	16	50 (33–67)	1.5 or 3T mpMRI at baseline, then bpMRI	Likert	2	Annual	Yes	One-step upgrade between diagnostic and repeat Bx for low- and intermediate-risk PCa and MRI stage progression	76% 89% 52% 96%	-PRECISE scores of 1–3 have high NPV, which may reduce the need for repeat Bx
Dieffenbacher et al,[6] 2019	Germany	2010–2018	158	Only 3 + 3	Initial sbx: 69 (64–75) Initial fusion bx: 69 (64–74)	Initial sbx: 6.2 (4.7–7.7) Initial fusion bx: 5.8 (4.5–7.0)	Initial sbx: 0.15 (0.09–0.22) Initial fusion bx: 0.15 (0.10–0.20)	100	0	Initial sbx: 12 (9–16) Initial fusion bx: 22 (20–25)	3T mpMRI	PI-RADs	2	12–24 mo	Yes	GS ≥ 3 + 4, PSA ≥ 10 ng/ml, ≥ 3 positive bx cores, PSA density >0.2 ng/ml, or clinical stage ≥ T2b	59% 90% 57% 91%	-No patients with PRECISE 1–2 (n = 57) are disqualified from AS -Repeat Bx only for PRECISE ≥ 3
Giganti et al,[7] 2020	UK	2005–2020	553	≤3 + 4	62 (56–67)	6.3 (4.7–8.4)	0.12 (0.09–0.2)	80	20	74.5 (53–98)	1.5 or 3T mpMRI	PI-RADs and Likert	1	12–24 mo, and based on clinical factors	Not for all	Histologic progression to GS ≥ 4 + 3 (GS 3) and/or initiation of active treatment	87% 77% 65% 92%	-PRECISE 1–3 cases: very low likelihood of clinical progression and many can avoid routine repeat Bx -PRECISE 4–5 cases show a trend to an increase in PSAD
O'Connor et al,[9] 2020	USA	2007–2020	391	≤3 + 4	63 (58–68)	5.38 (3.95–7.87)	0.10 (0.07–0.14)	73.4	26.6	35.6 (19.7–60.6)	3T mpMRI	In-house score and PI-RADs (after 2015)	2	12–24 mo	Yes	GG 1 to GG ≥ 2, GG1 to GG ≥ 3, GG2 to GG ≥ 3	53% 65% 67% / 64% 63% 59% / 38% 15% 32% / 76% 94% 86%	-PRECISE 1–3 cases: low probability of detecting progression form GG 1 to GG ≥ 3 -Elevated PSA density increases the risk of progression despite stable MRI

Osses et al,[11] 2020	Netherlands	2013–2019	111	Only 3 + 3	66 (60–70)	6.8 (5.1–9.1)	0.17 (0.1–0.25)	100	0	12	3T mpMRI	PI-RADs	1	12 mo	Yes	GG ≥ 2	-In MRI- men, limited value of Sbx at confirmatory bx; -In MRI + men, repeat Sbx is valuable	20% 87% 41% 70%	-No PRECISE 1–3 cases are upgraded at FU bx	100% 42% 66% 100%
Ullrich et al,[10] 2020	Germany	2011–2017	55	≤3 + 4	Mean 66 (SD 7)	7.3 (4.9–9.7)	0.17 (0.11–0.27)	76.4	23.6	19 (13–33)	3T mpMRI	PI-RADs	2	Median 19 (IQR:13–33) mo	Yes	One-step upgrade between diagnostic and repeat Bx for low- and intermediate-risk PCa				

N.B. The studies contain important differences from the inclusion criteria to the follow-up schedule, the most important of which are the exclusion of GS 3 + 4 disease, routine use of confirmatory biopsy, the absence of contrast at follow-up imaging, and use of the PI-RADS score (with two centers using only a Likert scoring system which is allowed by the PRECISE criteria).

AS, active surveillance; bpMRI, biparametric MRI; bx, biopsy; FU, follow-up; GG, Grade Group; GS, Gleason score; IQR, interquartile range; mo, months; mpMRI, multiparametric MRI; MRI, magnetic resonance imaging; n, number; NPV, negative predictive value; PCa, prostate cancer; PI-RADS, Prostate Imaging Reporting and Data System; PPV, positive predictive value; PRECISE, prostate cancer radiological estimation of change in sequential evaluation; PSAD, prostate-specific antigen density; Sbx, systematic biopsy; SD, standard deviation; T, tesla; yr, years.

LIMITATIONS

Systematic reviews have highlighted that the literature on MR imaging-led AS is predominantly retrospective, single-center, cohort studies, currently lacking in high-quality evidence or randomized controlled trials. The literature is heterogenous with variability in the populations enrolled, protocols employed, and the infrastructure and image acquisition within and between studies. Most studies have taken place in high-volume, academic centers, where imaging is analyzed and reviewed by a small number of expert genitourinary radiologists, limiting the generalisability of the results. Moreover, due to the need for long-term follow-up in AS populations and the relatively recent introduction of PRECISE in 2016, the system has typically been applied retrospectively. In addition, there are currently several limitations in the use of MR imaging for AS and also within the PRECISE recommendations[62] (**Fig. 10**).

Limitations of mpMRI in AS

- False positives and false negatives

A positive predictive value for MR imaging of 17%, 46%, and 75% has been reported for lesions with a PI-RADS score of 3, 4, and 5, respectively,[63,64] with false positives resulting from nonmalignant processes that mimic cancer,[65] technical issues such as artifacts from rectal air, improperly positioned endorectal coils or patient movement, iatrogenic causes (eg, post-biopsy changes), and unusual appearance of otherwise normal anatomic structures. These false positives can lead to interpretation errors and unnecessary biopsies. MR imaging also misses lesions, some of which are genuinely MR imaging occult, but there is a variation in negative predictive value,[66] which may also result from quality issues in patient preparation or acquisition.

- Optimal scan timing and growth thresholds to prompt additional biopsy or treatment are uncertain

The decision of when to perform imaging is not straightforward and ideally should be based on both baseline risk and biological changes during follow-up, as well as an assessment of the patient's suitability for treatment, taking into account comorbidities that may have developed during the surveillance period.[67] Moreover, the natural growth rate of PCa lesions and the threshold to rebiopsy or start active treatment are also unclear. Rais-Bahrami et al.[68] reviewed 153 patients with MR imaging and biopsies and recommended MR imaging to monitor small lesions at least once

Current limitations of PRECISE	Possible solutions

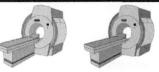

Interscan variability

- Scanner optimisation
- Normalisation (e.g., ADC values)
- MRI phantoms

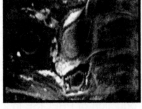

Suboptimal image quality

- Image quality assessment (e.g., PI-QUAL) should be included in the case report form

Likert	Meaning
1	Resolution of previous features suspicious on MRI
2	Reduction in volume and/or conspicuity of previous features suspicious on MRI
3	Stable MRI appearance: no new focal/diffuse lesions
4	Significant increase in size and/or conspicuity of features suspicious for prostate cancer
5	Definitive radiologic stage progression

PRECISE 1 and PRECISE 5 rarely utilised

Likert	Meaning
1	Resolution or reduction in volume and/or conspicuity of previous features on MRI
2	Stable MRI appearance: no new focal/diffuse lesions
3a	Significant increase in lesion size/conspicuity and/or radiologic stage progression up to T2c
3b	Radiologic stage progression to T3a or higher

- New 3-point scale

Reporting with PRECISE is time-consuming

- Implement dedicated PRECISE reporting software

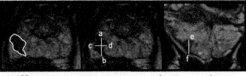

Different ways to measure lesion volume

- Always include the maximum diameter of lesion for consistency and reproducibility

Limited literature on clinical application of PRECISE

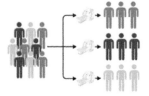

- Multi-centre studies using PRECISE

Fig. 10. Limitations of the current PRECISE recommendations and possible solutions. (Created with BioRender.com.)

every 2 years. It has been demonstrated that 11.6% of patients with no visible lesion on initial MR imaging develop a suspicious focus over a median follow-up of 3.6 years.[69] Morgan and colleagues[70] reported on 151 patients undergoing mpMRI at two-time points (median interval 1.9 years) and found that tumor volume increased measurably in 34.4% of patients after 2 years. While a cutoff of a 20% increase in maximum tumor diameter (on T2-weighted imaging) from baseline and a minimum absolute increase in diameter with a minimum size threshold of 3 mm have been proposed as a more objective definition of radiological progression.[57]

- Interscan variability debases quantitative measurements

The ADC has been proposed as a useful quantitative measure for lesion progression. Baseline ADC has also been shown to be strongly predictive of both adverse histology and time to deferred radical treatment in a prospective AS cohort with 9-year follow-up monitoring.[71] Furthermore, a change in ADC could be used to identify tumors with measurable growth, and a decreased ADC has been associated with pathologic progression.[70,72] A recent study demonstrated high interreader reproducibility of different ADC calculations from serial MR imaging scans of 30 AS patients, as well as a correlation between ADC values and radiologic changes.[73] However, interscan variability including different magnets, vendors, and coils, as well as the differences in diffusion-weighted imaging pulse sequences used by vendors, b values, and patient factors (eg, the presence of artifacts), can all impact results, and ADC values should preferably be normalized, for example, to noncancerous tissue or urine in the bladder (**Fig. 11**).[73,74]

- Resource availability, cost-effectiveness, and contrast risks

Expert genitourinary radiologists, MR imaging scanners, and contrast are not always available. Although a cost-effectiveness analysis suggests that an MR imaging-guided PCa diagnostic pathway would result in fewer patients needing biopsies, it was shown to be only 86% cost-effective if applied to all low-risk cases.[75] Potential solutions to reduce the cost include same-day MR imaging,[76] where imaging and biopsy are performed in the same visit, or the use of biparametric MR imaging.[77] There is still debate over the need for the dynamic contrast-enhanced sequences, and the PI-RADS committee position is that "in men at persistent (higher) risk [...] under AS who are being evaluated for fast PSA doubling times or changing clinical or pathologic status, contrast-enhanced MR imaging is also preferred."[78] Different AS studies have compared the use of biparametric MR imaging and multiparametric MR imaging.[79–81] One study, assessing whether biparametric MR imaging missed suspicious lesions, re-examined 101 patients with multiparametric MR imaging following biparametric MR imaging[81] and found that 4% of the population had PCa ($\geq$GG2) initially missed; however, the difference was not significant ($P = .13$). A secondary analysis from the PROMIS study[3] has demonstrated that dynamic contrast-enhanced sequences do not improve accuracy over T2-weighted imaging and diffusion-weighted imaging in detecting clinically significant PCa (defined as Gleason score $\geq 4 + 3$ or a maximum length of $\geq$6 mm), with an MR imaging sensitivity of 95% and 94% and specificity of 38% and 37% with and without contrast, respectively ($P > .05$). Although these results suggest that biparametric MR imaging could simplify scanning and reduce health care costs, more evidence (in particular, level 1 evidence) is required,[82] and studies such as the PRIME trial[83,84] are attempting to answer this question in the detection setting. In addition, the minor risk of gadolinium deposits in the brain or toxicity from multiple scans may concern patients.[85,86]

Limitations of PRECISE

- Difficulties in assessing lesion growth

Although PRECISE aims to standardize scan interpretation and reporting, recommendations are qualitative and do not include standardized thresholds for changes in lesion size or conspicuity. Tumor size and volume are important prognostic factors in PCa; however, variations in the size of prostatic lesions can occur due to interobserver and intraobserver variability in the visual grading of lesions as well as interscan variability. In addition, there is also an expected or natural rate of tumor growth, which is rarely considered but is expected as part of the natural history of low-grade tumors on AS. These variations make it difficult to distinguish between fluctuations due to technical factors and true radiological progression during AS.

- Variability in measuring lesions

In its current form, PRECISE offers no suggestions on the most accurate measurement for monitoring lesion size across serial MR imaging. It allows for lesion volume to be reported using several methods including planimetry, the ellipsoid

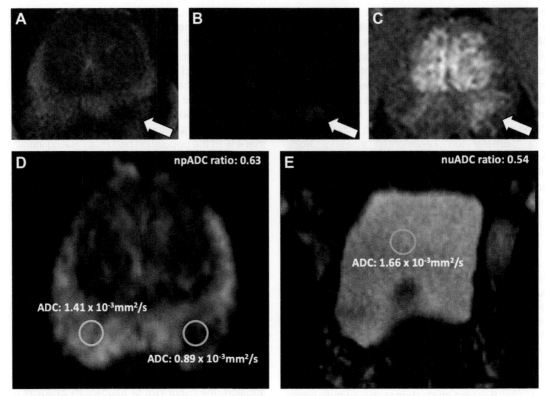

Fig. 11. Method for the normalization of apparent diffusion coefficient values. Multiparametric magnetic resonance imaging of a 71-year-old patient with biopsy-proven prostate cancer in the left peripheral zone between 4 and 5 o'clock. (*A*) T2-weighted, (*B*) diffusion-weighted, and (*C*) dynamic-contrast-enhanced imaging confirms the presence of the lesion (*arrows*). Three different regions of interest (of the same size and area) from the apparent diffusion coefficient map (*D–E*) were drawn on the lesion (orange circle) and normal prostatic tissue (blue circle) (*D*) and on the urine (green circle) in the bladder (*E*). These additional values were recorded and used to generate two parameters: the normalized prostatic ADC (npADC) and the normalized urinary ADC (nuADC) ratios, according to the formula: ADC (tumor)/ADC (reference).

formula, or with one or two diameters, which in turn permits inconsistencies and variability in reporting. We know that planimetry is the most accurate but time-consuming method. A recent study using a single, experienced genitourinary radiologist to report lesion volume for 196 AS patients found that the ellipsoid formula had the highest correlation with planimetry.[87] However, as acknowledged in PRECISE, a single diameter is likely to be the most reproducible one although no studies have been designed to confirm this. There is also debate about which sequence to measure the lesion on, and Le Nobin and colleagues[88] used RP samples to demonstrate that diffusion-weighted imaging may lead to tumor volumes being underestimated.

- Difficulties in assessing lesion conspicuity

Similarly, the current assessment of lesion conspicuity according to PRECISE is problematic. An increase or reduction in conspicuity will result in a change of PRECISE score. However, the visibility

of lesions is also affected by interobserver and interscan variability, as well as image quality, and certain conditions, as well as medications, can also have an impact. Lesion conspicuity is always assessed with reference to the prostate background, and in patients with prostatitis or benign prostatic hyperplasia, diffuse changes can make the delineation of tumor edges difficult.[89–92] Indeed, reporting background changes has been recommended to convey the potential for diagnostic uncertainty to clinicians.[93] In addition, the use of 5α-reductase inhibitors (eg, dutasteride) can impact lesion conspicuity. Using 40 patients randomized to dutasteride or placebo, the MAP-PED study[94] demonstrated that dutasteride can decrease the conspicuity on diffusion-weighted imaging but not necessarily on T2-weighted imaging (**Fig. 12**). Therefore, the size of a lesion could increase over time on T2-weighted imaging, but its conspicuity could decrease on diffusion-weighted imaging obfuscating the assessment of the PRECISE score for patients on 5α-reductase

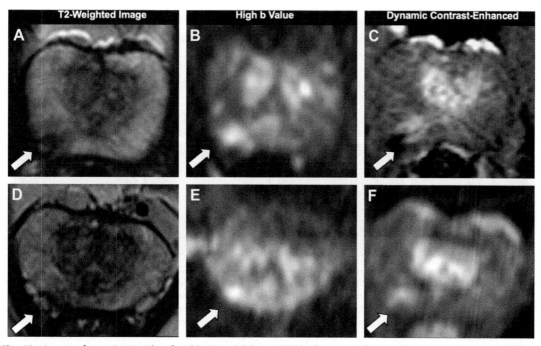

Fig. 12. A case of a patient with a focal lesion visible on MRI before and after starting a 5α-reductase inhibitor. (*A–C*) A 3T MR scan demonstrating a focal lesion (*arrow*) in the right peripheral zone between 7 and 8 o'clock extending toward the apex (Likert 4/5). The patient opted for AS and started daily dutasteride (0.5 mg) for 6 months as part of a trial. A 3 T MR scan after 6 months (*D–F*) shows that the lesion is less conspicuous and has reduced in size on the T2-weighted image (*D*), diffusion-weighted image (*E*), and dynamic contrast-enhanced (*F*) images.

inhibitors. This issue is particularly important for lesions in the peripheral zone, where diffusion-weighted imaging is the dominant sequence.

- Redundancy and points of confusion within the current scoring system

Presently, extremes in the PRECISE score are rarely reported. Caglic and colleagues[8] noted that the PRECISE scores of 1 and 5 were only assigned in 1.6% of their cohort of 295 AS patients. This effectively turns PRECISE into a three-point scoring system (ie, radiological improvement, stability, and progression). In addition, the overreporting of PRECISE 3 and PI-RADS 3 lesions by inexperienced radiologists to avoid missing clinically significant cancer may result in unnecessary biopsies and increased health care costs. There are also some areas of uncertainty within the current scoring system, for example, the growth of a lesion past the midline or appearance of a new lesion is classified as stage progression (eg, T2a to T2b or T2c), which, under the current system, is strictly defined as PRECISE 5 but, in practice, is often labeled as PRECISE 4. Moreover, the appearance of new lesions is not defined separately, and in practice,

these are often scored as PRECISE 4 (**Fig. 13**). However, this potentially leads to confusion if they are only PI-RADS 3 or possibly inflammatory "lesions" as well as if larger lesions on the same scan are stable or regress over time.

- Increased reporting time

Finally, reporting according to the PRECISE recommendations can be time-consuming in clinical practice, and this may be unfeasible given the increasing burden in prostate MR imaging reporting that radiologists face. One possible answer is to shorten the case report form, but this solution risks losing important clinical information. Technology and auto-populating template reports may also be a useful adjunct here and a study on a dedicated PRECISE software system, which provided a workflow to report step-by-step according to the recommendation, found a significant reduction in the reporting time at 6 months using the program.[95]

FUTURE DIRECTIONS

Moving forward, there is a need for better evidence on the use of MR imaging in AS to inform guidelines and clinical practice. Randomized

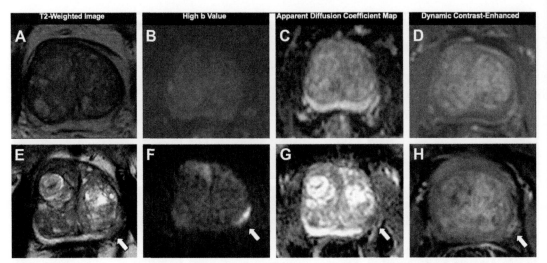

Fig. 13. A case of a new focal lesion appearing on magnetic resonance imaging. (*A–D*) A 1.5 T MR scan of a 62-year-old patient on active surveillance for invisible 1 mm Gleason 3 + 4 disease in the left posterior base (Likert 2/5). A subsequent 3T MR scan (*E–H*) demonstrates a 13 × 6 mm lesion (measured on the ADC map) in the left peripheral zone between 3 and 5 o'clock (*arrow*) (Likert 4/5). The PRECISE score was reported as 4 (ie, MR features suggesting disease progression), and a targeted biopsy of the lesion demonstrated 6 mm Gleason 3 + 4 disease.

controlled trials and multicenter studies are required to determine the threshold for radiological progression, appropriate intervals for MR imaging, and optimal triggers to start treatment before the widespread acceptance of fully MR imaging-based AS protocols. Our group at University College London are currently leading a multicenter validation of the PRECISE scoring system at an international level, and data will be available in the near future.

- Improvements in MR imaging acquisition

We must continue improving the diagnostic ability of MR imaging. Preliminary studies on 7T MR imaging have demonstrated higher spatial resolution than 1.5T and 3T[96] and can detect cancer in both the peripheral and transitional zones[97]; however, further research is required to determine its clinical utility.[9] We should also work to limit interscan variability by using standardized and optimized acquisition protocols, and anthropomorphic imaging phantoms may soon help to improve calibrating scanners.[98]

- Uniform standards for MR imaging reporting

Interreader variability could also be improved by teaching radiologists to report according to PRECISE. Studies have demonstrated a learning curve and that prognostic assessment of PCa is highly dependent on a radiologist's expertise. Indeed, higher rates of agreement have been found among expert reporters in prostate MR imaging, and teaching has been shown to improve performance.[99] A significant improvement in the accuracy of reporting and assessment of radiological change was demonstrated after 11 radiologists took part in a single dedicated teaching course on PRECISE.[100] Moreover, the widespread adoption of the PI-QUAL score (and its future iterations) for image quality should promote and standardize reporting of image-acquisition quality to ensure a basic standard has been met for all MR imaging scans.

- Adoption of artificial intelligence and radiomics

There is potential for artificial intelligence (AI) to assist in reporting serial prostate MR imaging. It may reduce the amount of time for evaluation of MR imaging scans and help less-experienced radiologists achieve similar PCa-detection performance to experts.[101] A recent systematic review revealed an average sensitivity of 84% and specificity of 61.5% for AI detecting PCa on MR imaging.[102] While Cacciamani and colleagues[103] pooled the results of five studies comparing the performance of radiologists and AI alone versus a combination of radiologists aided by a computer-aided diagnosis (CAD). The pooled sensitivity (89.1% vs 79.5%), specificity (78.1% vs 73.1%), and diagnostic odds ratio (29% vs 11%) were higher for the radiologists plus CAD than for radiologists alone. Deep learning AI systems, which use an algorithm to learn the underlying features of a given image and undergo a training process to provide a classification label as output, are also promising. Song and colleagues[104] used a deep-learning algorithm on 195 localized PCa patients and was able to detect PCa with a sensitivity of 87%, specificity of 90.6%, positive predictive value of 87%, and negative predictive value of 90.6%. However, further research is needed before AI tools can be adopted into clinical practice.

As an extension of AI, radiomics is a growing field where many MR imaging features are analyzed and used to predict histopathology and genetic signatures.[105] Hectors and colleagues found 14 radiomic features that correlated imaging with RP samples from 64 patients.[106] Sushentsev and colleagues developed a time series radiomics predictive model that analyzed longitudinal changes in tumor-derived radiomic features across 297 scans from 76 patients, combining time series radiomics and serial PSA density (area under the curve 0.86 [95% CI: 0.78–0.94]) that achieved comparable performance to expert-performed serial MR imaging analysis using the PRECISE scoring system (0.84 [0.76–0.93]).[107] Moreover, a recent systematic review found 57 articles on MR imaging radiomic features and concluded that there are good- to high-performance radiomics models for PCa detection and Gleason score discrimination.[108]

- An individualized risk-stratified approach to AS

A recent international consensus meeting identified developing a personalized risk-stratified approach as the most important priority in AS research.[109] Guidelines that recommend the same follow-up regime for all can result in overinvestigation and morbidity (ie, from repeat biopsy), and there is now a widely acknowledged need to risk-stratify AS follow-up events based on the evolution of a patient's disease characteristics and parameters rather than prespecified intervals. Following promising early outcomes, this approach is likely to continue evolving.

- Update and improve the PRECISE recommendations

Some limitations of the current PRECISE criteria should be addressed, and the recommendations should be updated. Standardizing the definitions of radiological progression, tumor volume measurement, and normal expected growth or fluctuations in the size of lesions should be a major focus of the next consensus meeting.

One suggestion could be to adopt a simplified three-point PRECISE score (where 1 = radiological improvement, 2 = radiological stability, and 3 = radiological progression) since studies have found higher interobserver reproducibility when reporting the absence or presence of radiological stability than the current PRECISE score.[54] Another aspect that should be addressed in the next iteration of PRECISE is the difference between visible and invisible PCa on mpMRI, as these are known to have different rates of progression during AS.[52] Finally, we encourage training courses and software to aid radiologists in adopting the updated recommendations.

In summary, the role of MR imaging in AS has recently been expanding. Studies suggest that it can improve the targeting accuracy of prostate biopsies, assist in the selection of eligible patients, and help to monitor PCa progression. The PRECISE recommendations standardize reporting of serial MR imaging scans for patients on AS, and their suggested case report form can be easily implemented into clinical practice. There is increasing evidence to support MR imaging-led AS, and the need for an individualized risk-stratified approach to AS has been identified. However, despite the promising results, there are some limitations to the current PRECISE criteria, which need to be addressed in a future update.

DISCLOSURE

All authors declare no conflict of interests and competing interests relevant to the article. C.E. is funded by the Brahm PhD Scholarship in memory of Chris Adams. T.B. acknowledges research support from the NIHR Cambridge Biomedical Research Centre (NIHR203312) and Cancer Research UK (Cambridge Imaging Centre grant number C197/A16465). C.M.M. is an NIHR research professor, and she also receives grant funding from Movember, Prostate Cancer UK, United Kingdom, Medical Research Council, United Kingdom, Cancer Research UK, United Kingdom, and the EAU Research Foundation, Netherlands. She has received proctor fees from Sonablate, study funding from SpectraCure, and speaker fees from Ipsen. F.G. is a recipient of the 2020 Young Investigator Award (20YOUN15) funded by the Prostate Cancer Foundation, United Kingdom/CRIS Cancer Foundation. F.G. reports consulting fees from Lucida Medical LTD outside of the submitted work.

CLINICS CARE POINTS

- MR imaging has become increasingly used to monitor disease progression for PCa patients on AS.

- In combination with blood markers and clinical factors, MR imaging may be used to determine the timing of follow-up biopsies for patients on AS.
- Adopting the PRECISE score and case report form help to standardize the reporting of serial MR imaging scans for patients on AS.
- The PRECISE recommendations encourage reporters to comment on changes in the size or conspicuity of prostate lesions across scans over time.
- Limitations with the current PRECISE criteria should be addressed in a future consensus meeting and the recommendations updated.

REFERENCES

1. NICE guideline for Prostate cancer: diagnosis and management. https://www.nice.org.uk/guidance/ng131/chapter/Recommendations#localised-and-locally-advanced-prostate-cancer. Accessed Feb 20, 2023.
2. Mottet N, van den Bergh RCN, Briers E, et al. EAU-EANM-ESTRO-ESUR-SIOG Guidelines on Prostate Cancer-2020 Update. Part 1: Screening, Diagnosis, and Local Treatment with Curative Intent. Eur Urol 2021;79(2):243–62.
3. Bosaily AE, Frangou E, Ahmed HU, et al. Additional Value of Dynamic Contrast-enhanced Sequences in Multiparametric Prostate Magnetic Resonance Imaging: Data from the PROMIS Study. Eur Urol 2020;78(4):503–11.
4. Kasivisvanathan V, Rannikko AS, Borghi M, et al. MRI-Targeted or Standard Biopsy for Prostate-Cancer Diagnosis. N Engl J Med 2018;378(19):1767–77.
5. Moore CM, Giganti F, Albertsen P, et al. Reporting Magnetic Resonance Imaging in Men on Active Surveillance for Prostate Cancer: The PRECISE Recommendations-A Report of a European School of Oncology Task Force. Eur Urol 2017;71(4):648–55.
6. Dieffenbacher S, Nyarangi-Dix J, Giganti F, et al. Standardized Magnetic Resonance Imaging Reporting Using the Prostate Cancer Radiological Estimation of Change in Sequential Evaluation Criteria and Magnetic Resonance Imaging/Transrectal Ultrasound Fusion with Transperineal Saturation Biopsy to Select Men on Active Surveillance. Eur Urol Focus 2021;7(1):102–10.
7. Giganti F, Stabile A, Stavrinides V, et al. Natural history of prostate cancer on active surveillance: stratification by MRI using the PRECISE recommendations in a UK cohort. Eur Radiol 2021;31(3):1644–55.
8. Caglic I, Sushentsev N, Gnanapragasam VJ, et al. MRI-derived PRECISE scores for predicting pathologically-confirmed radiological progression in prostate cancer patients on active surveillance. Eur Radiol 2021;31(5):2696–705.
9. O'Connor LP, Lebastchi AH, Horuz R, et al. Role of multiparametric prostate MRI in the management of prostate cancer. World J Urol 2021;39(3):651–9.
10. Ullrich T, Arsov C, Quentin M, et al. Multiparametric magnetic resonance imaging can exclude prostate cancer progression in patients on active surveillance: a retrospective cohort study. Eur Radiol 2020;30(11):6042–51.
11. Osses DF, Drost FH, Verbeek JFM, et al. Prostate cancer upgrading with serial prostate magnetic resonance imaging and repeat biopsy in men on active surveillance: are confirmatory biopsies still necessary? BJU Int 2020;126(1):124–32.
12. Cooperberg MR, Broering JM, Carroll PR. Time trends and local variation in primary treatment of localized prostate cancer. J Clin Oncol 2010;28(7):1117–23.
13. Hamdy FC, Donovan JL, Lane JA, et al. Fifteen-Year Outcomes after Monitoring, Surgery, or Radiotherapy for Prostate Cancer. N Engl J Med 2023;388(17):1547–58.
14. Choo R, Klotz L, Danjoux C, et al. Feasibility study: watchful waiting for localized low to intermediate grade prostate carcinoma with selective delayed intervention based on prostate specific antigen, histological and/or clinical progression. J Urol 2002;167(4):1664–9.
15. Klotz L. Active surveillance for low-risk prostate cancer. Curr Opin Urol 2017;27(3):225–30.
16. Tosoian JJ, Carter HB, Lepor A, et al. Active surveillance for prostate cancer: current evidence and contemporary state of practice. Nat Rev Urol 2016;13(4):205–15.
17. Loeb S, Folkvaljon Y, Curnyn C, et al. Uptake of Active Surveillance for Very-Low-Risk Prostate Cancer in Sweden. JAMA Oncol 2017;3(10):1393–8.
18. Timilshina N, Ouellet V, Alibhai SM, et al. Analysis of active surveillance uptake for low-risk localized prostate cancer in Canada: a Canadian multi-institutional study. World J Urol 2017;35(4):595–603.
19. Wilt TJ, Jones KM, Barry MJ, et al. Follow-up of Prostatectomy versus Observation for Early Prostate Cancer. N Engl J Med 2017;377(2):132–42.
20. Hamdy FC, Donovan JL, Lane JA, et al. 10-Year Outcomes after Monitoring, Surgery, or Radiotherapy for Localized Prostate Cancer. N Engl J Med 2016;375(15):1415–24.
21. Cooperberg MR, Cowan JE, Hilton JF, et al. Outcomes of active surveillance for men with intermediate-risk prostate cancer. J Clin Oncol 2011;29(2):228–34.

22. Klotz L, Vesprini D, Sethukavalan P, et al. Long-term follow-up of a large active surveillance cohort of patients with prostate cancer. J Clin Oncol 2015; 33(3):272–7.

23. Selvadurai ED, Singhera M, Thomas K, et al. Medium-term outcomes of active surveillance for localised prostate cancer. Eur Urol 2013;64(6): 981–7.

24. Lam TBL, MacLennan S, Willemse PM, et al. EAU-EANM-ESTRO-ESUR-SIOG Prostate Cancer Guideline Panel Consensus Statements for Deferred Treatment with Curative Intent for Localised Prostate Cancer from an International Collaborative Study (DETECTIVE Study). Eur Urol 2019;76(6): 790–813.

25. NCCN Guidelines Prostate Cancer. https://www. nccn.org/professionals/physician_gls/pdf/prostate. pdf. Accessed Feb 20, 2023. .

26. American Urological Association website: Clinically localised prostate cancer: AUA/ASTRO gudieline (2022). https://www.auanet.org/guidelines-and-quality/guidelines/clinically-localized-prostate-cancer-aua/astro-guideline-2022. Accessed Feb 20, 2023.

27. Bokhorst LP, Alberts AR, Rannikko A, et al. Compliance Rates with the Prostate Cancer Research International Active Surveillance (PRIAS) Protocol and Disease Reclassification in Noncompliers. Eur Urol 2015;68(5):814–21.

28. Welty CJ, Cowan JE, Nguyen H, et al. Extended followup and risk factors for disease reclassification in a large active surveillance cohort for localized prostate cancer. J Urol 2015;193(3):807–11.

29. Morash C, Tey R, Agbassi C, et al. Active surveillance for the management of localized prostate cancer: Guideline recommendations. Can Urol Assoc J 2015;9(5–6):171–8.

30. MpMRI for healthcare professionals. Prostate Cancer UK. https://prostatecanceruk.org/about-us/projects-and-policies/mpmri-for-healthcare-professionals. Accessed March 8, 2023.

31. Leake JL, Hardman R, Ojili V, et al. Prostate MRI: access to and current practice of prostate MRI in the United States. J Am Coll Radiol 2014;11(2): 156–60.

32. Fam MM, Yabes JG, Macleod LC, et al. Increasing Utilization of Multiparametric Magnetic Resonance Imaging in Prostate Cancer Active Surveillance. Urology 2019;130:99–105.

33. Quinn TP, Sanda MG, Howard DH, et al. Disparities in magnetic resonance imaging of the prostate for traditionally underserved patients with prostate cancer. Cancer 2021;127(16):2974–9.

34. Cole AP, Chen X, Langbein BJ, et al. Geographic Variability, Time Trends and Association of Preoperative Magnetic Resonance Imaging with Surgical Outcomes for Elderly United States Men with Prostate Cancer: A Surveillance, Epidemiology, and End Results-Medicare Analysis. J Urol 2022; 208(3):609–17.

35. Turkbey B, Rosenkrantz AB, Haider MA, et al. Prostate Imaging Reporting and Data System Version 2.1: 2019 Update of Prostate Imaging Reporting and Data System Version 2. Eur Urol 2019;76(3): 340–51.

36. Barentsz JO, Richenberg J, Clements R, et al. ESUR prostate MR guidelines 2012. Eur Radiol 2012;22(4):746–57.

37. Giganti F, Allen C, Emberton M, et al. Prostate Imaging Quality (PI-QUAL): A New Quality Control Scoring System for Multiparametric Magnetic Resonance Imaging of the Prostate from the PRECISION trial. Eur Urol Oncol 2020;3(5): 615–9.

38. Turkbey B, Mani H, Aras O, et al. Prostate cancer: can multiparametric MR imaging help identify patients who are candidates for active surveillance? Radiology 2013;268(1):144–52.

39. Baco E, Ukimura O, Rud E, et al. Magnetic resonance imaging-transectal ultrasound image-fusion biopsies accurately characterize the index tumor: correlation with step-sectioned radical prostatectomy specimens in 135 patients. Eur Urol 2015; 67(4):787–94.

40. Drost FH, Osses DF, Nieboer D, et al. Prostate MRI, with or without MRI-targeted biopsy, and systematic biopsy for detecting prostate cancer. Cochrane Database Syst Rev 2019;4(4):CD012663.

41. Rouviere O, Puech P, Renard-Penna R, et al. Use of prostate systematic and targeted biopsy on the basis of multiparametric MRI in biopsy-naive patients (MRI-FIRST): a prospective, multicentre, paired diagnostic study. Lancet Oncol 2019;20(1):100–9.

42. Stamatakis L, Siddiqui MM, Nix JW, et al. Accuracy of multiparametric magnetic resonance imaging in confirming eligibility for active surveillance for men with prostate cancer. Cancer 2013;119(18): 3359–66.

43. Marliere F, Puech P, Benkirane A, et al. The role of MRI-targeted and confirmatory biopsies for cancer upstaging at selection in patients considered for active surveillance for clinically low-risk prostate cancer. World J Urol 2014;32(4):951–8.

44. Guo R, Cai L, Fan Y, et al. Magnetic resonance imaging on disease reclassification among active surveillance candidates with low-risk prostate cancer: a diagnostic meta-analysis. Prostate Cancer Prostatic Dis 2015;18(3):221–8.

45. Bloom JB, Hale GR, Gold SA, et al. Predicting Gleason Group Progression for Men on Prostate Cancer Active Surveillance: Role of a Negative Confirmatory Magnetic Resonance Imaging-Ultrasound Fusion Biopsy. J Urol 2019;201(1): 84–90.

46. Klotz L, Loblaw A, Sugar L, et al. Active Surveillance Magnetic Resonance Imaging Study (ASIST): Results of a Randomized Multicenter Prospective Trial. Eur Urol 2019;75(2):300–9.

47. Klotz L, Pond G, Loblaw A, et al. Randomized Study of Systematic Biopsy Versus Magnetic Resonance Imaging and Targeted and Systematic Biopsy in Men on Active Surveillance (ASIST): 2-year Postbiopsy Follow-up. Eur Urol 2020;77(3):311–7.

48. Schoots IG, Nieboer D, Giganti F, et al. Is magnetic resonance imaging-targeted biopsy a useful addition to systematic confirmatory biopsy in men on active surveillance for low-risk prostate cancer? A systematic review and meta-analysis. BJU Int 2018;122(6):946–58.

49. Fujihara A, Iwata T, Shakir A, et al. Multiparametric magnetic resonance imaging facilitates reclassification during active surveillance for prostate cancer. BJU Int 2021;127(6):712–21.

50. Amin A, Scheltema MJ, Shnier R, et al. The Magnetic Resonance Imaging in Active Surveillance (MRIAS) Trial: Use of Baseline Multiparametric Magnetic Resonance Imaging and Saturation Biopsy to Reduce the Frequency of Surveillance Prostate Biopsies. J Urol 2020;203(5):910–7.

51. Shah S, Beckmann K, Van Hemelrijck M, et al. Guy's and St Thomas NHS Foundation active surveillance prostate cancer cohort: a characterisation of a prostate cancer active surveillance database. BMC Cancer 2021;21(1):573.

52. Stavrinides V, Giganti F, Trock B, et al. Five-year Outcomes of Magnetic Resonance Imaging-based Active Surveillance for Prostate Cancer: A Large Cohort Study. Eur Urol 2020;78(3):443–51.

53. Schoots IG, Petrides N, Giganti F, et al. Magnetic resonance imaging in active surveillance of prostate cancer: a systematic review. Eur Urol 2015;67(4):627–36.

54. Giganti F, Pecoraro M, Stavrinides V, et al. Interobserver reproducibility of the PRECISE scoring system for prostate MRI on active surveillance: results from a two-centre pilot study. Eur Radiol 2020;30(4):2082–90.

55. Turkbey B, Fotin SV, Huang RJ, et al. Fully automated prostate segmentation on MRI: comparison with manual segmentation methods and specimen volumes. AJR Am J Roentgenol 2013;201(5):W720–9.

56. Latifoltojar A, Appayya MB, Barrett T, et al. Similarities and differences between Likert and PIRADS v2.1 scores of prostate multiparametric MRI: a pictorial review of histology-validated cases. Clin Radiol 2019;74(11):895 e891–e895 e815.

57. Rajwa P, Pradere B, Quhal F, et al. Reliability of Serial Prostate Magnetic Resonance Imaging to Detect Prostate Cancer Progression During Active Surveillance: A Systematic Review and Meta-analysis. Eur Urol 2021;80(5):549–63.

58. Hettiarachchi D, Geraghty R, Rice P, et al. Can the Use of Serial Multiparametric Magnetic Resonance Imaging During Active Surveillance of Prostate Cancer Avoid the Need for Prostate Biopsies?-A Systematic Diagnostic Test Accuracy Review. Eur Urol Oncol 2021;4(3):426–36.

59. Chu CE, Cowan JE, Lonergan PE, et al. Diagnostic Accuracy and Prognostic Value of Serial Prostate Multiparametric Magnetic Resonance Imaging in Men on Active Surveillance for Prostate Cancer. Eur Urol Oncol 2022;5(5):537–43.

60. Chamorro Castillo L, Garcia Morales L, Ruiz Lopez D, et al. The role of multiparametric magnetic resonance in active surveillance of a low-risk prostate cancer cohort from clinical practice. Prostate 2023;83(8):765–72.

61. Thankapannair V, Keates A, Barrett T, et al. Prospective Implementation and Early Outcomes of a Risk-stratified Prostate Cancer Active Surveillance Follow-up Protocol. European Urology Open Science 2023;49:15–22.

62. Sanmugalingam N, Sushentsev N, Lee KL, et al. The PRECISE Recommendations for Prostate MRI in Patients on Active Surveillance for Prostate Cancer: A Critical Review. AJR Am J Roentgenol 2023. https://doi.org/10.2214/AJR.23.29518.

63. Park KJ, Choi SH, Kim MH, et al. Performance of Prostate Imaging Reporting and Data System Version 2.1 for Diagnosis of Prostate Cancer: A Systematic Review and Meta-Analysis. J Magn Reson Imag 2021;54(1):103–12.

64. Westphalen AC, McCulloch CE, Anaokar JM, et al. Variability of the Positive Predictive Value of PI-RADS for Prostate MRI across 26 Centers: Experience of the Society of Abdominal Radiology Prostate Cancer Disease-focused Panel. Radiology 2020;296(1):76–84.

65. Stavrinides V, Giganti F, Emberton M, et al. MRI in active surveillance: a critical review. Prostate Cancer Prostatic Dis 2019;22(1):5–15.

66. Sathianathen NJ, Omer A, Harriss E, et al. Negative Predictive Value of Multiparametric Magnetic Resonance Imaging in the Detection of Clinically Significant Prostate Cancer in the Prostate Imaging Reporting and Data System Era: A Systematic Review and Meta-analysis. Eur Urol 2020;78(3):402–14.

67. Light A, Lophatananon A, Keates A, et al. Development and External Validation of the STRATified CANcer Surveillance (STRATCANS) Multivariable Model for Predicting Progression in Men with Newly Diagnosed Prostate Cancer Starting Active Surveillance. J Clin Med 2022;12(1).

68. Rais-Bahrami S, Turkbey B, Rastinehad AR, et al. Natural history of small index lesions suspicious

for prostate cancer on multiparametric MRI: recommendations for interval imaging follow-up. Diagn Interv Radiol 2014;20(4):293–8.

69. Giganti F, Moore CM, Punwani S, et al. The natural history of prostate cancer on MRI: lessons from an active surveillance cohort. Prostate Cancer Prostatic Dis 2018;21(4):556–63.

70. Morgan VA, Parker C, MacDonald A, et al. Monitoring Tumor Volume in Patients With Prostate Cancer Undergoing Active Surveillance: Is MRI Apparent Diffusion Coefficient Indicative of Tumor Growth? AJR Am J Roentgenol 2017;209(3): 620–8.

71. Henderson DR, de Souza NM, Thomas K, et al. Nine-year Follow-up for a Study of Diffusion-weighted Magnetic Resonance Imaging in a Prospective Prostate Cancer Active Surveillance Cohort. Eur Urol 2016;69(6):1028–33.

72. Morgan VA, Riches SF, Thomas K, et al. Diffusion-weighted magnetic resonance imaging for monitoring prostate cancer progression in patients managed by active surveillance. Br J Radiol 2011;84(997):31–7.

73. Giganti F, Pecoraro M, Fierro D, et al. DWI and PRECISE criteria in men on active surveillance for prostate cancer: A multicentre preliminary experience of different ADC calculations. Magn Reson Imaging 2020;67:50–8.

74. Barrett T, Priest AN, Lawrence EM, et al. Ratio of Tumor to Normal Prostate Tissue Apparent Diffusion Coefficient as a Method for Quantifying DWI of the Prostate. AJR Am J Roentgenol 2015; 205(6):W585–93.

75. Gordon LG, James R, Tuffaha HW, et al. Cost-effectiveness analysis of multiparametric MRI with increased active surveillance for low-risk prostate cancer in Australia. J Magn Reson Imag 2017; 45(5):1304–15.

76. Tafuri A, Ashrafl AN, Palmer S, et al. One-Stop MRI and MRI/transrectal ultrasound fusion-guided biopsy: an expedited pathway for prostate cancer diagnosis. World J Urol 2020;38(4):949–56.

77. van der Leest M, Israel B, Cornel EB, et al. High Diagnostic Performance of Short Magnetic Resonance Imaging Protocols for Prostate Cancer Detection in Biopsy-naive Men: The Next Step in Magnetic Resonance Imaging Accessibility. Eur Urol 2019;76(5):574–81.

78. Schoots IG, Barentsz JO, Bittencourt LK, et al. PI-RADS Committee Position on MRI Without Contrast Medium in Biopsy-Naive Men With Suspected Prostate Cancer: Narrative Review. AJR Am J Roentgenol 2021;216(1):3–19.

79. Becker AS, Kirchner J, Sartoretti T, et al. Interactive, Up-to-date Meta-Analysis of MRI in the Management of Men with Suspected Prostate Cancer. J Digit Imag 2020;33(3):586–94.

80. Woo S, Suh CH, Kim SY, et al. Head-to-Head Comparison Between Biparametric and Multiparametric MRI for the Diagnosis of Prostate Cancer: A Systematic Review and Meta-Analysis. AJR Am J Roentgenol 2018;211(5):W226–41.

81. Thestrup KD, Logager V, Boesen L, et al. Comparison of bi- and multiparametric magnetic resonance imaging to select men for active surveillance. Acta Radiol Open 2019;8(8). 2058460119866352.

82. Giganti F, Kirkham A, Allen C, et al. Update on Multiparametric Prostate MRI During Active Surveillance: Current and Future Trends and Role of the PRECISE Recommendations. AJR Am J Roentgenol 2021;216(4):943–51.

83. Ng A, Khetrapal P, Kasivisvanathan V. Is It PRIME Time for Biparametric Magnetic Resonance Imaging in Prostate Cancer Diagnosis? Eur Urol 2022; 82(1):1–2.

84. Asif A, Nathan A, Ng A, et al. Comparing biparametric to multiparametric MRI in the diagnosis of clinically significant prostate cancer in biopsy-naive men (PRIME): a prospective, international, multicentre, non-inferiority within-patient, diagnostic yield trial protocol. BMJ Open 2023;13(4): e070280.

85. Fraum TJ, Ludwig DR, Bashir MR, et al. Gadolinium-based contrast agents: A comprehensive risk assessment. J Magn Reson Imag 2017;46(2): 338–53.

86. Ramalho J, Ramalho M. Gadolinium Deposition and Chronic Toxicity. Magn Reson Imag Clin N Am 2017;25(4):765–78.

87. Giganti F, Stavrinides V, Stabile A, et al. Prostate cancer measurements on serial MRI during active surveillance: it's time to be PRECISE. Br J Radiol 2020;93(1116):20200819.

88. Le Nobin J, Orczyk C, Deng FM, et al. Prostate tumour volumes: evaluation of the agreement between magnetic resonance imaging and histology using novel co-registration software. BJU Int 2014;114(6b):E105–12.

89. Eineluoto JT, Jarvinen P, Kenttamies A, et al. Repeat multiparametric MRI in prostate cancer patients on active surveillance. PLoS One 2017; 12(12):e0189272.

90. Walton Diaz A, Shakir NA, George AK, et al. Use of serial multiparametric magnetic resonance imaging in the management of patients with prostate cancer on active surveillance. Urol Oncol 2015; 33(5):202 e201–7.

91. Hotker AM, Njoh S, Hofer LJ, et al. Multi-reader evaluation of different image quality scoring systems in prostate MRI. Eur J Radiol 2023;161: 110733.

92. Hotker AM, Dappa E, Mazaheri Y, et al. The Influence of Background Signal Intensity Changes on

92   Englman et al

Cancer Detection in Prostate MRI. AJR Am J Roentgenol 2019;212(4):823–9.

93. Bura V, Caglic I, Snoj Z, et al. MRI features of the normal prostatic peripheral zone: the relationship between age and signal heterogeneity on T2WI, DWI, and DCE sequences. Eur Radiol 2021;31(7):4908–17.

94. Giganti F, Moore CM, Robertson NL, et al. MRI findings in men on active surveillance for prostate cancer: does dutasteride make MRI visible lesions less conspicuous? Results from a placebo-controlled, randomised clinical trial. Eur Radiol 2017;27(11):4767–74.

95. Giganti F, Allen C, Piper JW, et al. Sequential prostate MRI reporting in men on active surveillance: initial experience of a dedicated PRECISE software program. Magn Reson Imaging 2019;57:34–9.

96. Laader A, Beiderwellen K, Kraff O, et al. 1.5 versus 3 versus 7 Tesla in abdominal MRI: A comparative study. PLoS One 2017;12(11):e0187528.

97. Vos EK, Lagemaat MW, Barentsz JO, et al. Image quality and cancer visibility of T2-weighted magnetic resonance imaging of the prostate at 7 Tesla. Eur Radiol 2014;24(8):1950–8.

98. Bauer DF, Adlung A, Brumer I, et al. An anthropomorphic pelvis phantom for MR-guided prostate interventions. Magn Reson Med 2022;87(3):1605–12.

99. Brembilla G, Dell'Oglio P, Stabile A, et al. Interreader variability in prostate MRI reporting using Prostate Imaging Reporting and Data System version 2.1. Eur Radiol 2020;30(6):3383–92.

100. Giganti F, Aupin L, Thoumin C, et al. Promoting the use of the PRECISE score for prostate MRI during active surveillance: results from the ESOR Nicholas Gourtsoyiannis teaching fellowship. Insights Imaging 2022;13(1):111.

101. Giganti F, Panebianco V, Tempany CM, et al. Is Artificial Intelligence Replacing Our Radiology Stars in Prostate Magnetic Resonance Imaging? The Stars Do Not Look Big, But They Can Look Brighter. Eur Urol Open Sci 2023;48:12–3.

102. Syer T, Mehta P, Antonelli M, et al. Artificial Intelligence Compared to Radiologists for the Initial Diagnosis of Prostate Cancer on Magnetic Resonance Imaging: A Systematic Review and Recommendations for Future Studies. Cancers 2021;13(13).

103. Cacciamani GE, Sanford DI, Chu TN, et al. Is Artificial Intelligence Replacing Our Radiology Stars? Not Yet. Eur Urol Open Sci 2023;48:14–6.

104. Song Y, Zhang YD, Yan X, et al. Computer-aided diagnosis of prostate cancer using a deep convolutional neural network from multiparametric MRI. J Magn Reson Imag 2018;48(6):1570–7.

105. Sushentsev N, Rundo L, Blyuss O, et al. MRI-derived radiomics model for baseline prediction of prostate cancer progression on active surveillance. Sci Rep 2021;11(1):12917.

106. Hectors SJ, Cherny M, Yadav KK, et al. Radiomics Features Measured with Multiparametric Magnetic Resonance Imaging Predict Prostate Cancer Aggressiveness. J Urol 2019;202(3):498–505.

107. Sushentsev N, Rundo L, Abrego L, et al. Time series radiomics for the prediction of prostate cancer progression in patients on active surveillance. Eur Radiol 2023;33(6):3792–800.

108. Spohn SKB, Bettermann AS, Bamberg F, et al. Radiomics in prostate cancer imaging for a personalized treatment approach - current aspects of methodology and a systematic review on validated studies. Theranostics 2021;11(16):8027–42.

109. Moore CM, King LE, Withington J, et al. Best Current Practice and Research Priorities in Active Surveillance for Prostate Cancer-A Report of a Movember International Consensus Meeting. Eur Urol Oncol 2023;6(2):160–82.

Prostate Cancer Local Staging with Magnetic Resonance Imaging

Yue Lin, AB[a], Latrice A. Johnson, BS[a], Fiona M. Fennessy, MD, PhD[b],
Baris Turkbey, MD[a],*

KEYWORDS

- Prostatic neoplasms • Magnetic resonance imaging • Diagnostic imaging

KEY POINTS

- Multiparametric MRI (mpMRI) has become the preferred imaging modality for the local staging of prostate cancer and has been shown to provide additional information on the site and extent of disease compared to traditional clinical nomograms.
- The Prostate Imaging Reporting and Data System (PI-RADS) standardizes prostate mpMRI acquisition, interpretation, and reporting. It is used to characterize and assess focal intraprostatic lesions seen on mpMRI based on the probability of clinically significant cancer in treatment-naïve man.
- While mpMRI assessment of extra-prostatic extension and seminal vesicle invasion demonstrates moderate sensitivity and positive predictive value, it exhibits high specificity and negative predictive value. Utilizing standardized systematic evaluation methods can further enhance the accuracy of evaluating both extra-prostatic extension and seminal vesicle invasion.
- Utilizing mpMRI for surgical planning can help mitigate unfavorable surgical outcomes by identifying large index lesions that are often associated with positive surgical margins.

INTRODUCTION

Worldwide, prostate cancer is the most commonly diagnosed malignancy and the fifth leading cause of cancer death among men.[1] In the United States, it is the second leading cause of cancer deaths in men, in which African American men suffer from the highest incidence and mortality rates.[2] With prostate cancer affecting such a large majority of the male population, assessing the presence and extent of clinically significant prostate cancer and characterizing the risk of future progression is a priority. Over- or under-treatment can be avoided by accurately distinguishing low-versus high-risk cases and tailoring treatment accordingly.

Magnetic resonance imaging (MRI) has become increasingly used in detecting clinically significant prostate cancers and can facilitate the triage of patients for biopsy.[3] Additionally, MRI provides valuable information for staging tumor extent and monitoring treatment response.[4] Prostate MRI can aid in staging evaluation by verifying organ-confined status and establishing the location and extent of the tumor in patients being considered for radiation therapy or surgery.[5] It is often used for surgical planning, especially for defining presence of tumor in the neurovascular bundle and determining the need for nerve removal. While the practice of verifying organ-confined disease status with prostate MRI prior to nerve-sparing radical prostatectomy is well-supported by evidence,[6,7] it has yet to be fully integrated into major practice guidelines. According to the American College of Radiology (ACR) appropriateness criteria, prostate

[a] Molecular Imaging Branch, National Cancer Institute, National Institutes of Health, 10 Center Drive, MSC 1182, Building 10, Room B3B85, Bethesda, MD 20892, USA; [b] Department of Radiology, Brigham and Women's Hospital, Harvard Medical School, 75 Francis Street, Boston, MA 02115, USA
* Corresponding author. Molecular Imaging Branch, National Cancer Institute, National Institutes of Health, 10 Center Drive, MSC 1182, Building 10, Room B3B85, Bethesda, MD 20892.
E-mail address: turkbeyi@mail.nih.gov

Radiol Clin N Am 62 (2024) 93–108
https://doi.org/10.1016/j.rcl.2023.06.010
0033-8389/24/Published by Elsevier Inc.

MRI is recommended for all intermediate- and high-risk patients to assist in treatment planning.[8] Meanwhile, the updated guidelines from the European Association of Urology/European Association of Nuclear Medicine/European Society for Radiotherapy and Oncology/European Society of Urogenital Radiology/International Society of Geriatric Oncology (EAU-EANM-ESTRO-ESUR-SIOG) suggest prebiopsy prostate MRI for local staging for any risk group.[9] Given there is currently no consensus on how MRI should be deployed in clinical practice, in this review, we will describe the current data in the staging of local prostate cancer using MRI, specifically in the evaluation of extraprostatic extension (EPE), seminal vesicle invasion (SVI), and positive surgical margin (PSM).

MANAGEMENT OF LOCALLY ADVANCED PROSTATE CANCER

Patients with locally advanced prostate cancer and with high-risk features are advised to undergo definitive local therapy. Treatments for these patients typically includes external beam radiotherapy combined with long-term androgen deprivation therapy (ADT).[9,10] External beam radiotherapy combined with ADT provides patients with better survival outcomes compared to ADT alone and external beam radiotherapy alone.[10] Androgen deprivation therapy can be administered neoadjuvant, concurrently, or adjuvant when combined with radiation therapy.[11] For a subset of patients (such as being clinically node positive, having 2 out of 3 of the following criteria: clinical stage T3 or T4, PSA level of ≥40 ng/mL, or a Gleason score of ≥8), radiation and androgen deprivation therapy, along with a 2-year course of concurrent abiraterone acetate and prednisone may be recommended as well.[11,12] However, there are toxicities associated with long term continuous ADT, such as hot flashes, insomnia, and decreased libido.[13] For individuals at a very high risk, particularly those who are younger, radical prostatectomy in conjunction with extended pelvic lymph node dissection is another treatment option due to favorable cancer survival rates.[9] Studies indicate 5-year prostate-specific antigen (PSA) relapse–free survival rates ranging from 55% to 71% and 10-year prostate cancer-specific survival rates from 72% to 92%.[14–17] However, the most effective treatment for these patients is still currently being actively studied, and previous meta-analyses have reported inconsistent results regarding survival rates for different treatment options.[18,19] Nonetheless, it is important to note that the identification of EPE or SVI on MRI may lead to a discussion regarding the impact of T3 disease on pathology, the potential requirement for

adjuvant therapies, and possible consideration of nerve sparing of the ipsilateral bundle. Accurate local staging is, therefore, essential in deciding the optimal treatment strategy and prognosing patient outcomes.

THE PROSTATE IMAGING REPORTING AND DATA SYSTEM

The implementation of the Prostate Imaging Reporting and Data System (PI-RADS) has significantly enhanced the consistency and standardization of prostate cancer reporting.[20] PI-RADS is used to characterize and assess all focal intraprostatic lesions seen on multiparametric MRI (mpMRI). It offers a set of criteria to evaluate the likelihood that a lesion detected through mpMRI indicates clinically significant cancer. The guideline also includes technical standards for scanning hardware and protocols for image acquisition. To obtain the best images and results, PI-RADS guideline recommended acquiring images using 3 T scanners over 1.5 T. The use of an endorectal coil is optional but may be considered for better image quality. In addition to T2WI, obtained in the straight or oblique axial plane and at least one additional orthogonal plane, high-b-value DWI and DCE MRI should be routinely included in image acquisition protocols.

PI-RADS classifies prostate lesions on a five-point scale based on the probability of clinically significant cancer (**Fig. 1**). The primary sequence recommended for determining the category of the peripheral zone lesions is DWI (**Fig. 2**), while

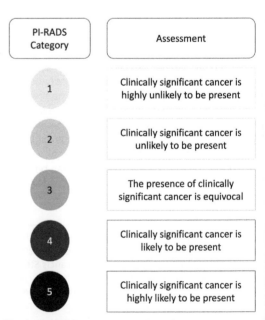

PI-RADS Category	Assessment
1	Clinically significant cancer is highly unlikely to be present
2	Clinically significant cancer is unlikely to be present
3	The presence of clinically significant cancer is equivocal
4	Clinically significant cancer is likely to be present
5	Clinically significant cancer is highly likely to be present

Fig. 1. PI-RADS assessment categories.

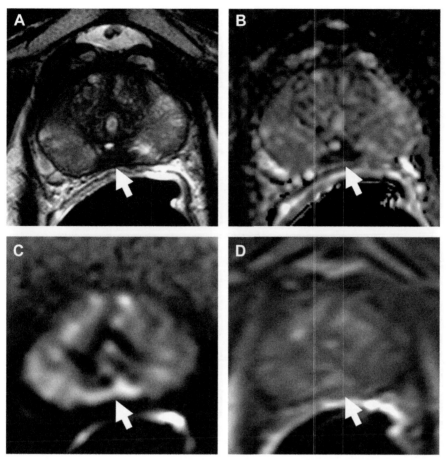

Fig. 2. Multiparametric MRI of a 74-year-old man with a serum prostate specific antigen level of 8.1 ng/mL. The lesion (*arrows*) was 1.3 cm in the midline apical-mid peripheral zone and assigned PI-RADS category 4. Targeted biopsy revealed Gleason score 7 (4 + 3) prostate adenocarcinoma. T2-weighted imaging (*A*), apparent diffusion coefficient map (*B*), high b-value (b = 1500 s/mm^2) diffusion-weighted imaging (*C*), and dynamic contrast enhanced imaging (*D*).

for transition zone lesions, T2WI is used (**Fig. 3**). In general, clinically significant cancer can be defined as a lesion that is predicted to have an International Society of Urologic Pathology (ISUP) Grade Group of 2 or higher, with either a volume ≥ 0.5 mL or EPE. Studies have found the cancer detection rates for PI-RADSv2 may be variable and category 3, 4, and 5 assessments in detecting clinically significant prostate cancer range from 12% to 23%, 39% to 60%, and 72% to 83%, respectively.[3,21,22] The differences in cancer detection rates may be due to intra- and inter-reader variability related to reader experiences and subjectivity.[23–25] However, some studies have shown the negative predictive value of PI-RADSv1 and v2 in detecting clinically significant cancer range from 86% to 91%.[26,27] Therefore, mpMRI of the prostate is generally an accurate test for ruling out clinically significant prostate cancer. PI-RADSv2.1 was refined and introduced in

2019. One meta-analysis with 11 studies showed the clinically significant cancer detection rates for PI-RADSv2.1 category 3, 4, and 5 assessment range from 13% to 27%, 43% to 61%, and 76% to 97%, respectively.[28] Its true detection performance is still under investigation, and large prospective studies are needed.[29] Radiologists should be aware of the inherent limitations of PI-RADS guidelines, specifically regarding the inconsistency in the published literature on the importance of a PI-RADS 3 lesion and the necessity of biopsies for all PI-RADS 3 lesions.[3,30]

EVALUATION OF EXTRA-PROSTATIC EXTENSION

For patients with prostate cancer, it is crucial to undergo a comprehensive risk assessment and staging process to ensure that they receive the best possible counseling and treatment. The American

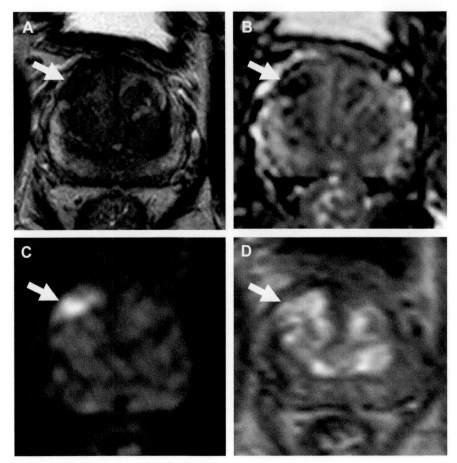

Fig. 3. Multiparametric MRI of a 62-year-old man with a serum prostate specific antigen level of 14.7 ng/mL. The lesion (*arrows*) was 1.5 cm in the right base anterior transition zone and assigned PI-RADS category 5. Targeted biopsy revealed Gleason score 7 (3 + 4) prostate adenocarcinoma. T2-weighted imaging (*A*), apparent diffusion coefficient map (*B*), high b-value (b = 1500 s/mm^2) diffusion-weighted imaging (*C*), and dynamic contrast enhanced imaging (*D*).

Joint Committee of Cancer (AJCC) tumor-node-metastasis (TNM) system, last revised in 2018, is the most commonly employed staging system for prostate cancer[31] (**Table 1**). Prostate cancer with EPE are staged as T3a according to the TNM staging system. The presence of EPE is associated with a higher risk of PSM, biochemical recurrence, metastatic disease, and lower survival rate after undergoing radical prostatectomy.[32,33]

On MRI scans, the prostatic capsule is mainly evaluated on axial T2W MRI since it has a higher spatial resolution compared to DWI and DCE images. The capsule appears as a hypointense rim surrounding the prostate gland (**Fig. 4**). It is best visible in the middle 70% to 80% of the prostate gland craniocaudally, whereas at the apex and base (ie, the inferior and superior-most portions of the gland), it is often difficult to visualize. EPE can generally be defined as the bulging of the capsule, irregular or ill-defined capsular surface,

thickened neurovascular bundle, or visible invasion of the surrounding structures (ie, bladder neck and rectal wall)[34] (**Fig. 5**). Pesapane and colleagues[35] suggested that MRI staging criteria of EPE can be based on the concept of a linear, stepwise progression of cancer growth. This concept allowed the researchers to define certain characteristics of EPE into stages of "early" and "late." The "early" stages include: disruption of the capsule, bulging of the contour that surrounds the prostate, and then eventually an irregular prostate margin. In the early stages, as the cancerous cells spread into the capsule, they disrupt the normal signal typically seen on the MRI. As tumor cells continue to grow beyond the capsule and beyond the smooth muscle of the prostate, it reflects on the MRI as an extension or "bulging" of the margin of the prostate contour. The "late" stages seen on T2WI include: a rise and fall of the contour surrounding the prostate, obliteration

Table 1
American Joint Committee on Cancer (AJCC) tumor-node-metastasis (TNM) Staging Manual

Primary Tumor (T)	
Clinical T (cT)	**cT Criteria**
T0	No evidence of primary tumor
T1	Clinically inapparent tumor not palpable
T1a	Incidental tumor in < 5% of tissue resected
T1b	Incidental tumor in > 5% of tissue resected
T1c	Tumor identified by needle biopsy found in one or both sides, but not palpable
T2	Tumor is palpable and confined within prostate
T2a	Tumor involves one-half of one side or less
T2b	Tumor involves more than one-half of one side but not both sides
T2c	Tumor involves both sides
T3	Extra-prostatic tumor that is not fixed or does not invade adjacent structures
T3a	Extra-prostatic extension (unilateral or bilateral)
T3b	Tumor invades seminal vesicle(s)
T4	Tumor invades external sphincter, rectum, bladder, levator muscles, and/or pelvic side wall
Tx	Primary tumor cannot be assessed
Pathologic T (pT)	**pT Criteria**
T2	Organ-confined
T3	Extra-prostatic extension
T3a	Extra-prostatic extension (unilateral or bilateral) or microscopic invasion of bladder neck
T3b	Tumor invades seminal vesicle(s)
T4	Tumor invades external sphincter, rectum, bladder, levator muscles, and/or pelvic side wall
Lymph Nodes (N)	**N Criteria**
N0	No positive regional lymph nodes
N1	Regional node metastases – including pelvic, hypogastric, obturator, iliac, and/or sacral
Nx	Regional nodes were not assessed
Distant Metastases (M)	**M Criteria**
M0	No distant metastasis
M1	Distant metastasis
M1a	Non-regional lymph nodes (outside true pelvis)
M1b	Bone(s)
M1c	Other site(s) with or without bone disease

of fat surrounding the prostate, and an obliteration of the angle between the rectum and the prostate. As the cancerous cells continue to grow, they extend past the prostate capsule, into the surrounding fat, and into the rectoprostatic angle. In the final stage of EPE, an overt macroscopic periprostatic mass is present.

At histopathology, EPE in prostate cancer denotes the spread of tumor cells beyond the fibromuscular pseudocapsule of the prostate gland and into the adjacent periprostatic soft tissues, such as the periprostatic fat.[36] A common criteria used to determine the extent of EPE was introduced by Epstein and colleagues[37] who

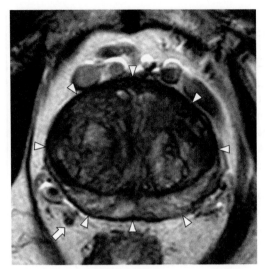

Fig. 4. Axial T2W MRI demonstrating mid prostate gland with prostatic capsule and neurovascular bundle. The prostatic capsule (*arrowheads*) appears as a hypointense rim surrounding the prostate gland. The neurovascular bundle (*arrow*) is a tubular structure located posterolateral to the prostatic capsule and adjacent to the peripheral zone. It mediates erectile function and continence. It is an expansion of the pelvic hypogastric plexus that contains the cavernous nerves of the penis and prostatic branches of the inferior vesical artery and prostatic veins.

characterized the extension as focal or established. Focal EPE extension was classified as a few cancerous glands outside of the protstate. Whereas established (or extensive) EPE was classified as cancerous cells present in more than a few glands.

This clarification in focal versus extensive EPE is important because extensive EPE is believed to be more frequently associated with PSM compared

to focal EPE.[38] The most understood mechanism of how these tumors cells extend from the parenchyma to the soft tissue is via perineural invasion. This mechanism is consistent with the fact that EPE is most often found at the posterolateral areas of the prostate.[39] There is very little capsule present in the base and apex of the prostate, so at these anatomic locations EPE is diagnosed when the cancer extended into the periprostatic fatty tissue.[34]

In cases where patients opt for surgery, the preoperative assessment of the location of pathologic EPE is crucial in determining the surgical approach to be taken. A wider excision with the removal of neurovascular bundles may be attempted to increase the likelihood of a negative margin.[40] However, while this more aggressive approach improves cancer control, it results in higher rates of urinary incontinence and erectile dysfunction.[41] It is important to closely examine the apex of the prostate. If cancer affects the external urethral sphincter, there is a risk during surgery of damaging the sphincter, which could lead to urinary continence. Additionally, the presence of a tumor in this area may impact the use of radiation therapy. Therefore, it is essential to have accurate assessment of pathologic EPE before treatment to optimize clinical decision-making and minimize the risk of side effects. Because EPE is difficult to determine intraoperatively, the diagnosis must be made preoperatively. This risk is traditionally assessed using nomograms, such as the Partin tables[42] or the Memorial Sloan Kettering Cancer Center [MSKCC] nomogram,[43] which consider clinical variables such as PSA levels, digital rectal exam, and Gleason score at biopsy. However, these traditional methods do not incorporate imaging modalities and have been found to be less effective than MRI in identifying the location and extent of EPE.[44,45] As a result, MRI can potentially

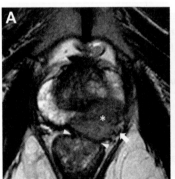
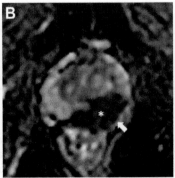
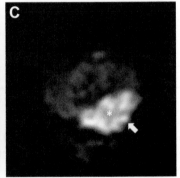

Fig. 5. MRI of a 67-year-old man with a serum prostate specific antigen level of 72.7 ng/mL. PI-RADS category 5 lesion (*asterisk*) in the left apical-mid peripheral zone with frank extra-prostatic extension (*arrows*) and possible rectal wall involvement (*arrowheads*). T2-weighted imaging (*A*), apparent diffusion coefficient map (*B*), and high b-value (b = 1500 s/mm^2) diffusion-weighted imaging (*C*).

improve the accuracy of EPE localization and help physicians and patients make more informed decisions regarding treatment options.

Standardized magnetic resonance imaging-based extra-prostatic extension evaluation

The PI-RADS guideline provides a brief overview of what radiologists should evaluate on mpMRI for EPE. The guideline suggests assessing features such as asymmetry or invasion of the neurovascular bundles, bulging prostatic contour, irregular or spiculated margin, obliteration of the rectoprostatic angle, tumor-capsule interface greater than 10 mm, breach of the capsule with evidence of direct tumor extension or bladder wall invasion.[20] However, there is little guidance on the utility or importance of these findings. Studies have evaluated the performance of the PI-RADS for detecting EPE and have found moderate sensitivity (ranging from 40% to 88%) and specificity (ranging from 75% to 83%).[46–49] One meta-analysis with 45 studies demonstrated a sensitivity of 61% and a specificity of 88% for MRI in detecting EPE.[50] In other words, the current data suggest that MRI has a high specificity but low sensitivity for EPE evaluation. Of note, one study found that PI-RADS categories 3 or less assessment could confidently rule out the presence of EPE irrespective of clinical risk group, with an overall sensitivity of 99% and negative predictive value of 98%.[51] The variations in the detection metrics are likely due to the lack of standardized EPE criteria from the PI-RADS guideline and the difference in readers experiences, with one study showing moderate inter-reader agreement ($\kappa = 0.45$).[46]

To address some of the shortcoming of PI-RADS on predicting EPE, few groups have reported use of systematic EPE evaluation methods.[52,53] One of these systems was developed at the National Cancer Institute (NCI) where it has been actively used for over a decade and half.[54] The NCI EPE grading system categorizes curvilinear contact length ≥ 1.5 cm or capsular bulge and irregularity seen on MRI as grade 1, both features together as grade 2, and frank capsular breach as grade 3 (Fig. 6). In the prospective study with 553 participants, a higher NCI EPE grade was associated with an increased risk of EPE at pathology. Grade 1, grade 2, and grade 3 had positive predictive value of 24%, 36%, and 66% for the detection of EPE on histopathology, respectively. Furthermore, clinical features combined with the grading system predicted pathologic EPE better than imaging alone, but the study did not specify how the clinical features can be incorporated into the scoring system.

Various studies have validated and compared the effectiveness of different MRI-based systems in assessing EPE, most commonly the NCI EPE grade, European Society of Urogenital Radiology (ESUR) score, Likert scale, and tumor capsule contact length.[55–57] These studies have found that all these MRI-based criteria demonstrated moderate diagnostic performance for EPE detection at pathology. Specifically, Park and colleagues evaluated all four MRI-based EPE criterias.[56] The area under the receiver operating characteristic curve (AUC, 0.77–0.85) and intra- and inter-reader agreement ($\kappa = 0.61$–0.74) for all of these systems were similar. The NCI EPE grade, however, demonstrated the highest correlation with histopathology (Spearman correlation coefficient of 0.42–0.55). The NCI EPE grade incorporates more objective parameters than the ESUR score and is further enhanced by including the measurement of tumor capsule contact length, which serves as a quantitative marker. As a result, the EPE grade is a more objective approach compared to the ESUR score and the Likert scale. Another study also showed the reader with less prostate imaging experience had lower sensitivity using the Likert scale and ESUR score compared to the NCI EPE grade, suggesting that the latter method is less reader experience dependent.[55] However, this is only reported in one study, and NCI EPE grade does include subjective criteria that may be affected by reader's experience (ie, capsular bulging and irregularity). One study by Reisaeter and colleagues found the inter-reader agreement for the NCI EPE grade and Likert scale was fair with weighted κ of 0.47 and 0.45, respectively.[57] Overall, the NCI EPE grade seems to perform as well as other systems but with the advantage of standardization. It is evident that combining clinical risk factors with imaging characteristics is necessary to improve the accuracy of predicting EPE and making informed treatment decisions.[44] Gandaglia and colleagues proposed a model to predict EPE using clinical variables with mpMRI and systematic biopsy results.[58] The study suggested the inclusion of mpMRI data may improve the discrimination of clinical models for EPE modestly (70%, 95% confidence interval [CI]: 65%–74% vs 67%, 95% CI: 61%–70%). An external validation of the model showed no significant performance improvement compared to the MSKCC model (72% vs 70%, $P = .3$), but a significant improvement compared to the Partin tables (72% vs 61%, $P < .001$).[59] Updated models that incorporate mpMRI information with greater generalizability and performance still need to be developed and investigated.

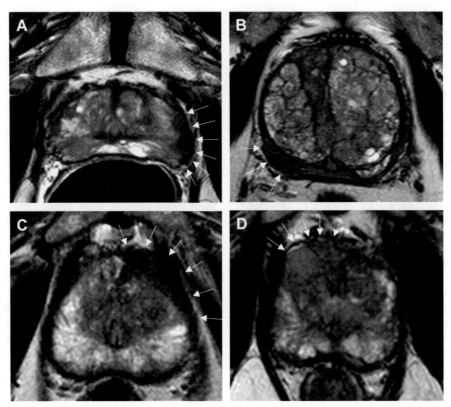

Fig. 6. Axial T2WIs with MRI-derived extra-prostatic extension (EPE) grade for the prediction of pathologic EPE. EPE grade 1 defined as either a curvilinear contact length ≥ 1.5 cm (*arrows, A*), or a capsular bulge or irregularity (*arrows, B*). EPE grade 2 is defined as curvilinear contact length ≥ 1.5 cm plus capsular bulge or irregularity (*arrows, C*). EPE grade 3 is defined as a well-defined breach of the prostate capsule with tumor extension into peri-prostatic space or invasion of adjacent anatomic structures (*arrows, D*).

The experience and expertise of the interpreting radiologist are also essential in the detection of EPE. Radiologists who are experienced in interpreting prostate MRI images are more likely to detect EPE accurately than those with less experience. Therefore, it is essential to have radiologists with specialized training and experience in interpreting prostate MRI scans to improve the detection of EPE.[60,61] Incorporating a standardized EPE reporting system such as the NCI EPE grade into PI-RADS would be a helpful first step to further improve the uniformity of mpMRI interpretations, and to transition from a overly simplistic binary assessment (ie, EPE present vs absent) to a probability risk assessment. If the grading system outcomes were placed as a footnote within reports, the grade would be readily associated with its corresponding quantitative risk of EPE. It is probable that enhancements in the consistency between readers can be achieved with the incorporation of artificial intelligence-based solutions that offer quantitative evaluations of EPE risk as well. Additionally, it is important for radiologists to recognize the limitations of mpMRI in predicting EPE. For example, even in cases of visible gross extension on mpMRI using the NCI EPE grade, only 66% were found to have EPE on pathologic examination, indicating potential false-positive results. Inflammation, desmoplastic reaction, or changes related to biopsy-induced trauma can contribute to such false positives. Moreover, the microscopic nature of EPE as a histopathological definition makes it challenging to accurately predict on mpMRI. However, positive predictive value may be influenced by disease prevalence and positive predictive value of mpMRI in detecting EPE, which could be as high as 89% in high-risk patients.[62] Nonetheless, it is crucial to approach the diagnosis of EPE with caution when using mpMRI.

EVALUATION OF SEMINAL VESICLE INVASION

SVI is another important factor for prognosis and local cancer staging due to an increased risk of lymph node metastasis.[63] SVI stages prostate cancer as T3b of the TNM staging system; tumors with SVI are classified as locally advanced and have very high risk for progression or recurrence.[64] Patients with SVI were found to have a 32% 7-year survival rate, while patients without SVI had a 67% 7-year survival rate.[65]

According to the ISUP Consensus, SVI is defined as the infiltration of tumor cells that did not originate from the seminal vesicles or ductus deferens present in the muscular layer on histopathology.[66] Mechanism of prostate cancer invasion into the seminal vesicle can be classified into three categories.[67] Type 1 was defined as a direct mechanism in which the prostate cancer spread along the ejaculatory duct and into the seminal vesicle. Type 2 was characterized as the spread of the cancer through the prostate capsule and into the seminal vesicle, in which Type 2A occurs between the base of the prostate and the seminal vesicle and type 2B occurs when the prostate cancer grows from the periprostatic nerve into the seminal vesicle. The least common mode of spread is Type 3 SVI, characterized by deposits of cancer in the seminal vesicle without any continuous primary cancer in the prostate. SVI can be identified by certain characteristics on MRI. These may include hypointense filling defects within SVs on T2W MRI with early contrast enhancement on DCE MRI and restricted diffusion (hypointense on ADC maps, hyperintense on high b DW MRI) within and/or along the seminal vesicle. Additionally, the obliteration of the angle between the base of the prostate and the seminal vesicle, as well as direct tumor extension from the base of the prostate into and around the seminal vesicle are among the MRI features of SVI[52] (Fig. 7). The PI-RADS guideline recommended that high spatial resolution T2WI is essential for the assessment of SVI.[20] Additionally, some studies have suggested that abstaining from ejaculation 3 or more days, especially in men older than 60 years, before undergoing an MRI examination may enhance seminal vesicle assessment. Abstinence from ejaculation showed a significant increase in T2W and ADC values in the peripheral zone (adjacent to seminal vesicles) and resulted in larger seminal vesicle volumes and lower rates of nondiagnostic evaluation and therefore might improve the evaluation of SVI.[68,69]

Similar to EPE evaluation, the risk of SVI was traditionally assessed using clinical nomograms, such as the Partin table[42] and Kattan nomogram.[70] These clinical monograms have moderate accuracy in detecting SVI.[30,71] Further studies have shown that MRI alone may perform similarly or superior to clinical assessments, and MRI plus clinical models can achieve the highest diagnostic accuracy for SVI detection.[44,72,73] A recent meta-analysis of the literature with 34 studies has shown

that, although mpMRI provides a low sensitivity (58%), the specificity is quite reliable for SVI detection (96%).[50] Additionally, in a study conducted by Kim and colleagues,[74] among a total of 1403 patients who underwent preoperative mpMRI, it was concluded that the sensitivity and specificity for corresponding pathologic SVI was 45% and 95%, respectively. Furthermore, one study showed that there is no huge variance in SVI interpretation for radiologists with different reading experiences.[75] SVI interpretation between a new radiologist and a senior radiologist showed a sensitivity of 18% versus 27%, a specificity of 97% versus 94%, a positive predictive value of 40% versus 32%, a negative predictive value of 92% versus 93%, and an overall accuracy of 90% versus 88%, respectively. Overall, current data suggest that mpMRI provides a low sensitivity but a high specificity for detecting SVI. Nonetheless, studies have suggested that mpMRI may be comparable to, or even superior to, traditional clinical monograms, rendering it a valuable asset for ruling in SVI, staging prostate cancer, and guiding treatment decisions.

Biparametric MRI (bpMRI) is becoming more popular as the current trend is moving toward prostate MRI without contrast agent.[76] This also raised questions regarding whether there is still a need for contrast agent for detecting SVI. In a retrospective study by Soylu and colleagues,[77] two radiologists estimated the likelihood of SVI in 3 image-viewing settings: T2WI alone, T2WI plus DWI, and T2WI plus DWI and DCE sequences. When reviewing T2WI alone, both radiologists achieved high specificity (93% and 94%) and high negative predictive value (94% and 95%) but only moderate sensitivity (52% and 59%) and positive predictive value (50% and 52%). The addition of DWI significantly improved specificity (97% and 98%) and positive predictive value (70% and 79%) for both radiologists. However, adding DCE showed no improvement, suggesting that DCE may not provide incremental value for the diagnosis of SVI. Christophe and colleagues[78] also demonstrated similar findings with AUC of 0.73 (95% CI: 0.66–0.83) for mpMRI and 0.76 (95% CI: 0.68–0.85) for bpMRI. Another more recent retrospective study showed conflicting results, however. Caglic and colleagues[79] found that mpMRI with DCE was better at detecting SVI and improved the inter-reader agreement compared to bpMRI without contrast. The AUC for mpMRI was 0.91 (95% CI: 0.84–0.96) and for bpMRI was 0.86 (95% CI: 0.78–0.92, P = .02), while the inter-reader agreement for the prediction of SVI was 0.75 (95% CI: 0.62–0.88) for mpMRI and 0.69 (95% CI: 0.57–0.81) for bpMRI. The

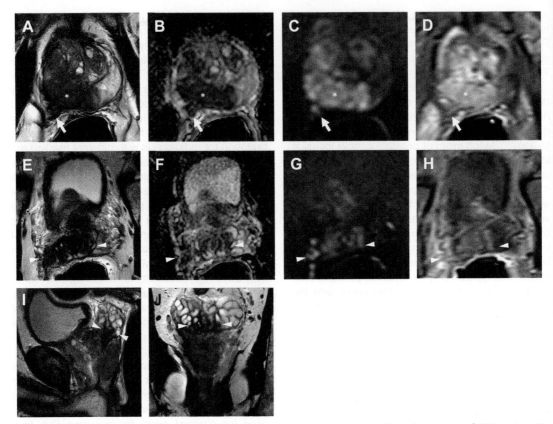

Fig. 7. Multiparametric MRI of a 51-year-old man with a serum prostate specific antigen level of 95.9 ng/mL. PI-RADS 5 lesion (*asterisk*) with frank capsular breach (*arrows*). Targeted biopsy of the lesion revealed Gleason score 10 (5 + 5) prostate adenocarcinoma. Seminal vesicles are invaded bilaterally (*arrowheads*). Targeted biopsy from the left and right seminal vesicles revealed Gleason score 7 (4 + 3) and Gleason score 8 (4 + 4) prostate adeno-carcinoma, respectively. Axial T2-weighted imaging of the prostate (*A*), apparent diffusion coefficient map of the prostate (*B*), high b-value (b = 1500 s/mm^2) diffusion-weighted imaging of the prostate (*C*), dynamic contrast enhanced imaging of the prostate (*D*), axial T2-weighted imaging of the seminal vesicles (*E*), apparent diffusion coefficient map of the seminal vesicles (*F*), high b-value (b = 1500 s/mm^2) diffusion-weighted imaging of the sem-inal vesicles (*G*), dynamic contrast enhanced imaging of the seminal vesicles (*H*), sagittal T2-weighted imaging of the seminal vesicles (*I*), and coronal T2-weighted imaging of the seminal vesicles (*J*).

discrepancy between studies may be due to the difference in patient selection and image acquisi-tion techniques. Caglic and colleagues examined biopsy naïve patients only whereas Soylu and col-leagues conducted their study in surgical patients, who likely have more advanced diseases and larger lesions on MRI. Soylu and colleagues also used endorectal coils while Caglic and colleagues did not. Both studies were retrospective with limited sample size. Larger prospective studies are needed to further evaluate how DCE sequence impact the detection of SVI.

Similar to categorical EPE grading systems, Jung and colleagues[80] proposed a 6-class grading sys-tem for the detection of SVI using T2WI morphologic features from exams performed on 1.5 T scanner with endorectal coil. Class 0 indicates normal find-ings whereas class 5 indicates apparent mass lesion with destructive architecture. For class 4 and 5 combined, the sensitivity was 71% with spec-ificity of 97%. This study was limited by its retro-spective nature and sample size of 217 patients. With the improvement of mpMRI and introduction of more advanced hardware, such as 3 T scanners, this system should be refined (such as incorporating other mpMRI pulse sequences) and validated in external cohorts. In conclusion, SVI is a crucial fac-tor in prostate cancer staging and prognosis, as it signifies a higher disease stage and worse out-comes. While traditional clinical nomograms have moderate accuracy in detecting SVI, mpMRI has been shown to be able to achieve higher overall diagnostic performance, making it a valuable tool for ruling in SVI and guiding treatment decisions. Despite mpMRI's low sensitivity, its high specificity for detecting SVI establishes it as a dependable diagnostic tool. Nonetheless, a standardized SVI grading system should be considered and developed to further improve the uniformity of SVI interpretations and performance of MRI in detecting SVI.

EVALUATION OF POSITIVE SURGICAL MARGIN

Prostate margin involvement status is an important determinant of patient outcome after radical prostatectomy. Around 20% to 30% of cases are reported to show a PSM for prostate cancer after prostatectomy.[81] In fact, the presence of a positive margin is associated with a higher risk for biochemical recurrence and patients should be followed closely.[82] While preventing PSM is one of the main objectives of prostatectomy, preserving the neurovascular bundles and membranous urethra is critical for preserving continence and potency. PSM is defined as tumor cells located at the edge of the tissue resected.[83] A study suggested that MRI lesions located at the apex are associated with a higher risk of PSM.[84] This might be due to the lack of a well-defined capsule at the prostatic apex and due to the absence of a clear boundary between the apex and the urethral sphincter. Posterolateral section is another commonly involved site (Fig. 8), and positive margin at this site may confer greater risk of biochemical recurrence when compared to those with negative surgical margins at this site.[85]

PSMs are often associated with the index and larger lesions.[86] As mpMRI can identify such lesions, the information obtained from mpMRI can be utilized during surgery to target large lesions to decrease the incidence of PSM. Furthermore, preoperative prostate mpMRI can identify patients with risk factors associated with PSMs and help surgical planning. In a recent retrospective study by Quentin and colleagues,[87] it was concluded that a large percentage of PSMs were located at the apical and posterior capsule. In this study, mpMRI visualized 80% of prostate cancer with PSM at the urethra and 100% at the bladder. The length of capsular contact was the best MRI predictor for PSM at the capsule. For tumors with PSMs at the apical urethra, the distance to the membranous urethra was the best MRI parameter. The highest accuracy was documented in cases where the distance between the prostate cancer and membranous urethra was ≤ 3.5 mm, indicating a high risk for PSMs at the urethra, and when the length of capsular contact was ≥ 22.5 mm, indicating a high risk for PSMs at the capsule. Similarly, Park and colleagues[88] developed a scoring system to estimate the risk of PSMs based on MRI features. The system assigned scores as follows: PI-RADS categories 1 to 2 received 0 points, categories 3 to 4 received 2 points, and category 5 received 3 points. Tumors located at the posterolateral side or apex were each assigned 1 point. Capsular contact length between 15 and 24 mm was given a score of 1, while lengths of ≥ 25 mm were scored 2. The cumulative score ranged from 0 to 7 points, with a higher score indicating an increased risk of PSM. The scoring system exhibited strong predictive performance for PSM in both the derivation (C statistics, 0.80) and validation (C statistics, 0.77) groups. By utilizing a cutoff score of ≥ 4 for predicting PSM, the sensitivity, specificity, positive predictive value, and negative predictive value were determined to be 63%, 72%, 51%, and 80%, respectively. It is important to note that

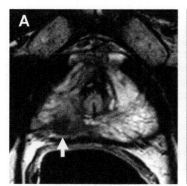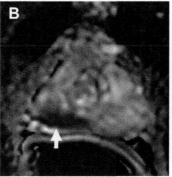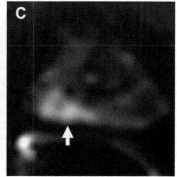

Fig. 8. Multiparametric MRI of a 71-year-old man with a serum prostate specific antigen level of 6.5 ng/mL. The lesion (arrows) was 1.8 cm in the right apical peripheral zone located in the posterolateral section and assigned PI-RADS category 5. Radical prostatectomy showed Gleason score 8 (4 + 4) prostate adenocarcinoma with extraprostatic extension. Positive surgical margins were also noted. T2-weighted imaging (A), apparent diffusion coefficient map (B), and high b-value (b = 1500 s/mm²) diffusion-weighted imaging (C).

one single-institution randomized trial with 438 patients did not show a clear reduction of PSM rate by performing MRI before surgery.[89] However, in this study, the observed frequency of PSM was roughly half of what was anticipated, which may have resulted in insufficient statistical power to establish a significant impact of MRI. Additionally, one meta-analysis suggested that while the decision-making process for determining the extent of resection during radical prostatectomy is significantly influenced by MRI, it is unclear whether preoperative MRI effectively reduces PSM rates.[90] Therefore, the impact of mpMRI on detecting PSM should be further explored.

In summary, PSM after radical prostatectomy remains as a significant concern as it is associated with an increased risk of early biochemical recurrence for which a close clinical follow-up is required. The utilization of preoperative mpMRI enables the assessment of both pelvic anatomy and tumor positioning, which can aid in mitigating unfavorable surgical outcomes like PSMs. The MRI features such as tumor-capsule contact length, PI-RADS category, and tumor location have been used to develop predictive scoring systems for PSM. However, the impact of mpMRI on reducing PSM rates is still unclear and warrants further investigation. Overall, the integration of mpMRI into clinical decision-making for prostate cancer management holds great value in improving clinical outcomes.

SUMMARY

Traditional methods of prostate cancer staging, such as digital rectal examination, serum PSA testing, and clinical nomograms, have limitations in their ability to provide a comprehensive evaluation of the extent and aggressiveness of the disease. Due to the ability of MRI to provide high spatial resolution and soft tissue contrast, it has emerged as a promising tool for preoperative local T-staging of prostate cancer. The specificity of mpMRI in detecting EPE and SVI has been shown to be excellent, while the sensitivity remains modest. The use of various scoring systems may improve EPE detection and provide uniformity in the assessment across various clinical settings. Information from preoperative MRI can guide treatment planning, including surgical resection and radiation therapy. Despite its potential benefits, the use of MRI for prostate cancer staging also has some limitations. One of the main drawbacks is the high cost of the imaging technique, which may not be feasible for some patients or healthcare systems. Additionally, the interpretation of MRI is highly dependent on the expertise of the radiologist, and the technique requires specialized training and equipment. With the increased focus on MR image quality and the introduction of the Prostate Imaging Quality (PI-QUAL) score system, more studies are needed to examine the potential effects of image quality on local staging. Furthermore, artificial intelligence-based solutions can provide consistent and objective image evaluation. Most of the current research focuses on the identification of intraprostatic lesions, but with the development of better algorithms, local staging using artificial intelligence models could be a possibility in the near future. Overall, the use of MRI for the local staging of prostate cancer represents a significant advance in the field of urologic oncology. As technology and imaging techniques continue to evolve, it is likely that MRI will play an increasingly important role in the diagnosis, staging, and management of prostate cancer. As such, it is important for clinicians and researchers to continue to explore the potential benefits and limitations of MRI in the local staging of prostate cancer, with the ultimate goal of improving patient care.

CLINICS CARE POINTS

- Extra-prostatic extension (EPE), seminal vesicle invasion (SVI), and positive surgical margin (PSM) indicate locally advanced disease and carry a worse clinical prognosis which can impact the choice of treatment.

- EPE can be visualized on multiparametric MRI (mpMRI) as bulging/irregularity of the capsule, broad curvilinear capsular contact length, or frank invasion of the surrounding structures.

- SVI can be identified on mpMRI as hypointense filling defects on T2WI and ADC maps, hyperintensity on high b value DWI, and early contrast enhancement on DCE within and/or along the seminal vesicle. Additional feature includes the obliteration of the angle between the base of the prostate and the seminal vesicle.

- PSM is associated with large index lesions, especially for those located at the apex and posterolateral section of the prostate.

- The current treatment options for patients with locally advanced high-risk prostate cancer are radiotherapy with androgen deprivation therapy or radical prostatectomy. However, research is still ongoing to identify the optimal treatment approach for these patients.

DISCLOSURE

Research support was provided by the NIH Medical Research Scholars Program, a public-private partnership supported jointly by the NIH and contributions to the Foundation for the NIH from the American Association for Dental Research and the Colgate-Palmolive Company.

REFERENCES

1. Rawla P. Epidemiology of Prostate Cancer. World J Oncol 2019;10(2):63–89.

2. Leslie SW, Soon-Sutton TL, R IA, et al. Prostate cancer. StatPearls. Treasure Island, FL: StatPearls Publishing; 2023.

3. Kasivisvanathan V, Rannikko AS, Borghi M, et al. MRI-Targeted or Standard Biopsy for Prostate-Cancer Diagnosis. N Engl J Med 2018;378(19): 1767–77.

4. Hricak H, Choyke PL, Eberhardt SC, et al. Imaging prostate cancer: a multidisciplinary perspective. Radiology 2007;243(1):28–53.

5. Murphy G, Haider M, Ghai S, et al. The expanding role of MRI in prostate cancer. AJR Am J Roentgenol 2013;201(6):1229–38.

6. Tan N, Margolis DJA, Mcclure TD, et al. Radical prostatectomy: value of prostate MRI in surgical planning. Abdom Imag 2012;37(4):664–74.

7. Caglic I, Kovac V, Barrett T. Multiparametric MRI - local staging of prostate cancer and beyond. Radiol Oncol 2019;53(2):159–70.

8. Expert Panel on Urologic I, Coakley FV, Oto A, et al. ACR Appropriateness Criteria((R)) Prostate Cancer-Pretreatment Detection, Surveillance, and Staging. J Am Coll Radiol 2017;14(5S):S245–57.

9. Mottet N, van den Bergh RCN, Briers E, et al. EAU-EANM-ESTRO-ESUR-SIOG Guidelines on Prostate Cancer-2020 Update. Part 1: Screening, Diagnosis, and Local Treatment with Curative Intent. Eur Urol 2021;79(2):243–62.

10. Chang AJ, Autio KA, Roach M, et al. High-risk prostate cancer-classification and therapy. Nat Rev Clin Oncol 2014;11(6):308–23.

11. Eastham JA, Auffenberg GB, Barocas DA, et al. Clinically Localized Prostate Cancer: AUA/ASTRO Guideline. Part III: Principles of Radiation and Future Directions. J Urol 2022;208(1):26–33.

12. Eastham JA, Auffenberg GB, Barocas DA, et al. Clinically Localized Prostate Cancer: AUA/ASTRO Guideline, Part II: Principles of Active Surveillance, Principles of Surgery, and Follow-Up. J Urol 2022; 208(1):19–25.

13. Horwitz EM, Bae K, Hanks GE, et al. Ten-year follow-up of radiation therapy oncology group protocol 92-02: a phase III trial of the duration of elective androgen deprivation in locally advanced prostate cancer. J Clin Oncol 2008;26(15):2497–504.

14. Stephenson AJ, Kattan MW, Eastham JA, et al. Prostate cancer-specific mortality after radical prostatectomy for patients treated in the prostate-specific antigen era. J Clin Oncol 2009;27(26):4300–5.

15. Eggener SE, Scardino PT, Walsh PC, et al. Predicting 15-year prostate cancer specific mortality after radical prostatectomy. J Urol 2011;185(3):869–75.

16. Spahn M, Joniau S, Gontero P, et al. Outcome predictors of radical prostatectomy in patients with prostate-specific antigen greater than 20 ng/ml: a European multi-institutional study of 712 patients. Eur Urol 2010;58(1):1–7 [discussion: 10–1].

17. Zwergel U, Suttmann H, Schroeder T, et al. Outcome of prostate cancer patients with initial PSA> or =20 ng/ml undergoing radical prostatectomy. Eur Urol 2007;52(4):1058–65.

18. Guy DE, Chen H, Boldt RG, et al. Characterizing Surgical and Radiotherapy Outcomes in Non-metastatic High-Risk Prostate Cancer: A Systematic Review and Meta-Analysis. Cureus 2021;13(8): e17400.

19. Wallis CJD, Saskin R, Choo R, et al. Surgery Versus Radiotherapy for Clinically-localized Prostate Cancer: A Systematic Review and Meta-analysis. Eur Urol 2016;70(1):21–30.

20. Turkbey B, Rosenkrantz AB, Haider MA, et al. Prostate Imaging Reporting and Data System Version 2.1: 2019 Update of Prostate Imaging Reporting and Data System Version 2. Eur Urol 2019;76(3): 340–51.

21. Westphalen AC, McCulloch CE, Anaokar JM, et al. Variability of the Positive Predictive Value of PI-RADS for Prostate MRI across 26 Centers: Experience of the Society o Abdominal Radiology Prostate Cancer Disease-focused Panel. Radiology 2020; 296(1):76–84.

22. Hofbauer SL, Maxeiner A, Kittner B, et al. Validation of Prostate Imaging Reporting and Data System Version 2 for the Detection of Prostate Cancer. J Urol 2018;200(4):767–73.

23. Greer MD, Shih JH, Lay N, et al. Interreader Variability of Prostate Imaging Reporting and Data System Version 2 in Detecting and Assessing Prostate Cancer Lesions at Prostate MRI. AJR Am J Roentgenol 2019;1–8. https://doi.org/10.2214/AJR.18.20536.

24. Smith CP, Harmon SA, Barrett T, et al. Intra- and interreader reproducibility of PI-RADSv2: A multireader study. J Magn Reson Imaging 2019;49(6): 1694–703.

25. Rosenkrantz AB, Ginocchio LA, Cornfeld D, et al. Interobserver Reproducibility of the PI-RADS Version 2 Lexicon: A Multicenter Study of Six Experienced Prostate Radiologists. Radiology 2016;280(3): 793–804.

26. Sathianathen NJ, Omer A, Harriss E, et al. Negative Predictive Value of Multiparametric Magnetic Resonance Imaging in the Detection of Clinically Significant Prostate Cancer in the Prostate Imaging Reporting and Data System Era: A Systematic Review and Meta-analysis. Eur Urol 2020;78(3): 402–14.

27. Moldovan PC, Van den Broeck T, Sylvester R, et al. What Is the Negative Predictive Value of Multiparametric Magnetic Resonance Imaging in Excluding Prostate Cancer at Biopsy? A Systematic Review and Meta-analysis from the European Association of Urology Prostate Cancer Guidelines Panel. Eur Urol 2017;72(2):250–66.

28. Oerther B, Engel H, Bamberg F, et al. Cancer detection rates of the PI-RADSv2.1 assessment categories: systematic review and meta-analysis on lesion level and patient level. Prostate Cancer Prostatic Dis 2022;25(2):256–63.

29. Yilmaz EC, Shih JH, Belue MJ, et al. Prospective Evaluation of PI-RADS Version 2.1 for Prostate Cancer Detection and Investigation of Multiparametric MRI-derived Markers. Radiology 2023;307(4): e221309.

30. Venderink W, van Luijtelaar A, Bomers JGR, et al. Results of Targeted Biopsy in Men with Magnetic Resonance Imaging Lesions Classified Equivocal, Likely or Highly Likely to Be Clinically Significant Prostate Cancer. Eur Urol 2018;73(3):353–60.

31. Buyyounouski MK, Choyke PL, McKenney JK, et al. Prostate Cancer - Major Changes in the American Joint Committee on Cancer Eighth Edition Cancer Staging Manual. Ca-a Cancer Journal for Clinicians 2017;67(3):246–53.

32. Mikel Hubanks J, Boorjian SA, Frank I, et al. The presence of extracapsular extension is associated with an increased risk of death from prostate cancer after radical prostatectomy for patients with seminal vesicle invasion and negative lymph nodes. Urol Oncol 2014;32(1):26.e1-7.

33. Tollefson MK, Karnes RJ, Rangel LJ, et al. The impact of clinical stage on prostate cancer survival following radical prostatectomy. J Urol 2013;189(5): 1707–12.

34. Rud E, Klotz D, Rennesund K, et al. Preoperative magnetic resonance imaging for detecting uni- and bilateral extraprostatic disease in patients with prostate cancer. World J Urol 2015;33(7):1015–21.

35. Pesapane F, Standaert C, De Visschere P, et al. T-staging of prostate cancer: Identification of useful signs to standardize detection of posterolateral extraprostatic extension on prostate MRI. Clin Imaging 2020;59(1):1–7.

36. Magi-Galluzzi C, Evans AJ, Delahunt B, et al. International Society of Urological Pathology (ISUP) Consensus Conference on Handling and Staging of Radical Prostatectomy Specimens. Working

group 3: extraprostatic extension, lymphovascular invasion and locally advanced disease. Mod Pathol 2011;24(1):26–38.

37. Epstein JI, Carmichael MJ, Pizov G, et al. Influence of capsular penetration on progression following radical prostatectomy: a study of 196 cases with long-term followup. J Urol 1993;150(1):135–41.

38. Chuang AY, Nielsen ME, Hernandez DJ, et al. The significance of positive surgical margin in areas of capsular incision in otherwise organ confined disease at radical prostatectomy. J Urol 2007;178(4): 1306–10.

39. Fleshner K, Assel M, Benfante N, et al. Clinical Findings and Treatment Outcomes in Patients with Extraprostatic Extension Identified on Prostate Biopsy. J Urol 2016;196(3):703–8.

40. Ward JF, Zincke H, Bergstralh EJ, et al. The impact of surgical approach (nerve bundle preservation versus wide local excision) on surgical margins and biochemical recurrence following radical prostatectomy. J Urol 2004;172(4 Pt 1):1328–32.

41. Loeb S, Smith ND, Roehl KA, et al. Intermediate-term potency, continence, and survival outcomes of radical prostatectomy for clinically high-risk or locally advanced prostate cancer. Urology 2007; 69(6):1170–5.

42. Eifler JB, Feng Z, Lin BM, et al. An updated prostate cancer staging nomogram (Partin tables) based on cases from 2006 to 2011. BJU Int 2013;111(1):22–9.

43. Cagiannos I, Karakiewicz P, Eastham JA, et al. A preoperative nomogram identifying decreased risk of positive pelvic lymph nodes in patients with prostate cancer. J Urol 2003;170(5):1798–803.

44. Rayn KN, Bloom JB, Gold SA, et al. Added Value of Multiparametric Magnetic Resonance Imaging to Clinical Nomograms for Predicting Adverse Pathology in Prostate Cancer. J Urol 2018;200(5):1041–7.

45. Augustin H, Fritz GA, Ehammer T, et al. Accuracy of 3-Tesla magnetic resonance imaging for the staging of prostate cancer in comparison to the Partin tables. Acta Radiol 2009;50(5):562–9.

46. Boesen L, Chabanova E, Logager V, et al. Prostate cancer staging with extracapsular extension risk scoring using multiparametric MRI: a correlation with histopathology. Eur Radiol 2015;25(6):1776–85.

47. Schieda N, Quon JS, Lim C, et al. Evaluation of the European Society of Urogenital Radiology (ESUR) PI-RADS scoring system for assessment of extraprostatic extension in prostatic carcinoma. Eur J Radiol 2015;84(10):1843–8.

48. Baco E, Rud E, Vlatkovic L, et al. Predictive value of magnetic resonance imaging determined tumor contact length for extracapsular extension of prostate cancer. J Urol 2015;193(2):466–72.

49. Bittencourt LK, Litjens G, Hulsbergen-van de Kaa CA, et al. Prostate Cancer: The European Society of Urogenital Radiology Prostate Imaging

Reporting and Data System Criteria for Predicting Extraprostatic Extension by Using 3-T Multiparametric MR Imaging. Radiology 2015;276(2):479–89.

50. de Rooij M, Hamoen EH, Witjes JA, et al. Accuracy of Magnetic Resonance Imaging for Local Staging of Prostate Cancer: A Diagnostic Meta-analysis. Eur Urol 2016;70(2):233–45.

51. Alessi S, Pricolo P, Summers P, et al. Low PI-RADS assessment category excludes extraprostatic extension (>= pT3a) of prostate cancer: a histology-validated study including 301 operated patients. Eur Radiol 2019;29(10):5478–87.

52. Barentsz JO, Richenberg J, Clements R, et al. ESUR prostate MR guidelines 2012. Eur Radiol 2012;22(4): 746–57.

53. Costa DN, Passoni NM, Leyendecker JR, et al. Diagnostic Utility of a Likert Scale Versus Qualitative Descriptors and Length of Capsular Contact for Determining Extraprostatic Tumor Extension at Multiparametric Prostate MRI. AJR Am J Roentgenol 2018;210(5):1066–72.

54. Mehralivand S, Shih JH, Harmon S, et al. A Grading System for the Assessment of Risk of Extraprostatic Extension of Prostate Cancer at Multiparametric MRI. Radiology 2019;290(3):709–19.

55. Asfuroglu U, Asfuroglu BB, Ozer H, et al. Which one is better for predicting extraprostatic extension on multiparametric MRI: ESUR score, Likert scale, tumor contact length, or EPE grade? Eur J Radiol 2022;149:110228.

56. Park KJ, Kim MH, Kim JK. Extraprostatic Tumor Extension: Comparison of Preoperative Multiparametric MRI Criteria and Histopathologic Correlation after Radical Prostatectomy. Radiology 2020;296(1):87–95.

57. Reisaeter LAR, Halvorsen OJ, Beisland C, et al. Assessing Extraprostatic Extension with Multiparametric MRI of the Prostate: Mehralivand Extraprostatic Extension Grade or Extraprostatic Extension Likert Scale? Radiol Imaging Cancer 2020;2(1):e190071.

58. Gandaglia G, Ploussard G, Valerio M, et al. The Key Combined Value of Multiparametric Magnetic Resonance Imaging, and Magnetic Resonance Imaging-targeted and Concomitant Systematic Biopsies for the Prediction of Adverse Pathological Features in Prostate Cancer Patients Undergoing Radical Prostatectomy. Eur Urol 2020;77(6):733–41.

59. Diamand R, Ploussard G, Roumiguie M, et al. External Validation of a Multiparametric Magnetic Resonance Imaging-based Nomogram for the Prediction of Extracapsular Extension and Seminal Vesicle Invasion in Prostate Cancer Patients Undergoing Radical Prostatectomy. Eur Urol 2021;79(2): 180–5.

60. Wibmer A, Vargas HA, Donahue TF, et al. Diagnosis of Extracapsular Extension of Prostate Cancer on Prostate MRI: Impact of Second-Opinion Readings by Subspecialized Genitourinary Oncologic Radiologists. AJR Am J Roentgenol 2015;205(1):W73–8.

61. Tay KJ, Gupta RT, Brown AF, et al. Defining the Incremental Utility of Prostate Multiparametric Magnetic Resonance Imaging at Standard and Specialized Read in Predicting Extracapsular Extension of Prostate Cancer. Eur Urol 2016;70(2):211–3.

62. Somford DM, Hamoen EH, Futterer JJ, et al. The predictive value of endorectal 3 Tesla multiparametric magnetic resonance imaging for extraprostatic extension in patients with low, intermediate and high risk prostate cancer. J Urol 2013;190(5): 1728–34.

63. Stone NN, Stock RG, Parikh D, et al. Perineural invasion and seminal vesicle involvement predict pelvic lymph node metastasis in men with localized carcinoma of the prostate. J Urol 1998;160(5):1722–6.

64. Mohler JL, Antonarakis ES, Armstrong AJ, et al. Prostate Cancer, Version 2.2019, NCCN Clinical Practice Guidelines in Oncology. J Natl Compr Canc Netw 2019;17(5):479–505.

65. Potter SR, Epstein JI, Partin AW. Seminal vesicle invasion by prostate cancer: prognostic significance and therapeutic implications. Rev Urol 2000;2(3): 190–5.

66. Berney DM, Wheeler TM, Grignon DJ, et al. International Society of Urological Pathology (ISUP) Consensus Conference on Handling and Staging of Radical Prostatectomy Specimens. Working group 4: seminal vesicles and lymph nodes. Mod Pathol 2011;24(1):39–47.

67. Billis A, Teixeira DA, Stelini RF, et al. Seminal vesicle invasion in radical prostatectomies: Which is the most common route of invasion? Int Urol Nephrol 2007-11-23 2007;39(4):1097–102.

68. Medved M, Sammet S, Yousuf A, et al. MR Imaging of the Prostate and Adjacent Anatomic Structures before, during, and after Ejaculation: Qualitative and Quantitative Evaluation. Radiology 2014; 271(2):452–60.

69. Kabakus IM, Borofsky S, Mertan FV, et al. Does Abstinence From Ejaculation Before Prostate MRI Improve Evaluation of the Seminal Vesicles? AJR Am J Roentgenol 2016;207(6):1205–9.

70. Koh H, Kattan MW, Scardino PT, et al. A nomogram to predict seminal vesicle invasion by the extent and location of cancer in systematic biopsy results. J Urol 2003;170(4):1203–8.

71. Wang L, Hricak H, Kattan MW, et al. Prediction of seminal vesicle invasion in prostate cancer: incremental value of adding endorectal MR imaging to the Kattan nomogram. Radiology 2007;242(1): 182–8.

72. Grivas N, Hinnen K, de Jong J, et al. Seminal vesicle invasion on multi-parametric magnetic resonance imaging: Correlation with histopathology. Eur J Radiol 2018;98:107–12.

73. Lim B, Choi SY, Kyung YS, et al. Value of clinical parameters and MRI with PI-RADS(V2) in predicting seminal vesicle invasion of prostate cancer. Scand J Urol 2021;55(1):17–21.

74. Kim JK, Lee HJ, Hwang SI, et al. Prognostic value of seminal vesicle invasion on preoperative multiparametric magnetic resonance imaging in pathological stage T3b prostate cancer. Sci Rep 2020; 10(1):5693.

75. Riney JC, Sarwani NE, Siddique S, et al. Prostate magnetic resonance imaging: The truth lies in the eye of the beholder. Urol Oncol 2018;36(4):159 e1–e159 e5.

76. Belue MJ, Yilmaz EC, Daryanani A, et al. Current Status of Biparametric MRI in Prostate Cancer Diagnosis: Literature Analysis. Life 2022;12(6):804.

77. Soylu FN, Peng YH, Jiang YL, et al. Seminal Vesicle Invasion in Prostate Cancer: Evaluation by Using Multiparametric Endorectal MR Imaging. Radiology 2013;267(3):797–806.

78. Christophe C, Montagne S, Bourrelier S, et al. Prostate cancer local staging using biparametric MRI: assessment and comparison with multiparametric MRI. Eur J Radiol 2020;132:109350.

79. Caglic I, Sushentsev N, Shah N, et al. Comparison of biparametric versus multiparametric prostate MRI for the detection of extracapsular extension and seminal vesicle invasion in biopsy naive patients. Eur J Radiol 2021;141doi. https://doi.org/10.1016/j.ejrad.2021.109804.

80. Jung DC, Lee HJ, Kim SH, et al. Preoperative MR imaging in the evaluation of seminal vesicle invasion in prostate cancer: pattern analysis of seminal vesicle lesions. J Magn Reson Imaging 2008;28(1):144–50.

81. Herlemann A, Cowan JE, Carroll PR, et al. Community-based Outcomes of Open versus Robot-assisted Radical Prostatectomy. Eur Urol 2018; 73(2):215–23.

82. Iczkowski KA, Lucia MS. Frequency of Positive Surgical Margin at Prostatectomy and Its Effect on Patient Outcome. Prostate Cancer 2011;2011. Artn 673021.

83. Cheng L, Slezak J, Bergstralh EJ, et al. Preoperative prediction of surgical margin status in patients with prostate cancer treated by radical prostatectomy. J Clin Oncol 2000;18(15):2862–8.

84. Yao A, Iwamoto H, Masago T, et al. The role of staging MRI in predicting apical margin positivity for robot-assisted laparoscopic radical prostatectomy. Urol Int 2014;93(2):182–8.

85. Eastham JA, Kuroiwa K, Ohori M, et al. Prognostic significance of location of positive margins in radical prostatectomy specimens. Urology 2007;70(5):965–9.

86. Karavitakis M, Ahmed HU, Abel PD, et al. Margin status after laparoscopic radical prostatectomy and the index lesion: implications for preoperative evaluation of tumor focality in prostate cancer. J Endourol 2012;26(5):503–8.

87. Quentin M, Schimmoller L, Ullrich T, et al. Pre-operative magnetic resonance imaging can predict prostate cancer with risk for positive surgical margins. Abdominal Radiology 2022;47(7):2486–93.

88. Park MY, Park KJ, Kim MH, et al. Preoperative MRI-based estimation of risk for positive resection margin after radical prostatectomy in patients with prostate cancer: development and validation of a simple scoring system. Eur Radiol 2021;31(7): 4898–907.

89. Rud E, Baco E, Klotz D, et al. Does preoperative magnetic resonance imaging reduce the rate of positive surgical margins at radical prostatectomy in a randomised clinical trial? Eur Urol 2015;68(3): 487–96.

90. Kozikowski M, Malewski W, Michalak W, et al. Clinical utility of MRI in the decision-making process before radical prostatectomy: Systematic review and meta-analysis. PLoS One 2019;14(1):e0210194.

Targeted Prostate Biopsies—What the Radiologist Needs to Know

Daniel N. Costa, MD[a,b,*], Debora Z. Recchimuzzi, MD[a], Nicola Schieda, MD[c]

KEYWORDS

- Prostate cancer • Biopsy • Imaging-pathology • US • MR imaging

KEY POINTS

- Systematic or template ultrasound-guided biopsy of the prostate frequently detects indolent and misses clinically significant prostate cancer.
- Different imaging modalities, image registration techniques, and anatomic accesses can be used to target a suspicious region identified within the prostate on MR imaging. It is important for radiologists to be familiar with the principles, advantages, and disadvantages of these various approaches.
- Ultrasound-guided fusion biopsies are less expensive, more readily available and can include synchronous systematic biopsy; whereas, MR-guided in-bore biopsies can target areas more precisely, particularly small lesions in challenging locations or in men that underwent previous prostatic instrumentation.
- A process of data reconciliation after targeted biopsy to identify potential misses related to inadequate lesion sampling or image misinterpretation is important.

INTRODUCTION

Prostate biopsies are essential for the diagnosis and management of patients with suspected prostate cancer (PCa).[1] The broad spectrum of disease aggressiveness requires accurate pretreatment risk stratification and is inferred from predictive models revolving around biopsy findings, including cancer grade, number of positive cores, and cancer core length in biopsy fragments.[2,3]

Until recently, prostate biopsies were performed using an ultrasound (US)-guided, anatomy-based approach.[1] In this systematic sampling, the biopsy operator uses an US system to locate and sample different regions of the prostate, frequently using a 12-core template. Because of its nontargeted nature, this approach frequently misses or underestimates clinically significant cancers (usually defined as International Society of Urogenital Pathology—ISUP Grade Group 2 or higher) and contributes to overdiagnosis by identifying indolent tumors (ISUP Grade Group 1), which do not necessarily require treatment.[4] Consequently, it can lead to suboptimal assessment of the disease volume, extent, and aggressiveness, resulting in increased uncertainty and potential undertreatment of men with significant cancers. For these reasons, alternative biopsy approaches have emerged in recent years.

The incorporation of multiparametric MR imaging as a prostate biopsy triage and planning tool has transformed the landscape of PCa detection. Combining the anatomic information from T2-weighted imaging, the functional information from diffusion-weighted and dynamic contrast-enhanced imaging, and supported by the common

a Department of Radiology, University of Texas Southwestern Medical Center, 2201 Inwood Road, Dallas, TX 75390, USA; b Department of Urology, University of Texas Southwestern Medical Center, 2201 Inwood Road, Dallas, TX 75390, USA; c Department of Medical Imaging, The Ottawa Hospital, 1053 Carling Avenue, Room C159, Ottawa, Ontario K1Y 4E9, Canada
* Corresponding author. 2201 Inwood Road, Dallas, TX 75390.
E-mail address: Daniel.Costa@UTSouthwestern.edu

Radiol Clin N Am 62 (2024) 109–120
https://doi.org/10.1016/j.rcl.2023.06.011
0033-8389/24/© 2023 Elsevier Inc. All rights reserved.

prostate imaging reporting and data system (PI-RADS)[5] language, multiparametric MR imaging has enabled targeted biopsies to improve the detection and characterization of PCas. In the randomized controlled PROMIS trial,[4] multiparametric MR imaging revealed a higher detection rate (93%) of clinically significant PCa than systematic biopsies (48%). Moreover, the negative predictive value of MR imaging (95%) was significantly higher than that of systematic biopsy (78%). Finally, MR imaging avoided biopsies in one-quarter of the patients. Similarly, the multicenter randomized controlled PRECISION trial[6] found that targeted biopsies of MR imaging-visible lesions detected clinically significant cancers in more men than transrectal ultrasound (TRUS)-guided biopsy (52% vs 39%), with a 30% lower risk of overdiagnosis. These findings were validated by the more recently published, population-based GÖTE-BORG-2 trial.[7] Consequently, revised guidelines—such as the American Urologic Association and the Society of Abdominal Radiology joint recommendation to obtain a multiparametric MR imaging before biopsy for all men[8]—supported broader adoption of prebiopsy imaging, a phenomenon that has been observed in the Medicare[9] and private insurance[10] population.

As targeted biopsies become the new standard of care, it is imperative for radiologists to be familiar with the principles, advantages, and disadvantages of the different techniques available for targeting an MR imaging-visible suspicious lesion, the topic discussed in this article.

TARGETED BIOPSY TECHNIQUES

Three approaches have been described to perform targeted biopsies of suspicious lesions identified on prostate MR imaging: (1) cognitive MR imaging–US fusion, (2) software-assisted MR imaging–US fusion, and (3) direct MR-guided in-bore biopsy[11] (Table 1). A transrectal or a transperineal route can be chosen with any of these techniques.

Cognitive MR imaging–US Fusion Biopsy

The earliest and simplest method to adapt a prostate biopsy practice to incorporate information from MR imaging and obtain targeted biopsy of MR imaging-visible lesions is through cognitive fusion biopsy. In cognitive fusion, the US operator attempts to identify lesions detected on MR imaging in order to perform targeted biopsy. In some cases, this may include directly visualizing the same lesion seen on MR imaging and US in the same location (Fig. 1) or, geographically landmarking to a particular location using anatomic

references including the seminal vesicles, prostate apex, and benign prostatic hyperplasia nodules. After cognitive fusion is performed, the US operator will obtain targeted core biopsies of the lesion(s) with or without additional core biopsies of the adjacent sextants (sometimes referred to as the "penumbra").[12]

Advantages of cognitive fusion biopsy are as follows: (1) cost (cognitive fusion biopsy is less expensive and can be performed using existing biopsy equipment), (2) low training (most existing US operators can perform cognitive fusion biopsy), (3) speed (cognitive fusion biopsy is fast, where MR imaging review, cognitive registration, and additional biopsies can be performed quickly), and (4) concurrent systematic or template biopsy can be performed with targeted biopsy. Disadvantages of cognitive fusion biopsy relate mainly to poor US visibility, which includes nonvisibility of the MR imaging lesion decreasing operator confidence. In many cases of cognitive fusion biopsy, an MR imaging lesion may not be visible on US. This may occur even with good US visibility of the gland. Experienced operators are more likely to identify an MR imaging target cognitively, perhaps not at first but with a "second-look" using anatomic landmarks, which improves targeting accuracy.[13] Yet, even with good technique and experience, an MR imaging lesion frequently is not well seen on US. In one study, only two-fifths of all MR imaging lesions on MR imaging and two-thirds of PI-RADS 5 lesions were visible on US.[14] Low-US visibility of prostate MR imaging detected lesions may be related to dense calcifications in the peripheral zone obscuring visibility or, for deeper lesions located in the transition zone, the end-fire transducer configuration of endocavitary transrectal US probes and near-field restrictions of the linear component of endocavitary TRUS probes used for transperineal biopsy. The use of ultrahigh frequency endocavitary TRUS probes (ie, micro-US performed at 29 MHz) improves visibility of lesions but remains challenging for anterior lesions in the transition zone.[15]

Software-assisted MR imaging–US Fusion Biopsy

To address the challenges of cognitive fusion biopsy, software-based fusion techniques were developed and introduced to clinical practice. These software fusion techniques vary by vendor; however, generally follow some basic steps (Fig. 2) and enable a registration of the MR imaging and US images with varying operator control and refinement to localize lesions detected at MR

Table 1
Advantages and disadvantages of the different targeting approaches

		Advantages	Disadvantages
Fusion	Cognitive biopsy	Quick, office-based procedure No additional technology	Target lesions are not seen during biopsy Highly operator dependent Impossibility of reconciliation
	Software-assisted biopsy	Quick, office-based procedure Ease of performing concurrent systematic biopsy Potential superior image registration	High costs for acquiring technology Dependent on operator experience Multiple steps that may hinder registration accuracy
MR-guided in-bore biopsy		Direct visualization of target during biopsy Ability to confirm needle placement in the lesion Small number of cores Potential for super selective targeting of the most aggressive component of heterogenous lesions Precise targeting of small lesions in difficult to reach locations An option for patients with no rectal access	Higher cost Longer duration Limited availability No systematic sampling

imaging for targeted biopsy (**Fig. 3**). MR imaging–US registration can be performed using rigid or elastic registration. In rigid registration, rotational differences between MR imaging and US can be corrected; whereas, for elastic registration, differences related to the US itself (spatial deformation of the prostate) can be corrected. The differences between rigid and elastic registration in clinical practice may be small because a 2018 meta-analysis on the topic[16] did not note any significant difference in cancer detection comparing the 2 techniques. Registration of MR imaging and US images forms one component of the software fusion process, which also uses continuous tracking of the movement of the US probe during the procedure. Tracking of the US probe is typically performed through software, which uses 3D organ-based segmentation tracking, positional sensing encoders attached to a mechanical arm, or electromagnetic sensors.[17] Registration of MR imaging and US images forms one component of the software fusion process, which also uses continuous tracking of the movement of the US

probe during the procedure. Tracking of the US probe is typically performed through software, which uses 3D organ-based segmentation tracking, positional sensing encoders attached to a mechanical arm, or electromagnetic sensors.[17] Registration of MR imaging and US images forms one component of the software fusion process, which also uses continuous tracking of the movement of the US probe during the procedure. Tracking of the US probe is typically performed through software, which uses 3D organ-based segmentation tracking, positional sensing encoders attached to a mechanical arm, or electromagnetic sensors.[17]

Advantages of software fusion systems include many of the advantages of cognitive fusion (eg, the ability to perform concurrent systematic or template biopsy and relatively easy to use with minimal training); however, software fusion systems have the disadvantages of an initial purchasing cost of equipment, which may have limited or no use for other general US applications, and added time to the procedure, which depends on

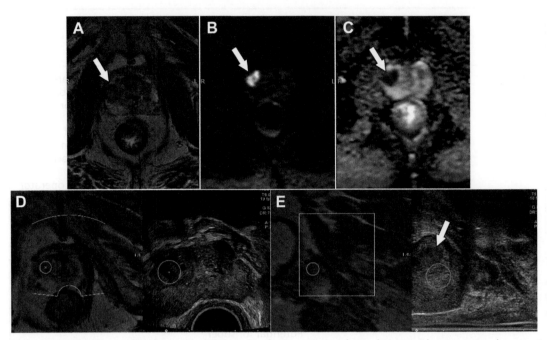

Fig. 1. Image visibility on US informed by MR imaging findings during fusion biopsy with transperineal access. A 66-year-old biopsy-naïve man with elevated PSA (7.5 ng/mL) underwent multiparametric MR imaging, which revealed a PI-RADS 5 lesion in the right anterior midgland, seen on the axial T2-weighted images (*A*), diffusion-weighted images (*B*), and ADC map (*C*). The patient was referred for a fusion MR imaging–TRUS biopsy with transperineal access. The previously acquired diagnostic MR imaging is dynamically reformatted to show a cross-section image corresponding to the real-time US image (*D*: axial view; *E*: sagittal view). The real-time TRUS images (*D, E*) are shown with an overlay of the suspicious lesion (*region of interest outlined in pink*) detected by the prebiopsy diagnostic MR imaging. Note the mismatch between the target projection (pink outline) and the hypoechoic lesion seen on the US image (*arrow* in *E*). The identification of the US-visible lesion on integration with the MR imaging findings improves the sampling accuracy. Biopsy revealed grade group 4 adenocarcinoma.

the type of software fusion and tracking. For institutions where biopsy is performed by operators who are unfamiliar with MR imaging, a learning curve exists[18] and a separate segmentation task may be added to the radiologist interpreting the MR imaging. Compared with cognitive fusion, however, software fusion provides the operator an opportunity to sample an MR imaging target, which may be totally occult on US and generally provides the operator with increased confidence regarding geographic targeting. Accuracy of fusion systems have been reported to range from 1.2 mm to 2.92 mm.[19,20]

MR-Guided In-Bore Biopsy

In this technique, the biopsy is performed directly while the patient is on the MR scanner using an MR-compatible device. After patient is positioned, a needle guide is placed in the rectum or juxtaposed to the perineal region, prebiopsy images are obtained to identify the target and inform the position changes required to align the needle guide and the lesion and tissue is sampled. **Fig. 3** further details the imaging elements of an in-bore biopsy procedure.

The main advantage is the direct visualization of the suspicious lesion, the needle guide, and the biopsy needle before, during, and after tissue sampling. This allows for precise sampling accuracy, real-time identification of unexpected suboptimal sampling and prompt operator response with adjustments to optimize subsequent additional samples.[21,22] This distinctive feature makes the method an excellent option, for example, to target very small lesions in challenging locations, such as thin peripheral, subcapsular lesions, which can be more susceptible to image misregistration in US-based biopsies. It also mitigates the potential impact of motion (gross patient motion, subtle and involuntary motion, or changes in the anatomy secondary to the introduction and repositioning of the biopsy devices)-related interference in the image registration across modalities. The acquisition

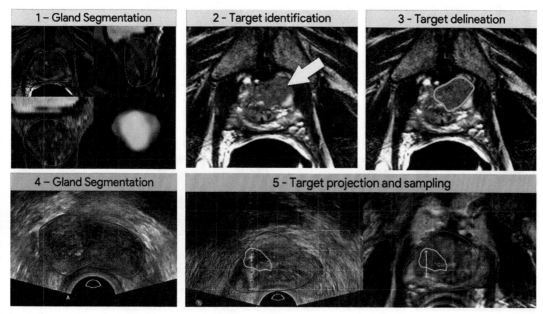

Fig. 2. Steps of a software-assisted fusion biopsy. A 69-year-old man with elevated PSA and systematic biopsy revealing small volume grade group 1 PCa. Before the confirmatory biopsy, the MR imaging is interpreted and processed, in this case revealing a PI-RADS 5 left anterior apex lesion. The boundaries of the prostate are outlined using a semiautomated segmentation tool (*1*). When a suspicious area is identified (*arrow* in *2*), it is delineated as a target (outlined in *3*). During US-guided (TRUS) biopsy, a volumetric US image of the prostate is acquired and used to again determine the boundaries the prostate (purple outline in *4*). This data set enables registration of images across the modalities, allowing to project the MR imaging-visible lesion on the US screen (green outline in *5*). Many fusion systems provide a reformatted MR image (*bottom right*) equivalent to the real-time US image obtained during the examination. Biopsy revealed grade group 3 PCa.

of MR images with excellent anatomic display and soft tissue contrast during the procedure provides other less-known advantages over the more traditional US guidance. By being able to properly show the relevant anatomy along with the interventional instrument, in-bore biopsies can be applied to a broader range of clinical scenarios. For example, suspected recurrent local PCa recurrence in the prostatectomy bed or changes in the prostate architecture secondary to previous procedures (eg, focal therapy) may preclude accurate gland segmentation on MR imaging and US and thus compromise the precision of MR imaging-US imaging registration. Suspicious lesions can be best seen with MR imaging in these scenarios and targeted with the in-bore method. In addition, at our institution, we have also achieved targeting of regional metastatic disease in selected cases. Disadvantages of in-bore biopsies include higher cost, access to MR imaging, and longer procedure time. In-bore biopsies also typically require the use of conscious sedation, which requires the use of adequately trained staff and patient monitoring equipment further increasing procedure time and potentially limiting access. Use of US before MR imaging to perform nerve block or use of intrarectal US gel for analgesia could also be trialed.[23] In-bore MR imaging-guided biopsies require expertise in the interpretation of prostate MR imaging to ensure accurate targeting because the images acquired during the procedure may not be of comparable quality and do not conform to standard planes familiar to the nonexpert radiologist and so, in general, are typically performed by experienced radiologists. Moreover, because systematic sampling is not routinely performed during in-bore biopsies, MR imaging-invisible lesions would be missed with this approach.

Comparison of the Targeting Accuracy of the Different Techniques

There are conflicting data in the literature regarding which targeting technique is the most precise. The FUTURE trial,[24] for example, did not reveal a significant difference in cancer detection rates among the 3 techniques available. Despite intuitive expectations that software-assisted fusion would be more accurate than cognitive fusion, particularly for lesions that are not well seen on US, there is paucity of evidence to support this observation.[25] Of 9 studies comparing these 2 US-based fusion

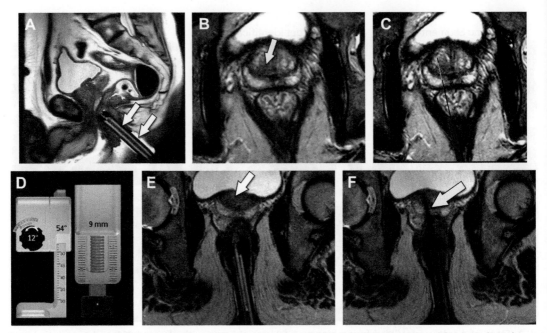

Fig. 3. Imaging steps of an in-bore biopsy. A 64-year-old patient with elevated PSA, referred for an in-bore biopsy after a negative MR imaging–TRUS fusion biopsy of a PI-RADS 4 lesion. After localizer images, the in-bore MR-guided biopsy begins with sagittal T2W images (A) to assess the location of the needle guide (*arrows* in A). Then, axial T2W images (B) are obtained and correlated with the prebiopsy diagnostic MR imaging examination to identify the suspicious region; in this case a 13-mm PI-RADS 4 lesion in the right midgland posterior transition zone (*arrow* in B). After the system has been calibrated and the target (*green region of interest* in C) chosen, the system proposes changes to the needle guide position coordinates (D). After these changes are made, prefiring axial oblique T2W images along the long axis of the needle guide (E) are obtained to determine the proper alignment between the needle guide and the lesion (*arrow* in E). After needle is placed and the biopsy gun is fired, images are obtained (F) to confirm that the needle (*arrow* in F) has properly sampled the region of interest. Biopsy revealed grade group 2 PCa.

approaches,[26–34] most did not show a significant difference while some[26,28–31,33] showed a higher cancer-detection rate with software-assisted fusion compared with cognitive fusion. This superiority appeared more relevant in men with small lesions[28,33] or lesions in the anterior gland.[26,28,29] Comparisons between sampling accuracy of in-bore versus software-assisted fusion biopsies also have conflicting data. A randomized study[35] did not reveal a significant difference in cancer detection rates between these 2 techniques. Conversely, some studies have shown higher detection of clinically significant cancers,[22,36–38] a stronger concordance between preoperative and postoperative cancer grade,[39] and a higher per-core percentage of cancer[40] assessed by in-bore biopsies compared with MR imaging–TRUS fusion biopsies, suggesting a potential improved sampling accuracy with the in-bore approach.

Transrectal Versus Transperineal Access

Both transrectal and transperineal needle biopsy routes can be pursued in the office setting for US-guided biopsy using local analgesia and both can be performed using any of the 3 targeting strategies previously discussed. Some institutions, however, prefer to perform transperineal biopsies under general anesthesia or with conscious sedation in a hospital setting. Additionally, it should be noted that in-bore biopsies can be performed using a transgluteal route, which can be advantageous in men without rectal access.

Both transrectal and transperineal US-based techniques require insertion of an US probe in the rectum, with the transrectal needle approach using an end-fire probe and the transperineal needle approach using 2 side-fire high-frequency and curvilinear arrays. In the transrectal approach, the biopsy needle is mounted to the transrectal US probe and follows an oblique path along the probe through the rectal wall and into the prostate. Transrectal needle biopsy is more familiar to most operators, is fast, less expensive, and generally well tolerated by patients.[41] The main drawback of the transrectal approach is urinary sepsis. Infection rates related to transrectal prostate biopsy range from 0.7% to 7.0%[42]; moreover,

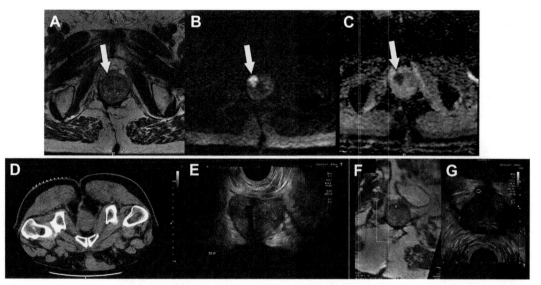

Fig. 4. Transperineal US-guided biopsy in a patient without the rectum. A 54-year-old man after abdominoperineal resection for colorectal cancer with increasing PSA. Multiparametric MR imaging revealed a PI-RADS 5 lesion in the right anterior transition zone, seen on the axial T2-weighted images (*A*), diffusion-weighted images (*B*), and ADC map (*C*). The patient was referred for a CT-guided prostate biopsy (*D*), and biopsy was negative for PCa. Second attempt with transperineal access was achieved by placing endocavitary probe into the perineal fossa (*E*) and successfully using the software-assisted fusion (*F, G*). The real-time US image (*G*) is shown with an overlay of the suspicious lesion (*region of interest outlined in pink*) detected by the prebiopsy diagnostic MR imaging. Biopsy revealed grade group 2 PCa.

prophylactic use of preprocedural antibiotics including fluoroquinolones are undesirable and may lead to increased bacterial resistance.

Increasingly, the transperineal needle approach is becoming more recognized as a potential alternative to transrectal needle biopsy due to its substantially lower, near zero percent, infection rate.[43] With transperineal biopsy, the biopsy needle traverses through the perineal body following a direct path into the prostate gland, avoiding the rectum entirely. The transperineal biopsy can be performed "free-hand" or mounted onto the probe using a needle-guide to assist operators. A brachytherapy grid can also be used to assist users but is not mandatory. Due to low-infection rates, preprocedural antibiotic coverage can be reduced to a single dose of a first-generation cephalosporin (or sulphonamide if allergic)[43] and more recently, centers have begun to abandon preprocedural antibiotic coverage entirely.[44] Drawbacks of the transperineal biopsy relate mainly to increased procedural time and increased procedural pain scores,[45] the latter historically requiring that the procedure be performed with sedation, compared with the transrectal needle approach. Our experience is that although the transperineal needle biopsy procedure time is longer compared with the transrectal needle

biopsy, the difference can be minimized with experience and will become less significant in patients in whom only targeted biopsy or targeted + focal saturation biopsies are performed. Other complications including rectal bleeding, urinary retention, and hematuria have varied reported rates for both transrectal and transperineal needle biopsy; however, in a 2019 meta-analysis were shown to be lower or comparable using transperineal biopsy.[45] Yield of targeted biopsy comparing transrectal and transperineal fusion prostate biopsy is an area under active investigation.

Biopsy Template

An ongoing debate in the field of prostate biopsy is the ideal number and distribution of cores obtained during a targeted US-based biopsy. There is no consensus regarding eliminating, keeping, or modifying the concomitant systematic sampling. In general, however, the biopsy strategy includes at least 2 core biopsies from the target and, in some cases, a higher number (eg, 4 or 5). In one study, the first 2 core biopsies had the highest cancer yield, although in ~10% of patients clinically significant cancer was detected only in the third or fourth biopsy.[46] In another study, increasing the number of samples per index lesion

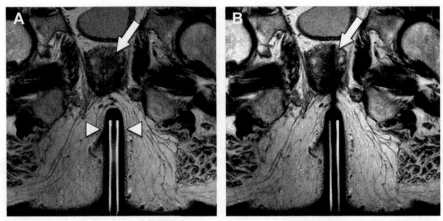

Fig. 5. Transperineal in-bore biopsy in a patient without the rectum. A 83-year-old patient with a history of abdominoperineal resection for colorectal cancer, elevated PSA, and prebiopsy diagnostic MR imaging (not shown) revealing a PI-RADS 5 lesion in the left anterior apex of the prostate. Prefiring axial oblique T2W image (*A*) reveals the optimal alignment of the needle guide (*arrowhead*) and the suspicious lesion (*arrow*), and postfiring repeat imaging confirms adequate lesion sampling. Biopsy revealed grade group 2 PCa.

from 1 to 3 and from 3 to 5 led to higher detection of clinically significant cancers (6.4% and 2.4%, respectively).[47] We suggest obtaining a higher number of core biopsies and oversampling the vicinity of the target (ie, penumbra) [as has been suggested[48]] particularly for instances of initially negative ISUP Grade Group 1 PCa in a patient with high clinical suspicion of clinically significant cancer, transition zone lesions or where the biopsy target is not well seen on US. The low yield of contralateral systematic sampling is increasingly reported in the literature[49] and motivated some institutions to adopt a modified template to include regional sampling near the target in lieu of the contralateral sampling.[50]

Because of time constraints, systematic sampling usually is not performed during in-bore biopsies, and few studies have assessed the incremental value of additional cores in that approach. In one study,[51] clinically significant PCa not detected by preceding cores was detected by the second, third, fourth, and fifth cores in 6%, 4%, 1%, and 0% of the lesions, respectively.

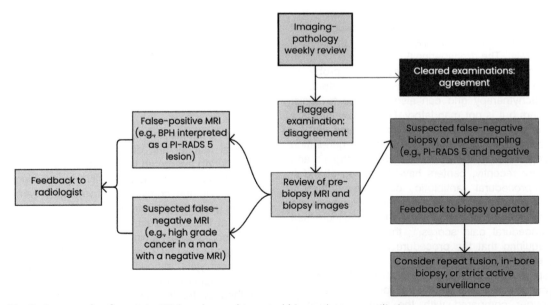

Fig. 6. An example of prostate MR imaging and targeted biopsy data reconciliation.

Patients Without Rectal Access

A challenging clinical scenario is presented by men with elevated prostate-specific antigen (PSA) serum levels and without rectal access.[52] In these patients, although possible, US-guided biopsies are difficult due to the limited acoustic window offered by the transperineal US guidance. Authors have had some success in sampling the prostate using the transrectal US probe applied to the prostate fossa where visualization of the prostate can be achieved and even software fusion attempted (**Fig. 4**). The sampling accuracy of the in-bore MR-guided approach is not negatively impacted, and both transperineal (**Fig. 5**) and transgluteal routes can be used.

IMAGING-PATHOLOGY RECONCILIATION

Accurate targeted biopsies require precise placement of the biopsy needle into the region of interest, and management of patients with negative-targeted biopsy can be a challenging clinical scenario. Therefore, a process of data reconciliation after biopsy to identify potential misses related to inadequate lesion sampling or image misinterpretation is of paramount importance.[53] Some institutions have already successfully implemented multidisciplinary team discussion of biopsy results and imaging findings (**Fig. 6**). Options include immediate repeat biopsy or PSA surveillance (with or without a repeat MR imaging or biopsy).[53–55] Studies reviewing repeat (ie, second-round) MR imaging-targeted biopsy have reported a wide range in clinically significant PCa detection. A minisystematic review on the topic in 2022 including 9 studies and 485 patients reported any PCa and clinically significant PCa detection percentages of 0% to 80% and 0% to 20% for PI-RADS 3 lesions and 15% to 86% and 8% to 57% for PI-RADS 4 or 5 lesions.[56] Clinical or imaging markers to identify which lesions harbor undiagnosed PCa and which do not and, thus, which patients should undergo repeat biopsy are lacking. In one study, growth of a lesion on MR imaging was the only significant predictor of subsequent PCa detection at second-round biopsy,[54] and in another study, persistence of PIRADS 4 or 5 at repeat MR imaging was a predictor of cancer on repeat biopsy.[57]

SUMMARY

Different imaging modalities, image registration techniques, and anatomic accesses can be used to target a suspicious region identified within the prostate. It is important for radiologists to be familiar with the principles, advantages, and disadvantages of these various approaches.

Currently, it seems premature to state definitively which strategy is better. More research is needed to explore factors that providers and patients must consider, including availability, learning curve, reproducibility, and cost.

CLINICS CARE POINTS

- The use of risk assessment with MRI before biopsy and MRI-targeted biopsy is superior to standard transrectal ultrasound-guided biopsy in men at clinical risk for prostate cancer.

DISCLOSURE

The authors have no commercial or financial conflicts of interest or funding source related to this submission.

REFERENCES

1. Shariat SF, Roehrborn CG. Using biopsy to detect prostate cancer. Rev Urol 2008;10(4):262–80.
2. Chun FK, Karakiewicz PI, Briganti A, et al. Prostate cancer nomograms: an update. Eur Urol 2006; 50(5):914–26 [discussion: 926].
3. Ross PL, Scardino PT, Kattan MW. A catalog of prostate cancer nomograms. J Urol 2001;165(5):1562–8.
4. Ahmed HU, El-Shater Bosaily A, Brown LC, et al. Diagnostic accuracy of multi-parametric MRI and TRUS biopsy in prostate cancer (PROMIS): a paired validating confirmatory study. Lancet 2017;389(10071):815–22.
5. Prostate Imaging and Reporting and Data System: Version 2.1. American College of Radiology; 2019. Available at: https://www.acr.org/-/media/ACR/Files/RADS/PI-RADS/PIRADS-V2-1.pdf. Accessed 6 11, 2021.
6. Kasivisvanathan V, Rannikko AS, Borghi M, et al. MRI-targeted or standard biopsy for prostate-cancer diagnosis. N Engl J Med 2018;378(19): 1767–77.
7. Hugosson J, Mansson M, Wallstrom J, et al. Prostate cancer screening with PSA and MRI followed by targeted biopsy only. N Engl J Med 2022;387(23): 2126–37.
8. Bjurlin MA, Carroll PR, Eggener S, et al. Update of the standard operating procedure on the use of multiparametric magnetic resonance imaging for the diagnosis, staging and management of prostate cancer. J Urol 2020;203(4):706–12.
9. Rosenkrantz AB, Hemingway J, Hughes DR, et al. Evolving use of prebiopsy prostate magnetic

resonance imaging in the medicare population. J Urol 2018;200(1):89–94.

10. Kim SP, Karnes RJ, Mwangi R, et al. Contemporary trends in magnetic resonance imaging at the time of prostate biopsy: results from a large private insurance database. Eur Urol Focus 2021;7(1):86–94.

11. Costa DN, Pedrosa I, Donato F Jr, et al. MR imaging-transrectal US fusion for targeted prostate biopsies: implications for diagnosis and clinical management. Radiographics 2015;35(3):696–708.

12. Padhani AR, Schoots IG, Giannarini G. Re: targeted prostate biopsy: umbra, penumbra, and value of perilesional sampling. Eur Urol 2022;82(1):143–4.

13. John S, Cooper S, Breau RH, et al. Multiparametric magnetic resonance imaging - Transrectal ultrasound-guided cognitive fusion biopsy of the prostate: clinically significant cancer detection rates stratified by the prostate imaging and data reporting system version 2 assessment category. Can Urol Assoc J 2018;12(12):401–6.

14. van de Ven WJ, Sedelaar JP, van der Leest MM, et al. Visibility of prostate cancer on transrectal ultrasound during fusion with multiparametric magnetic resonance imaging for biopsy. Clin Imaging 2016; 40(4):745–50.

15. Klotz L, Lughezzani G, Maffei D, et al. Comparison of micro-ultrasound and multiparametric magnetic resonance imaging for prostate cancer: a multicenter, prospective analysis. Can Urol Assoc J 2021;15(1):E11–6.

16. Venderink W, de Rooij M, Sedelaar JPM, et al. Elastic versus rigid image registration in magnetic resonance imaging-transrectal ultrasound fusion prostate biopsy: a systematic review and meta-analysis. Eur Urol Focus 2018;4(2):219–27.

17. Verma S, Choyke PL, Eberhardt SC, et al. The current state of MR imaging-targeted biopsy techniques for detection of prostate cancer. Radiology 2017;285(2):343–56.

18. Meng X, Rosenkrantz AB, Huang R, et al. The institutional learning curve of magnetic resonance imaging-ultrasound fusion targeted prostate biopsy: temporal improvements in cancer detection in 4 years. J Urol 2018;200(5):1022–9.

19. Xu S, Kruecker J, Turkbey B, et al. Real-time MRI-TRUS fusion for guidance of targeted prostate biopsies. Comput Aided Surg 2008;13(5):255–64.

20. Natarajan S, Marks LS, Margolis DJ, et al. Clinical application of a 3D ultrasound-guided prostate biopsy system. Urol Oncol 2011;29(3):334–42.

21. Giganti F, Moore CM. A critical comparison of techniques for MRI-targeted biopsy of the prostate. Transl Androl Urol 2017;6(3):432–43.

22. Costa DN, Goldberg K, Leon AD, et al. Magnetic resonance imaging-guided in-bore and magnetic resonance imaging-transrectal ultrasound fusion targeted prostate biopsies: an adjusted comparison of clinically significant prostate cancer detection rate. Eur Urol Oncol 2019;2(4):397–404.

23. Quentin M, Arsov C, Ullrich T, et al. Comparison of analgesic techniques in MRI-guided in-bore prostate biopsy. Eur Radiol 2019;29(12):6965–70.

24. Wegelin O, Exterkate L, van der Leest M, et al. The FUTURE trial: a multicenter randomised controlled trial on target biopsy techniques based on magnetic resonance imaging in the diagnosis of prostate cancer in patients with prior negative biopsies. Eur Urol 2019;75(4):582–90.

25. Wegelin O, van Melick HHE, Hooft L, et al. Comparing three different techniques for magnetic resonance imaging-targeted prostate biopsies: a systematic review of in-bore versus magnetic resonance imaging-transrectal ultrasound fusion versus cognitive registration. is there a preferred technique? Eur Urol 2017;71(4):517–31.

26. Puech P, Rouviere O, Renard-Penna R, et al. Prostate cancer diagnosis: multiparametric MR-targeted biopsy with cognitive and transrectal US-MR fusion guidance versus systematic biopsy–prospective multicenter study. Comparative study multicenter study research support, Non-U.S. Gov't. Radiology 2013;268(2):461–9.

27. Delongchamps NB, Peyromaure M, Schull A, et al. Prebiopsy magnetic resonance imaging and prostate cancer detection: comparison of random and targeted biopsies. J Urol 2013;189(2):493–9.

28. Wysock JS, Rosenkrantz AB, Huang WC, et al. A prospective, blinded comparison of magnetic resonance (MR) imaging-ultrasound fusion and visual estimation in the performance of MR-targeted prostate biopsy: the PROFUS trial. Eur Urol 2014;66(2):343–51.

29. Lee DJ, Recabal P, Sjoberg DD, et al. Comparative effectiveness of targeted prostate biopsy using magnetic resonance imaging ultrasound fusion software and visual targeting: a prospective study. J Urol 2016;196(3):697–702.

30. Hamid S, Donaldson IA, Hu Y, et al. The smarttarget biopsy trial: a prospective, within-person randomised, blinded trial comparing the accuracy of visual-registration and magnetic resonance imaging/ultrasound image-fusion targeted biopsies for prostate cancer risk stratification. Eur Urol 2019;75(5):733–40.

31. Khoo CC, Eldred-Evans D, Peters M, et al. A comparison of prostate cancer detection between visual estimation (cognitive registration) and image fusion (software registration) targeted transperineal prostate biopsy. J Urol 2021;205(4):1075–81.

32. Cool DW, Zhang X, Romagnoli C, et al. Evaluation of MRI-TRUS fusion versus cognitive registration accuracy for MRI-targeted, TRUS-guided prostate biopsy. AJR Am J Roentgenol 2015;204(1):83–91.

33. Yamada Y, Shiraishi T, Ueno A, et al. Magnetic resonance imaging-guided targeted prostate biopsy: comparison between computer-software-based

fusion versus cognitive fusion technique in biopsy-naive patients. Int J Urol 2020;27(1):67–71.

34. Stabile A, Dell'Oglio P, Gandaglia G, et al. Not all multiparametric magnetic resonance imaging-targeted biopsies are equal: the impact of the type of approach and operator expertise on the detection of clinically significant prostate cancer. Eur Urol Oncol 2018;1(2):120–8.

35. Arsov C, Rabenalt R, Blondin D, et al. Prospective randomized trial comparing magnetic resonance imaging (MRI)-guided in-bore biopsy to MRI-ultrasound fusion and transrectal ultrasound-guided prostate biopsy in patients with prior negative biopsies. Eur Urol 2015;68(4):713–20.

36. Ramos F, Korets R, Fleishman A, et al. Comparative effectiveness of magnetic resonance imaging-ultrasound fusion versus in-bore magnetic resonance imaging-targeted prostate biopsy. Urology 2023;171:164–71.

37. Venderink W, van der Leest M, van Luijtelaar A, et al. Retrospective comparison of direct in-bore magnetic resonance imaging (MRI)-guided biopsy and fusion-guided biopsy in patients with MRI lesions which are likely or highly likely to be clinically significant prostate cancer. World J Urol 2017;35(12):1849–55.

38. Prince M, Foster BR, Kaempf A, et al. In-bore versus fusion MRI-targeted biopsy of PI-RADS category 4 and 5 lesions: a retrospective comparative analysis using propensity score weighting. AJR Am J Roentgenol 2021;217(5):1123–30.

39. Costa DN, Cai Q, Xi Y, et al. Gleason grade group concordance between preoperative targeted biopsy and radical prostatectomy histopathologic analysis: a comparison between in-bore MRI-guided and MRI-transrectal US fusion prostate biopsies. Radiol Imaging Cancer 2021;3(2):e200123.

40. Del Monte M, Cipollari S, Del Giudice F, et al. MRI-directed biopsy for primary detection of prostate cancer in a population of 223 men: MRI In-Bore vs MRI-transrectal ultrasound fusion-targeted techniques. Br J Radiol 2022;95(1131):20210528.

41. Grummet J, Pepdjonovic L, Huang S, et al. Transperineal vs. transrectal biopsy in MRI targeting. Transl Androl Urol 2017;6(3):368–75.

42. Liss MA, Ehdaie B, Loeb S, et al. An update of the american urological association white paper on the prevention and treatment of the more common complications related to prostate biopsy. J Urol 2017;198(2):329–34.

43. Stefanova V, Buckley R, Flax S, et al. Transperineal prostate biopsies using local anesthesia: experience with 1,287 patients. Prostate cancer detection rate, complications and patient tolerability. J Urol 2019;201(6):1121–6.

44. Gunzel K, Magheli A, Baco E, et al. Infection rate and complications after 621 transperineal MRI-TRUS fusion biopsies in local anesthesia without standard antibiotic prophylaxis. World J Urol 2021;39(10):3861–6.

45. Xiang J, Yan H, Li J, et al. Transperineal versus transrectal prostate biopsy in the diagnosis of prostate cancer: a systematic review and meta-analysis. World J Surg Oncol 2019;17(1):31.

46. Kenigsberg AP, Renson A, Rosenkrantz AB, et al. Optimizing the number of cores targeted during prostate magnetic resonance imaging fusion target biopsy. Eur Urol Oncol 2018;1(5):418–25.

47. Zhang M, Milot L, Khalvati F, et al. Value of increasing biopsy cores per target with cognitive MRI-targeted transrectal US prostate biopsy. Radiology 2019;291(1):83–9.

48. Tschirdewahn S, Wiesenfarth M, Bonekamp D, et al. Detection of significant prostate cancer using target saturation in transperineal magnetic resonance imaging/transrectal ultrasonography-fusion biopsy. Eur Urol Focus 2021;7(6):1300–7.

49. Freifeld Y, Xi Y, Passoni N, et al. Optimal sampling scheme in men with abnormal multiparametric MRI undergoing MRI-TRUS fusion prostate biopsy. Urol Oncol 2019;37(1):57–62.

50. Hagens MJ, Fernandez Salamanca M, Padhani AR, et al. Diagnostic performance of a magnetic resonance imaging-directed targeted plus regional biopsy approach in prostate cancer diagnosis: a systematic review and meta-analysis. Eur Urol Open Sci 2022;40:95–103.

51. Subramanian N, Recchimuzzi DZ, Xi Y, et al. Impact of the number of cores on the prostate cancer detection rate in men undergoing in-bore magnetic resonance imaging-guided targeted biopsies. J Comput Assist Tomogr 2021;45(2):203–9.

52. Costa DN, Menard A, Moore C, et al. The global reading room: MRI-targeted prostate biopsy after proctocolectomy. AJR Am J Roentgenol 2022. https://doi.org/10.2214/AJR.22.27619.

53. Costa DN, Kay FU, Pedrosa I, et al. An initial negative round of targeted biopsies in men with highly suspicious multiparametric magnetic resonance findings does not exclude clinically significant prostate cancer-Preliminary experience. Urol Oncol 2017;35(4):149 e15–21.

54. Chelluri R, Kilchevsky A, George AK, et al. Prostate cancer diagnosis on repeat magnetic resonance imaging-transrectal ultrasound fusion biopsy of benign lesions: recommendations for repeat sampling. J Urol 2016;196(1):62–7.

55. Montorsi F, Stabile A, Gandaglia G, et al. Followup of men with PI-RADS 4 or 5 abnormality on prostate magnetic resonance imaging and nonmalignant

pathological findings on initial targeted prostate biopsy. Letter. J Urol 2021;206(5):1335.

56. Grivas N, Lardas M, Espinos EL, et al. Prostate cancer detection percentages of repeat biopsy in patients with positive multiparametric magnetic resonance imaging (prostate imaging reporting and data system/likert 3-5) and negative initial biopsy. A mini systematic review. Eur Urol 2022; 82(5):452–7.

57. Meng X, Chao B, Chen F, et al. Followup of men with PI-RADS(TM) 4 or 5 abnormality on prostate magnetic resonance imaging and nonmalignant pathological findings on initial targeted prostate biopsy. Reply. J Urol 2021;205(5):1528–9.

MR Imaging-Guided Prostate Cancer Therapies

Daniel A. Adamo, MD[a], Bernadette Marie Greenwood, MSc, RT(R)(MR)(ARRT)[b],
Pejman Ghanouni, MD, PhD[c], Sandeep Arora, MBBS[d],*

KEYWORDS

- Prostate cancer • MR imaging-guided • Focal therapy • Cryoablation • Laser ablation • TULSA
- HIFU

KEY POINTS

- MR imaging-guided interventions are a growing therapeutic option for men diagnosed with prostate cancer.
- Proper patient selection is the key in evaluation for focal therapy, with ideal candidates having low- to intermediate-risk disease, good life expectancy, and concordance of an MR imaging visible lesion with pathologic mapping.
- Ablative treatment options include cryoablation, laser ablation, and therapeutic ultrasound.
- MR imaging-guidance provides exceptional soft tissue resolution of the growing iceball during cryoablation.
- Laser ablation and high intensity ultrasound ablation take advantage of MR thermometry for temperature mapping. High intensity ultrasound can be delivered transrectally or transurethrally for ablative therapy.

INTRODUCTION TO MR IMAGING-GUIDED PROSTATE THERAPY

Treatment of men with low-risk and intermediate-risk prostate cancer (PCa) is controversial. Traditional therapies such as surgery and radiation therapy (RT) have significant side-effect profiles, as well as varying rates of biochemical recurrence.[1] Focal therapy (FT) for prostate cancer has become an emerging alternative for the treatment of localized disease due to the lower rates of side effects compared with traditional treatments. Recent advances have established a clear role for MR imaging in the diagnosis of PCa.[2,3] However, the role of MR imaging in PCa therapy is less well delineated, but MR imaging-guided therapies continue to gain traction.

The purpose of this review is to describe the current state of MR imaging-guided therapies, focusing on our experience with MR imaging-guided cryoablation (CA), laser ablation, transrectal high intensity focused ultrasound (HIFU) and transurethral high-intensity-directional ultrasound(HIDU). **Table 1** summarizes the four different treatment modalities. General anesthesia is typically preferred for all modalities, as patient motion can cause significant imaging artifact with MR imaging monitoring. Laser ablation uses very fast heating and can often be performed under conscious sedation and local anesthesia. The choice of treatment modality is based on operator comfort, patient preference, equipment availability, and considerations as listed in **Table1**.

a Mayo Clinic, 200 1st Street Southwest, Rochester, MN 55905, USA; b Halo Diagnostics, 74785 Hwy 111, Suite 101, Indian Wells, CA 92210, USA; c Department of Radiology, Stanford University, Lucas Center for Imaging, 1201 Welch Road, Room P267, Stanford, CA 94305, USA; d Yale University School of Medicine, Department of Radiology & Biomedical Imaging, 330 Cedar Street, TE-2, PO Box 208042, New Haven, CT 06520-8042, USA
* Corresponding author.
E-mail address: sandeep.arora@yale.edu

Radiol Clin N Am 62 (2024) 121–133
https://doi.org/10.1016/j.rcl.2023.06.012

Table 1
A comparative table of the four described treatment modalities. Real-time MR imaging monitoring is performed during all procedures

Procedure (In-Bore MR imaging)	Route/Method of Delivery	Energy	Ablation Extent	Monitoring	Safety Features	Limitations/ Precautions
Cryoablation	Transperineal or Transrectal insertion of cryoprobes in to the prostate	Cold argon gas to freeze tissue	Whole-gland, partial gland, focal	Iceball visualization	Visualization of ice growth during freeze, urethral warming, temperature monitoring, active heating and injection of protective media, widening of recto prostatic space with injectables for posterior lesions	1. Narrow space of pelvis may make it hard to control spherical iceball edge to avoid critical structures while delivering adequate dose to the tumor—safety precautions may help mitigate 2. Multiple rectal punctures for multiple probes
Laser ablation	Transperineal or Transrectal insertion of laser fibers in to the prostate	LASER to heat tissue	Focal, partial gland	MR thermometry/ dosimetry	Fluid cooling system: only active tip is light-emitting, safety cursors with automatic shut off placed at critical structures, continuous bladder irrigation for tumors near bladder neck, widening of recto prostatic space with injectables for posterior lesions	1. Charring/carbonization of tissue may happen with treatments >2 min. Charring prevents the effective transfer of heat to more peripheral tissue, thereby limiting the effective size of the ablation zone 2. Overheating above 90°C and inadequate cooling between ablations can also cause carbonization 3. Multiple rectal punctures may be needed with the same sheath

HIFU	Intraluminal placement of therapeutic ultrasound transducer in rectum, delivery of energy through the rectal wall to prostate	High-intensity-focused ultrasound to heat tissue	Focal, partial gland	MR thermometry/dosimetry	Rectal cooling, Foley catheter, critical structures such as anterior rectal wall and prostate capsule are contoured and actively monitored	1. ≥2 mm calcification within 5 mm of the rectal wall or calcification measuring ≥5mm located between the target and the transducer 2. Treatment margin >4 cm from rectal wall or >focal length of transducer which is >6 cm
HIDU	Intraluminal placement of urinary applicator with therapeutic ultrasound elements built in the urethra, delivery of energy through the urethra in to the prostate	High-intensity directional ultrasound to heat tissue	Whole-gland, partial gland, focal	MR thermometry/dosimetry	Urethral and rectal cooling, T(edge) at capsule set at 55° Celsius—which is neuroprotective, conformal heating	1. >3 cm treatment margin from urethra 2. Calcification >3 mm between urethral and tumor may be a contraindication 3. 2–3 mm of prostate tissue adjacent to urethra does not get adequate dose as urethra is actively cooled

Abbreviation: HIFU, high-intensity focused ultrasound; HIDU, high-intensity directional ultrasound.

Cryoablation

Percutaneous CA of the prostate gland was first described in 1966, with the first whole-gland CA with ultrasound guidance described in 1993, and first recognized as a therapeutic option for PCa by the American Urological Association (AUA) in 1996.[4–6] Initially, CA predominantly used ultrasound guidance; however, this technique has several limitations, notably in monitoring the growing iceball. Gangi and colleagues described the first MR imaging-guided CA in 2011.[7] Recent advances in both CA devices as well as increasing in-bore MR capabilities have made MR imaging-guided CA an increasingly viable therapeutic option. The benefits of MR imaging guidance include exquisite visualization of the growing iceball, which is solid and has ultra-short T1 and T2 relaxation times, resulting in exceptional contrast compared with surrounding soft tissue structures.[8] In addition, guidance with MR imaging allows for imaging in multiple planes, which is extremely valuable when ablating in the confined space of the pelvis with adjacent critical structures, including the rectum and ureters.

Procedural technique

The proper placement of cryoprobes is naturally critical to ensure complete coverage of the tumor as well as avoidance of critical neighboring structures. Needle guidance may be accomplished with the use of various targeting systems, which often use a grid system, and some of which include robotic guidance.[9] Other interventional MR imaging systems have the capability for real-time MR imaging guidance allowing for precise needle placement.[10] Needle placement may be performed transrectal or transperineal, with the transperineal approach becoming more commonly used due to lower risk of infection relative to a transrectal approach. At an author's institution (DAA), the procedure is done under general anesthesia in the interventional MR imaging suite containing a 1.5 T magnet, with the patients placed in the semi-frog-legged position. A grid is placed against the patient's perineum, and diagnostic MR images are obtained. Using the grid as a guide, multiple cryo-needles are placed into the prostate gland in a manner to cover the entire tumor with good margins of iceball coverage. Once the needles are in place, a dual-lumen urethral warmer is placed. Saline is continually instilled through the urethral warmer for thermal protection to prevent urethral sloughing. Sequential real-time axial T2-weighted or proton density images are obtained to monitor the iceball growth to ensure adequate tumoral coverage as well as monitor for growth near critical structures (Fig. 1). Depending on the type and vendor of cryoprobes used, the solid hypointense iceball represents a spectrum of temperatures with typical isothermic data suggesting temperatures of $-40°C$ near the center and $0°C$ at the periphery. The lethal thermal effect is a function of both time and temperature, though lethal ablation typically occurs very rapidly at temperatures below $-30°C$.[11] A minimum of 5 mm margin of iceball coverage beyond the expected margin of the tumor is suggested as best practice for proper coverage.[12] Typically, three separate "freeze–thaw" cycles are performed, with the cryoprobes actively thawed during the thawing period. The duration of each freeze cycle is variable but typically lasts 8 to 10 minutes.

During active freezing, iceball growth is sequentially monitored for avoidance of adjacent critical structures. This includes monitoring the external urinary sphincter at the apex to preserve urinary continence, the ureters near the base and seminal vesicles, as well as the rectum posteriorly. Other techniques may be performed for thermal protection of these adjacent critical structures, most commonly saline hydro displacement of the rectum. If possible, the neurovascular bundle should be spared to preserve erectile function.

Patients are typically discharged the same day with a Foley catheter in place. After a successful voiding trial, the Foley catheter is removed 2 to 3 days postprocedure. After the procedure, patients are followed with serum prostate-specific antigen (PSA) levels at 3- and 6-month postprocedure and with multiparametric MR (mpMR) imaging at 6 months.

Patient selection

Widespread screening with serum PSA has led to both overdiagnosis and overtreatment of prostate cancer, especially in patients with low-risk or favorable intermediate-risk disease. Although there are well-established guidelines for the treatment of high-risk disease, treatment of those with low- and favorable intermediate-risk disease is debated.[13] As such, a proper patient selection is critical when considering a patient for FT. Our institution requires consensus management at a multidisciplinary review performed in conjunction with urologists and often medical and radiation oncologists. An international Delphi consensus panel gave recommendations on patient selection for FT, notably concluding that patients should have a high-quality mpMR imaging, MR imaging-targeted biopsies with systemic biopsy, low- or intermediate-risk cancers with Gleason score $\leq$ 4 + 3, tumors less than 1.5 mL, good life expectancy, PSA De $\leq$ 1 ng/ml, among other factors.[14] Patients often opt for FT in hopes of avoiding the

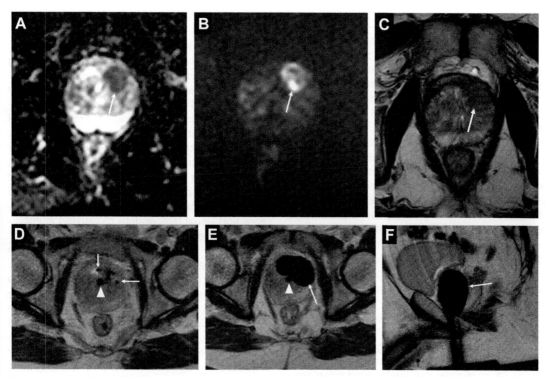

Fig. 1. Axial DWI (*b* = 1600) (*A*) images from a 69-year-old patient with biopsy-proven Gleason 3 + 4 adenocarcinoma demonstrating a focal hyperintense lesion in the left anterior transition with corresponding hypointensity on apparent diffusion coefficient (ADC) map (*B*) and hypointensity on the axial T2-weighted images (*C*). Initial axial proton density (PD)-weighted image (*D*) obtained during MR imaging-guided CA demonstrate cryo-probe placement (*arrows*) as well as placement of the urethral warmer (*arrowhead*). Subsequent axial (*E*) and sagittal (*F*) PD-weighted images demonstrate iceball growth with excellent coverage of the tumor.

untoward effects of whole gland therapies such as surgery and radiation, notably erectile dysfunction and urinary incontinence.

Outcomes and experience

As a relatively new technique, little is known about long-term outcomes of MR Imaging-guided CA for prostate cancer. A few of the early studies reported on oncologic outcomes for whole gland therapy, however, these studies were often small, retrospective, and had somewhat limited follow-up.[7,15] Although prostate cancer is often multifocal, the natural history and prognosis of the cancer are mainly dictated by the "index lesion," which tends to be the largest and highest-grade lesion.[16,17] Drawing on this principle, FT seeks to primarily target the index lesion, with preservation of the remaining prostate gland, thus minimizing untoward side effects and improving quality of life.[18] Several studies have demonstrated focal CA as a primary treatment, but these have largely relied on ultrasound guidance rather the MR imaging guidance.[19,20] Further data are needed to evaluate the long-term oncologic outcomes of MR imaging-guided CA as FT for primary PCa.

Although there is no consensus on the salvage treatment of recurrent PCa following RT, many patients often undergo androgen deprivation therapy (ADT).[21] ADT, however, carries a significant side effect profile, and patients often seek alternative therapies, including CA. Salvage CA after RT has shown promise in several studies; in a recent study, biochemical recurrence-free survival was achieved in 81% of who underwent salvage CA following RT.[22]

Robust data are also lacking regarding complications and side effects of CA, especially performed with MR imaging-guidance. Data from studies looking at ultrasound-guided whole-gland CA suggest modest complication rates, including a study by Roberts and colleagues, which showed that urinary incontinence occurred in 9.8%, and erectile dysfunction occurred in 20.1% of the patients, both of which are favorable compared with whole gland therapy such as radical prostatectomy.[23] As the procedural technique has been refined, the rate of erectile dysfunction has decreased compared with prior studies.[24] Data on complication rates from FT versus whole gland therapy is lacking, but intuitively FT would compare similarly or favorably.

MR Imaging-Guided Laser Ablation

Laser FT, also called focal laser ablation (FLA) or laser interstitial thermal therapy of prostate cancer, uses light energy harnessed at levels sufficient to induce tissue death. The acronym "laser" stands for light amplification by stimulated emission of radiation. Lasers have been used in medicine for decades for various applications, including ablation of bone, liver, kidney, and brain tissues.[25]

MR imaging-guided laser ablation is possible because raw MR imaging data used to create MR imaging images can also be used to measure phase shifts along a gradient and converted via Arrhenius modeling to generate temperature maps for near real-time updated thermometry. Proton resonance thermal mapping proton resonance frequency (PRF) exploits the measurement of water proton resonant frequency at a baseline reference and over time with change due to alterations in temperature.[26] **Fig. 2** illustrates a prostate thermal map, magnitude image, graph demonstrating temperature change over time and irreversible damage estimate. The irreversible damage estimate is the cumulative representation of tissue necrotization. It is worth mentioning that background noise, motion, and flow can create artifacts.

There are several commercially available laser fibers and planning platforms cleared by the Food and Drug Administration (FDA) for coagulation necrosis of soft tissue.[27,28] These devices operate between 980 and 1064 nm and are compatible with magnets of 1.5 and 3.0 T. The specifications of the fibers vary regarding the energy-emitting tip length of the fiber. This is important as it is a consideration during surgical planning to achieve the appropriate size and shape of ablative treatment based on the size, location, and geometry of the target tumor. Our experience has been with Visualase (Medtronic, Minneapolis, MN, USA) and Clinical Laserthermia AB (Lund, Sweden).

Visualase fibers are saline-cooled and available in 1 and 1.5 cm lengths of energy emitting tip, and the Clinical Laserthermia Systems (CLS) AB fibers are available in 1 mm radial, 2.5 cm and 1.5 cm energy emitting tips. The primary difference between Visualase fibers and CLS fibers is that the Visualase system has a cooling applicator into which the laser fiber is inserted before advancement into the tumor, which ensures cooling along the length of the fiber with the exception of the energy-emitting tip. The cooling pump must be run during each treatment when the Visualase is used, and the tubing must be free of any air bubbles. The system also requires the use of a titanium stiffener inside the applicator at the time of initial insertion and location confirmation. Once the location is

established, the stiffener is removed, and the laser fiber is placed. This process is repeated for each new puncture location.

The CLS fiber is "naked" and has no cooling applicator. It is inserted through an MR imaging-compatible cannula which is placed over a stylet and advanced to the target location. Once the tumor location is reached and confirmed with MR imaging, the stylet is replaced with the CLS fiber. The cannula and fiber can be retracted together for serial treatments along the length of a target, but the stylus must be replaced and reinserted for each new puncture. Because there is no fluid cooling system, a careful placement of safety cursors and visual temperature monitoring is important to prevent overheating and overtreatment.

The laser fiber connects to the laser via sub miniature version A (SMA) adapter and is run from the laser box outside the MR imaging scan room into the operative area, anchored to the floor with tape. If the cooled system is used, the pump remains outside the MR imaging scan room, and the length of tubing is taped to the floor along with the fiber to reach the patient. All computer equipment remains outside the MR imaging scan room.

At the time of tumor board, a multidisciplinary team determines which laser fiber should be used to achieve the best clinical outcome for the patient in terms of oncologic control and preservation of urologic and sexual function. Regardless of which fiber is chosen, the user has the ability to sculpt the area of desired coagulation necrosis while protecting vital structures with safety cursors, creating boundaries against structures such as the neurovascular bundles, rectal wall, and external urethral sphincter. The placement of the safety cursors limits temperature relative to the reference image so that if temperatures exceed a preset threshold of 45° C, the system shuts off automatically.[29]

Although these fibers can be used both transperineally and transrectally, our experience, having done the first-in-human treatment in May, 2010 (NCT 02243033),[30] is limited exclusively to transrectal delivery using the Philips Invivo DynaTRIM device (Philips, Best, the Netherlands) with DynaLOC software (Philips, Best, the Netherlands) for planning and MR imaging-compatible instruments.

Before the procedure, depending on the location of the tumor, a 16 French three-way catheter may be placed by a urologist for continuous bladder irrigation specifically for apical tumors. The patient then lies prone on the MR imaging table, and lidocaine jelly is administered transrectally. A transrectal needle guide is placed in the rectum and attached to a positioner, DynaTRIM.

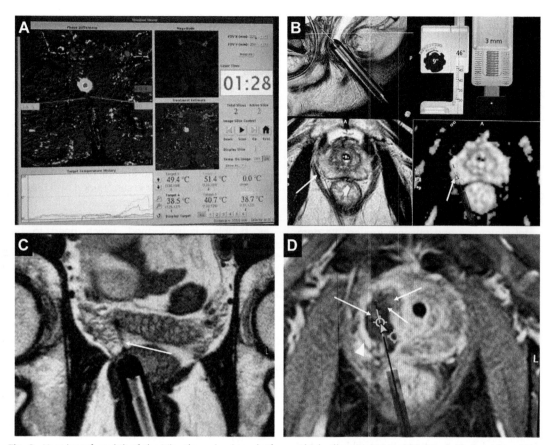

Fig. 2. User interface (*A*) of the Visualase viewing platform which allows intraoperative monitoring of temperature and assessment of tissue necrotization. A cursor (*arrow*) placed on the T2-weighted axial image (*B*) allows the software to adjust and display the coordinates need for angulation A-P, R-L, and insertion/retraction to achieve desired target location. Right-sided periprostatic nerve block (*C*) of 10 cc 0.25% Marcaine via transrectal needle (*arrow*) which is both anesthetic and serves the purpose of hydro dissection to protect neurovascular bundles (NVBs) and rectal wall. Post-contrast T1-weighted axial image (*D*) demonstrating central hypointense coagulation necrosis (*arrows*) and a rim of hyperemia (*arrowhead*) of the treated area.

The device Is calibrated with DynaLOC planning software to determine its location in three-dimensional space after acquisition of a localizer scan in the sagittal plane. The DynaTRIM hardware allows angulation of the device anterior, posterior, and left to right as well as insertion and retraction. These adjustments are guided by the software and the judgment of the performing physician based on image guidance. The software numerically displays the suggested adjustments and generates a planned trajectory of the instrument with a graphic overlay (**Fig. 2**B) for reference.

General anesthesia is not required for this procedure as it is performed in an outpatient setting under conscious sedation. Bilateral periprostatic nerve blocks are performed with 0.25% Marcaine (**Fig. 2**C) and intravenous versed and fentanyl are administered by a sedation nurse. After axial T2-weighted images and axial diffusion-weighted

images (DWI) are acquired, a comparison is made to the preoperative multiparametric prostate MR imaging (mpMR imaging) of the biopsy-proven malignancy; then a titanium coaxial needle is introduced under MR imaging guidance into the tumor.

Before tissue ablation, the introducer sheath must be pulled back to expose the energy-emitting tip. A test dose is administered to visualize the laser fiber tip on the thermometry image. Once the tip is identified in the proper location, the energy is increased to treatment levels sufficient to induce coagulation necrosis.[30] The operator can switch between displayed planes or display multiple planes to monitor treatment (**Fig. 2**). Most tumors require multiple treatments of approximately 2 minutes using a 15-W laser to achieve thorough ablation of the MR imaging-visible tumor and a sufficient margin of 0.7 to 1 cm surrounding it. It is important that no treatment exceed 2 minutes in the same location as the carbonization of tissue or the applicator tip may induce char. This can cause leakage of cooling saline or breakage of the applicator or fiber.

During the course of treatment, the laser fiber can be removed and reinserted or simply retracted to begin a new treatment at a more distal location. Therefore, it is important to plan the surgical strategy to minimize the number of rectal wall punctures.

Device recalls related to safety resulted in modifications to instructions for use, and it is important to consider strategies to avoid injury and complication.

- Place low-temperature safety cursors over vital structures and observe irreversible damage estimation real time.
- Prevent charring and possible fiber damage by minimizing the duration of ablation with a maximum of 2-minute treatment.
- Balance the rate of cooled saline flow on the Visualase system with energy level to optimize areas of ablation.
- Take advantage of automatic shutoff feature by placing safety cursors near vital structures, especially neurovascular bundles and rectal wall.
- Always allow the system to cool down between ablations to avoid carbonization.

Once the tumor has been thoroughly ablated, MR images are acquired after intravenous gadolinium-based contrast is administered to assess the volume of coagulation necrosis (Fig. 2D). In order to minimize marginal recurrence rates, our strategy is to ablate a .7 to 1 cm margin around the MR imaging visible tumor. These larger ablations necessitate the insertion of a Foley catheter during postoperative recovery for a period of 10 to 14 days.

Nothing spoils good results as much as follow-up.

B. Ramana[31]

Our research protocol requires mpMR imaging and targeted biopsy at 6 months. It also requires mpMR imaging at 1 year and annually thereafter, along with serum PSA and standardized surveys, including Patient Health Questionnaire-9, International Prostate Symptom Score, and Sexual health Inventory for Men at each visit. It is our hope that with others we can build a registry of outcomes through the Focal Therapy Society to continue measuring the outcomes of laser FT. We intend to continue providing minimally invasive therapy to our patients and follow them closely to minimize the morbidity of whole gland therapy.

Transrectal MR Imaging-Guided High-Intensity Focused Ultrasound

The ExAblate 2100 prostate device (INSIGHTEC, Haifa, Israel) is an FDA-approved transrectal MR imaging-guided device used for the focal treatment of PCa index lesions. The ExAblate system is integrated with general electruc (GE) MR imaging scanners and provides real-time PRF thermometry of the target area. The system comprises a beam-steerable endorectal phased-array transducer containing 990 elements and operating at 2.3 MHz (up to 30 W). The transducer is surrounded by a balloon filled with circulating chilled degassed water to protect the rectal wall.[32,33] Imaging surveillance of any air bubbles is performed, which need to be removed if present.

After induction of general anesthesia, patients are positioned in the lithotomy position on the MR imaging table, and the transducer is placed along with a Foley catheter. Multiplanar T2WI and DWI are acquired for treatment planning (Fig. 3D). After identifying the tumor and critical structures, including the anterior rectal wall and prostate capsule, contour mapping of the treatment zone (tumor contour + treatment margins) is done. Tumor margins are set at 5 mm but are user-adjustable to account for sensitive, nontarget structures, such as the urethra, urethral sphincter, bladder wall, rectal wall, and neurovascular bundles. Subsequently, the integrated treatment software develops a therapeutic plan, including energy levels as well as sonication numbers, size, shape, and overlap. A single sonication creates an area of ablation which is cylindrical and measures 2 mm in diameter by 8 mm in anterior-posterior dimension. The software calculates and plans the required number of sonications to completely cover the treatment zone. This can be modified by the operator. Baseline thermometry images are initially obtained with the water in the balloon at 37 °C, then the water is chilled to 15 °C, and thermometry images are reacquired to establish the baseline anterior-posterior temperature gradient across the prostate gland for subsequent calculation of thermal dose (3). Pretreatment micro-sonications are performed to confirm the appropriate treatment field with MR thermometry. Acoustic energy is then sequentially titrated to temperatures sufficient for tissue ablation (approximately 60°C–70 °C) guided by real-time MR-based temperature feedback of the treated region (Fig. 4). Between each sonication, updated anatomic imaging is obtained to allow for modification of the treatment plan if needed to account for any motion or treatment-induced changes in the gland

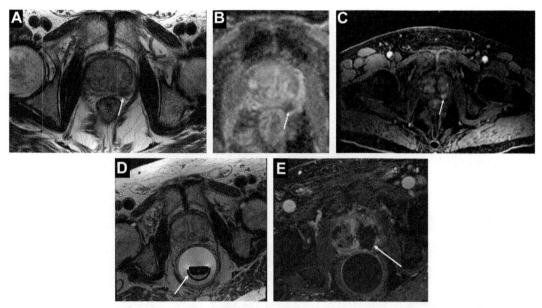

Fig. 3. Axial T2-weighted images (*A*) from a 73-year-old patient with biopsy-proven Gleason 4 + 3 adenocarcinoma demonstrating a hypointense lesion in the posterolateral left peripheral zone (*arrows*), with corresponding hypointensity on ADC map (*B*) and enhancement on post-contrast T1-weighted images (*C*). T2-weighted images on the day of treatment (*D*) demonstrate the transrectal ultrasound probe in place (*arrow*) directed toward the hypointense lesion. Following therapy, post-contrast T1-weighted images (*E*) demonstrate non-perfused volume covering the tumor (*arrow*).

volume. Sonications are swept across the region of treatment slice-by-slice until the user-defined tumor and treatment margin were covered by an adequate thermal dose. Focal re-treatment may be performed if the thermometry suggests an area of undertreatment. Post-procedurally, a contrast-enhanced MR imaging is performed to visualize the non-perfused volume (NPV) and to confirm treatment completion (**Fig. 3**E).

Major criteria for patient exclusion are as follows:

1. Calcifications detected by pre-therapy computed tomography (CT) scan measuring ≥ 2 mm and within 5 mm of the rectal wall, or measuring ≥ 5 mm and located between the target and the sonication array.
2. Anterior margin of an index lesion ≥ 40 mm from the rectal wall or beyond the focal length (60 mm) of the transducer as measured on MR imaging.

In the study which led to FDA approval of this device, 101 patients were treated.[34] Most cancers were grade group 2 (79 [78%] of 101). At 24 months, 78 of 89 men (88%) had no evidence of grade group ≥ 2 PCa in the treated area. There was no evidence of grade group ≥ 2 cancer anywhere in the prostate in 59 of 98 men (60%) at 24-month combined biopsy. Among the men

who had functional erections at baseline, 69% (40) responded to survey at 24-month follow-up with 18% of these reporting grade 1 erectile dysfunction, 28% grade 2%, and 10% grade 3. No significant change was observed in urinary symptoms from baseline to 24 months. No rectal toxicity was noted. No grade 4 or 5 treatment-related adverse events were reported, and only one grade 3 adverse event (urinary tract infection) was reported. There were no treatment-related deaths.

Transurethral MR Imaging-Guided High-Intensity Directional Ultrasound

Transurethral ultrasound ablation (TULSA) is a minimally invasive treatment modality that allows the transmission of mechanical energy in the form of ultrasound waves through intact urethral mucosa toward targeted prostate tissue. The energy is absorbed in the targeted tissue leading to temperature increase causing coagulative necrosis in targeted prostate tissue (benign or malignant). TULSA can be used for whole-gland, partial-gland, or focal ablation and is done under general anesthesia.

Major inclusion considerations for TULSA are.

1. The maximum treatable distance of this device is 3 cm, that is, the outer margin of the lesion

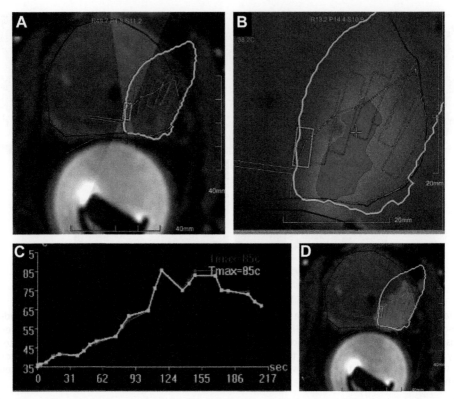

Fig. 4. Treatment planning images (*A*) obtained during MR-guided transrectal HIFU demonstrate prostate contour (blue) with region of treatment contour (yellow) and sonications used to cover region of treatment (green boxes). The ultrasound beam shape is also depicted for the subspot sonication (blue hourglass). The thermal dose volume is also demonstrated (green contour). MR thermometry images (*B*) during individual subspot sonication demonstrate the 70°C threshold (red). A temperature versus time graph (*C*) shows the temperatures of a single voxel (red) and a 3 × 3 group of voxels (green). Final images (*D*) show the thermal dose (green) encompassing the planned region of treatment.

should be no more than 3 cm from the center of the urethra with the urinary applicator (UA) in place.

2. The presence of calcifications in the treatment beam path may be a contraindication to therapeutic US, depending on their location and size. For TULSA, the size of calcification, which can be successfully managed if in between the UA and a lesion, is 3 mm.

The TULSA-PRO system incorporates an UA, robotic positioning system, and an endorectal cooling device (ECD).[32] The UA is a 22 Fr rigid tube with a soft coudé tip. The UA has a linear array that incorporates 10 individual transducers of 5 mm length. The transducers emit high-intensity ultrasound directly into the adjacent prostate tissue. ECD has a balloon that fixes the rectum and decreases rectal gas. Pores in the ECD allow injection of lubricant and removal of air. Cooled fluid flowing through the transducer (sterile water) and the ECD (water with manganese chloride

and surfactant) protect 1 to 2 mm of periurethral tissue and the rectal wall from thermal damage, respectively. The robotic positioning system provides linear and rotational motion of the UA in the urethra.

The procedure can be performed in a 1.5 or 3 T MR imaging scanner (Phillips or Siemens) using a 32-channel anterior/posterior cardiac coil array. MR imaging thermometry is performed with an echoplanar imaging sequence that is temperature-sensitive, using a proton-resonance frequency shift-induced phase difference sequence. Directional therapy is displayed on thermometry as a "flame" shape. Thermometry feedback maps use a feedback algorithm to adjust the transducer's rotation and each element's frequency/power. Tmax of the flame is set to 87 °C to prevent progression to boiling. In the periphery of the prostate, 2 mm inside the edge/capsule, the temperature is controlled at 57 °C, to ensure adequate cytotoxic dose to prostate tissue while ensuring the absence of significant dose to neurovascular bundle and other critical structures

(**Fig. 5**C). After the treatment of an angular sector, the robotic positioning system algorithmically rotates the transducer through each subsequent angular sector to complete the ablation volume. Dose and temperature maps are monitored during treatment.

After device insertion and registration under MR imaging guidance, the ablation volume is defined using high-resolution 2D T2W imaging with MR thermometry, obtained perpendicular to the transducer and centered across each individual element to completely cover MR-visible lesions (**Fig. 5**). The prostate boundary within the ablation volume is drawn to avoid the neurovascular bundle, the rectal wall, and the bladder neck/urethral sphincter. Continuous MR thermometry during treatment provides closed-loop feedback control (**Fig. 5**C). The areas of prostate tissue which did not get an adequate dose are re-treated. Re-treatment may also be needed due to prostate swelling during the procedure or unexpected motion. After completing treatment, post-contrast axial T1-weighted images provide an

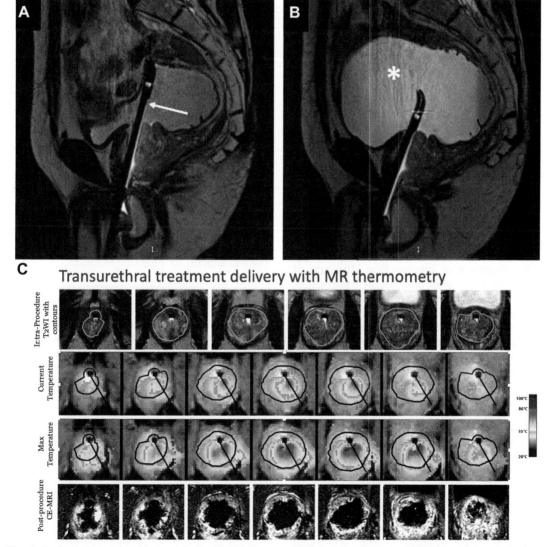

Fig. 5. Sagittal T2-weighted images during TULSA therapy (*A*) demonstrate proper placement of the urethral applicated device (*arrow*) in a patient with history of abdominoperineal resection. Sagittal T2-weighted images after addition of 200 mL of saline (*star*) into the bladder (*B*) significantly decreased impact of artifact from bowel motion on the prostate. Multiple intraprocedural images (*C*) including T2-weighted images with contours (first row), current temperature map images (second row), maximum temperature images (third row) demonstrate the treatment zone, with postprocedural contrast-enhanced T1-weighted images following treatment (fourth row) showing coverage of the intended treatment zone.

assessment of the acute NPV (see **Fig. 5**C). The patient is discharged home the same day of the procedure with a Foley catheter that is usually removed in 7 days.[33]

Medications used before, during, and after TULSA treatment are.

1. Antibiotics: A single dose is given intraprocedurally as well as a course postprocedurally for up to 1 week for prophylaxis.
2. NSAID (Toradol) and corticosteroid (Decadron): Preprocedure IV injection to decrease prostate swelling during the procedure.
3. During GA, a paralytic drip (rocuronium) is used to minimize any accidental spasmodic muscular contraction, as any motion may lead to treatment pause and redrawing of contours.
4. Glucagon IV and IM injections are used to decrease bowel motion.
5. Pain control: Almost all patients are managed with over the counter (OTC) oral medications.
6. Flomax (tamsulosin—alpha blocker) is used for up to 1 month to improve urine flow as post-treatment swelling resolves.
7. Ditropan (oxybutynin—anticholinergic): Patient may experience some bladder spasms during the immediate posttreatment procedure for which Ditropan may be prescribed.

A systematic review was recently published on the TULSA usage.[35] This included 224 patients in 10 studies with up to a 5-year follow-up, mostly for the treatment of primary PCa. The rate of salvage treatment after one TULSA treatment of primary PCa was 7% to 17%. Continence and potency preservation rates ranged from 92% to 100% and from 75% to 98%, respectively. Grade III adverse events were incurred by 13/224 men (6%), with no rectal injury/fistula or Grade IV complication.

SUMMARY

FT for prostate cancer continues to grow in patients with low-to-intermediate risk disease. The use of MR imaging for PCa therapy will likely continue to expand in the future. The ability of real-time imaging to monitor therapeutic outcomes is the main advantage of performing such therapies with MR imaging guidance. However, these therapies require significant investments in procedural time, availability, and equipment cost. As these therapies continue to grow, we anticipate these difficulties to be mitigated with increased procedural experience. Additional research is needed to understand the long-term oncologic outcomes of MR imaging-guided PCa interventions.

CLINICS CARE POINTS

- MR imaging-guided therapy for prostate cancer is a growing alternative to traditional whole gland therapies such as radical prostatectomy and radiation therapy
- Proper patient selection is paramount, and those most suited for focal therapy are those with localized, low- to intermediate-risk prostate cancer.
- Multiple modalities of treatment are available, including cryoablation, laser ablation, high-intensity-focused ultrasound, and transurethral ultrasound ablation.
- Studies on long-term oncologic outcomes and side effects are lacking, but MR-guided minimally invasive procedures are likely to continue to grow in utility.

DISCLOSURE

D. A. Adamo has nothing to disclose. B. M. Greenwood is an officer/employee and shareholder of HALO Diagnostics with one ultrasound (US) patent pending. P. Ghanouni is an advisor for SonALAsense, Profound Medical, INSIGHTEC, a shareholder in SonALAsense, and consultant for Histiosonics. S. Arora performs research and clinical trial support for Profound Medical.

REFERENCES

1. Cornford P, van den Bergh RCN, Briers E, et al. EAU-EANM-ESTRO-ESUR-SIOG Guidelines on Prostate Cancer. Part II-2020 Update: Treatment of Relapsing and Metastatic Prostate Cancer. Eur Urol 2021;79(2):263–82.
2. Kasivisvanathan V, Rannikko AS, Borghi M, et al. MRI-Targeted or Standard Biopsy for Prostate-Cancer Diagnosis. N Engl J Med 2018;378(19): 1767–77.
3. Padhani AR, Barentsz J, Villeirs G, et al. PI-RADS Steering Committee: The PI-RADS Multiparametric MRI and MRI-directed Biopsy Pathway. Radiology 2019;292(2):464–74.
4. Onik GM, Cohen JK, Reyes GD, et al. Transrectal ultrasound-guided percutaneous radical cryosurgical ablation of the prostate. Cancer 1993;72(4): 1291–9.
5. Ritch CR, Katz AE. Prostate cryotherapy: current status. Curr Opin Urol 2009;19(2):177–81.
6. Gonder MJ, Soanes WA, Shulman S. Cryosurgical treatment of the prostate. Invest Urol 1966;3(4): 372–8.

7. Gangi A, Tsoumakidou G, Abdelli O, et al. Percutaneous MR-guided cryoablation of prostate cancer: initial experience. Eur Radiol 2012;22(8):1829–35.

8. Morrison PR, Silverman SG, Tuncali K, et al. MRI-guided cryotherapy. J Magn Reson Imaging 2008; 27(2):410–20.

9. van den Bosch MR, Moman MR, van Vulpen M, et al. MRI-guided robotic system for transperineal prostate interventions: proof of principle. Phys Med Biol 2010;55(5):N133–40.

10. Thomas C, Springer F, Rothke M, et al. In vitro assessment of needle artifacts with an interactive three-dimensional MR fluoroscopy system. J Vasc Interv Radiol 2010;21(3):375–80.

11. Littrup PJ, Jallad B, Vorugu V, et al. Lethal isotherms of cryoablation in a phantom study: effects of heat load, probe size, and number. J Vasc Interv Radiol 2009;20(10):1343–51.

12. Overduin CG, Jenniskens SFM, Sedelaar JPM, et al. Percutaneous MR-guided focal cryoablation for recurrent prostate cancer following radiation therapy: retrospective analysis of iceball margins and outcomes. Eur Radiol. Nov 2017;27(11):4828–36.

13. Masic S, Washington SL 3rd, Carroll PR. Management of intermediate-risk prostate cancer with active surveillance: never or sometimes? Curr Opin Urol 2017;27(3):231–7.

14. Tay KJ, Scheltema MJ, Ahmed HU, et al. Patient selection for prostate focal therapy in the era of active surveillance: an International Delphi Consensus Project. Prostate Cancer Prostatic Dis 2017;20(3): 294–9.

15. Kinsman KA, White ML, Mynderse LA, et al. Whole-Gland Prostate Cancer Cryoablation with Magnetic Resonance Imaging Guidance: One-Year Follow-Up. Cardiovasc Intervent Radiol 2018;41(2):344–9.

16. Andreoiu M, Cheng L. Multifocal prostate cancer: biologic, prognostic, and therapeutic implications. Hum Pathol. Jun 2010;41(6):781–93.

17. Eggener SE, Scardino PT, Carroll PR, et al. Focal therapy for localized prostate cancer: a critical appraisal of rationale and modalities. J Urol 2007; 178(6):2260–7.

18. Nomura T, Mimata H. Focal therapy in the management of prostate cancer: an emerging approach for localized prostate cancer. Adv Urol 2012;2012: 391437.

19. Ward JF, Jones JS. Focal cryotherapy for localized prostate cancer: a report from the national Cryo On-Line Database (COLD) Registry. BJU Int 2012; 109(11):1648–54.

20. Durand M, Barret E, Galiano M, et al. Focal cryoablation: a treatment option for unilateral low-risk prostate cancer. BJU Int 2014;113(1):56–64.

21. Artibani W, Porcaro AB, De Marco V, et al. Management of Biochemical Recurrence after Primary Curative Treatment for Prostate Cancer: A Review. Urol Int 2018;100(3):251–62.

22. Tan WP, Kotamarti S, Ayala A, et al. Oncological and Functional Outcomes for Men Undergoing Salvage Whole-gland Cryoablation for Radiation-resistant Prostate Cancer. Eur Urol Oncol 2023. https://doi.org/10.1016/j.euo.2023.02.007.

23. Roberts CB, Jang TL, Shao YH, et al. Treatment profile and complications associated with cryotherapy for localized prostate cancer: a population-based study. Prostate Cancer Prostatic Dis 2011;14(4): 313–9.

24. Barqawi AB, Huebner E, Krughoff K, et al. Prospective Outcome Analysis of the Safety and Efficacy of Partial and Complete Cryoablation in Organ-confined Prostate Cancer. Urology 2018;112:126–31.

25. Khalkhal E, Rezaei-Tavirani M, Zali MR, et al. The Evaluation of Laser Application in Surgery: A Review Article. J Lasers Med Sci 2019;10(Suppl 1): S104–11.

26. Odeen H, Parker DL. Magnetic resonance thermometry and its biological applications - Physical principles and practical considerations. Prog Nucl Magn Reson Spectrosc 2019;110:34–61.

27. U. S. Food and Drug Administration. Dept. of Health and Human Services. (2007). 510(k) Premarket Notification. https://www.accessdata.fda.gov/scripts/cdrh/cfdocs/cfpmn/pmn.cfm?ID=K071328.

28. U. S. Food and Drug Administration. Dept. of Health and Human Services. (2021). 510(k) Premarket Notification. . https://www.accessdata.fda.gov/cdrh_docs/pdf20/K201466.pdf.

29. U. S. Food and Drug Administration. Dept. of Health and Human Services. (2007). 510(k) Summary: p.14. . https://www.accessdata.fda.gov/cdrh_docs/pdf8/k081656.pdf.

30. U.S. National Library of Medicine. ClinicalTrials.gov Phase II Laser Focal Therapy of Prostate Cancer (LITT or FLA). . https://clinicaltrials.gov/ct2/show/NCT02243033.

31. Roberts WC. Facts and ideas from anywhere. SAVE Proc 2009;22(4):377–84.

32. Masoom SN, Sundaram KM, Ghanouni P, et al. Real-Time MRI-Guided Prostate Interventions. Cancers 2022;14(8). https://doi.org/10.3390/cancers14081860.

33. Sundaram KM, Chang SS, Penson DF, et al. Therapeutic Ultrasound and Prostate Cancer. Semin Intervent Radiol 2017;34(2):187–200.

34. Ehdaie B, Tempany CM, Holland F, et al. MRI-guided focused ultrasound focal therapy for patients with intermediate-risk prostate cancer: a phase 2b, multicentre study. Lancet Oncol 2022;23(7):910–8.

35. Dora C, Clarke GM, Frey G, et al. Magnetic Resonance Imaging-Guided Transurethral Ultrasound Ablation of Prostate Cancer: A Systematic Review. J Endourol 2022;36(6):841–54.

Evaluation of Prostate Cancer Recurrence with MR Imaging and Prostate Imaging for Recurrence Reporting Scoring System

Martina Pecoraro, MD[a], Ailin Dehghanpour, MD[a], Jeeban Paul Das, MD[b],
Sungmin Woo, MD, PhD[b], Valeria Panebianco, MD[a],*

KEYWORDS

- Magnetic resonance imaging • Prostate cancer • Prostate cancer recurrence
- Prostate imaging for local recurrence reporting • Standardization • Structured reporting

KEY POINTS

- MR imaging is accurate to identify prostate cancer local recurrence with an area under the curve (AUC) ranging from 0.77 (95% confidence interval CI: 0.63, 0.90) to 0.92 (95% CI: 0.83, 1.00) after radiation therapy and 0.80 (95% CI: 0.67, 0.92) to 0.88 (95% CI: 0.79, 0.99) after radical prostatectomy.
- Prostate Imaging for local Recurrence Reporting (PI-RR) advises using the same MR imaging equipment, and imaging protocol as outlined in the Prostate Imaging-Reporting and Data System (PI-RADS) version 2.1.
- The PI-RR scoring system is designed to provide a standardized approach to evaluate prostate cancer recurrence on MR imaging, which can aid in treatment planning to guide the choice of further diagnostic testing or to help determine whether salvage therapy is appropriate or not.
- Prostate cancer recurrence has specific MR imaging semeiotics after radical prostatectomy and radiation therapy.
- After radical prostatectomy, dynamic contrast-enhanced imaging (DCE) is the dominant sequence for interpreting recurrence. In contrast, after radiation therapy, DCE and diffusion-weighted imaging can both be the dominant sequence for interpreting recurrence.

INTRODUCTION

Rising prostate specific antigen (PSA) levels may occur in men with prostate cancer (PCa) who undergo whole-gland treatment with curative intent. The reported percentage of patients experiencing PSA recurrence after treatment ranges from 27% to 53%, varying based on factors such as cancer stage and treatment type.[1] For men who experience biochemical failure, identifying those who may benefit from local salvage therapy is critical.[2]

Imaging Modalities and Prostate Cancer Recurrence

Both MR imaging and radionuclide imaging are used to assess local recurrence and distant metastases. Multiple clinical studies have demonstrated the accuracy of magnetic resonance (MR) imaging in detecting local PCa recurrence. Prostate MR imaging combines anatomic data from T1-weighted (T1WI) and T2-weighted imaging (T2WI) with functional data from diffusion-weighted imaging (DWI)

[a] Department of Radiological Sciences, Oncology and Pathology, Sapienza University, Policlinico Umberto I, Viale Regina Elena 324, Rome 00161, Italy; [b] Department of Radiology, Memorial Sloan Kettering Cancer Center, 1275 York Avenue, New York, NY 10065, USA
* Corresponding author.
E-mail address: Valeria.panebianco@uniroma1.it

Radiol Clin N Am 62 (2024) 135–159
https://doi.org/10.1016/j.rcl.2023.06.013
0033-8389/24/© 2023 Elsevier Inc. All rights reserved.

and dynamic contrast-enhanced imaging (DCE), enabling the differentiation between normal post-treatment changes and possible recurrence sites.[3–6]

In daily clinical practice, MR imaging is often the preferred method for evaluating suspicion of local disease recurrence. Several studies have investigated the diagnostic accuracy of MR imaging for detecting local recurrence after initial treatment, with promising results.[7,8]

A nonsystematic review that evaluated the diagnostic performance of various imaging techniques for detecting PCa recurrence concluded that MR imaging can successfully differentiate between locally recurrent tumors and residual healthy or scar tissue, making it the most reliable diagnostic method for assessing local relapse in PCa.[9]

In a systematic review aimed at examining the effectiveness of MR imaging in detecting local recurrence of PCa after radical prostatectomy (RP) and radiotherapy (RT), findings suggested that MR imaging is currently the most dependable imaging modality for detecting local recurrence in patients with biochemical failure. Indeed, authors found an accuracy ranging from 89% to 94%, sensitivity from 86% to 98%, and specificity from 75% to 100%.[10] This is especially advantageous when PSA levels are low, as it potentially allows for early diagnosis facilitating prompt changes in patients' management.[10]

In 2021, a group of experts in genitourinary radiology established the Prostate Imaging for Recurrence Reporting (PI-RR) system.[11] The purpose of the PI-RR system is to provide an international consensus-based guideline to standardize image acquisition, interpretation, and structured reporting of MR imaging for instances of suspected PCa local recurrence following whole-gland curative therapies. The ultimate purpose of PI-RR is to improve the management of patients with recurrent PCa by improving diagnostic performance and to enable early personalized treatment tailored to individual patient disease. The aim of this pictorial review is to provide an overview on the criteria for imaging in the setting of prostate cancer relapse and to be practical guide for recurrence detection and PI-RR categorization.

Guidelines Recommendations on Imaging

National comprehensive cancer network guidelines

The National Comprehensive Cancer Network (NCCN) guidelines suggest that conventional imaging such as computed tomography (CT) or MR imaging may not be necessary before performing prostate specific membrane antigen (PSMA)-positron emission tomography (PET) to detect micrometastatic disease in patients at both initial staging and in the context of biochemical recurrence. This is because PSMA-PET tracers have shown increased sensitivity and specificity in comparison to conventional imaging. The NCCN recommends that PSMA-PET/CT or PSMA-PET/MRI imaging can be used as a front-line imaging tool for these patients and may even be more effective than conventional imaging.[12]

American Association of Urology guidelines

Based on the American Association of Urology (AUA) guidelines, no clear indication to imaging is provided. It is noted that novel PET tracers are more sensitive than traditional 18F deoxyglucose PET imaging in identifying PCa recurrence and metastases when PSA levels are low (less than 2.0 ng/mL). MR imaging with DCE imaging is able to define sites of local recurrence and improve salvage radiation therapy (sRT) targeting and the need to add adjuvant therapies. It is also stated that advanced/molecular imaging tests may improve the detection of metastatic lesions, but their effect on patient outcomes and overall survival have not been completely established.[13]

American Society of Clinical Oncology guidelines

According to the American Society of Clinical Oncology (ASCO) guidelines, in case of biochemical recurrence, conventional imaging (such as CT, bone scans, and/or prostate MR imaging) should be used as the first-line test. When conventional imaging fails to detect metastases and local therapy is not feasible, the use of next-generation imaging technologies is not recommended. When, instead, salvage local therapy is deemed appropriate and conventional imaging is negative, patients should be directed to next generation imaging including whole-body MR imaging, and choline- or PSMA-PET/CT.[14]

MR Imaging Protocol Acquisition and Patients' Preparation

PI-RR documents advises using the same MR imaging equipment, and imaging procedures as outlined in PI-RADS version 2.1.[15]

The minimum acquisition protocol consists of high-resolution T2WI in 3 planes (axial, coronal, and/or sagittal) along with DWI and DCE. To detect the presence of blood products, lymph nodes involvement, and bone metastasis, a T1W image is employed. The sequences must encompass the whole prostate gland or vesicourethral anastomosis, seminal vesicles, and pelvic nodes. To attain appropriate spatial resolution and signal-to-noise ratio, it is recommended to use a 1.5 or

3 T scanner. When using a 1.5 T scan, acquisition parameters should be modified slightly to reduce resolution while maintaining signal-to-noise ratio. A multichannel phased array body surface coil with at least 16 channels is recommended. For a reference to recommended settings, refer to **Table 1**.

T2-weighted imaging

T2W images display the prostate gland anatomy and vesicourethral anastomosis optimally, and are employed for locating tumors, in addition to evaluating their size and morphology. Fast-spin-echo (FSE) or turbo-spin-echo (TSE) sequences, either 2Dimensional (D) or 3D, should be acquired with a slice thickness of 3 mm–no gap–and a small field of view (FOV) (eg, ~20 cm for 3T, ~25 cm for 1.5 T) to attain adequate spatial resolution with an acceptable signal-to-noise ratio. For patients treated with RP, it is recommended to acquire 3 orthogonal T2WI including sagittal images to better visualize areas at higher risk of relapse, such as the vesicourethral anastomosis, residual seminal vesicles, and the entire posterior wall of the bladder, unless 3D images are acquired.

Diffusion-weighted imaging

An axial spin-echo planar imaging sequence with fat saturation is recommended. A standard DWI sequence is acquired with several b values, ranging from b50 to 100, b400 to 500, b800, and a high b value of at least b1400 s/mm^2. The apparent diffusion coefficient (ADC) map for DWI is always computed using multiple b values that are less than 1000 s/mm^2. Owing to brachytherapy seed or fiducial marker implants, and surgical clips, causing susceptibility artifacts, DWI may be less useful in detecting a local recurrence after low-dose RT (eg, brachytherapy seeds) and RP, especially when open surgery is the technique of choice, in which generally the number of clips used is higher than robotic-assisted procedures.[16]

Dynamic contrast-enhancement MR imaging

DCE reflects tissue vascularity and microvessel permeability, and it is the dominant sequence for local recurrence detection in patients treated surgically. Images are acquired in the pre-contrast phase as well as during injection of a gadolinium-based contrast agent. The contrast agent is administered using an injector system at a rate of 3 mL/s. To illustrate early enhancement of the tumor recurrence, a high temporal resolution of less than 15 seconds is needed. To avoid recurrence misinterpretation due to inflammatory changes related to RT itself, MR imaging should be performed at least after 3 months from the last RT treatment.[17,18]

Patient preparation

According to PI-RADS v2.1 recommendations, there is no consensus concerning patient preparation issues.[15,19] Nonetheless, a preparation enema in the hours before the examination could be advantageous. In a recently published scoping review, a preparatory enema proved to have the highest yield in terms of improving image quality and reducing artifacts.[20]

MR Imaging Semeiotics of Post-treatment Anatomy and Tumor Recurrence

Post-treatment anatomy

After radical prostatectomy A commonly employed method for RP is the retropubic approach, which may be carried out via open, laparoscopic, or robot-assisted means.[21] The procedure consists of the complete removal of the prostate, the seminal vesicles, and the ampullary segments of the vas deferens, followed by the establishment of a vesicourethral anastomosis. On the axial plane, an increase of fat tissue surrounding descended bladder base and the cranial aspect of the levator ani sling filling the space of the resected prostate can be appreciated.[22] Immediately after surgery, a slightly hyperintense signal on T2WI with early enhancement after contrast injection may be observed in the surgical bed, which represents the presence of inflammatory granulation tissue and should not be mistaken for residual neoplastic tissue. Fibrotic scar tissue typically forms along the surgical planes, appearing as smooth and hypointense on T2WI, with absent or late modest post-contrast enhancement. The vesicourethral anastomosis is expected to appear smooth, with absent or thin symmetric curvilinear post-contrast enhancement; central urothelial enhancement is normal. The bladder neck typically takes on a tapered or funnel-like morphology down to the anastomosis.[22] Retained seminal vesicles are observed in approximately 20% of patients who undergo RP, visualized as a linear low/intermediate signal on both T1W and T2W imaging.[23] Surgical clips and enhancing linear veins are commonly visualized at the seminal vesicle beds.[22,24]

After radiotherapy Post-radiation prostate gland becomes atrophic and fibrotic, resulting in a small and diffusely hypointense gland on T2WI with loss of zonal differentiation.[25] Post-radiation atrophy and fibrosis in the transition zone, where benign prostatic hyperplasia (BPH) may have been seen pre-treatment, also contribute to uniformity of the gland's post-treatment signal intensity (SI) on T2WI. If a recurrent lesion is large or peripheral, an asymmetric contour abnormality may be the only detectable feature on T2WI.[26] The seminal vesicles also appear reduced in volume. To

Table 1
Optimal MR imaging acquisition parameters on 3 and 1.5 T scanners

	T2WI			DWI	DCE
3 T scanner					
Sequence	Sagittal	Coronal	Axial	Axial	Axial
	Fast recovery fast spin echo (FRFSE)			Echo planar imaging (EPI)	Gradient-echo
TE (ms)	101	101	134	75	1
TR (ms)	5590	5000	6000	4300	3
Number of averages	6	6	6	2 (b = 50); 6 (b = 800); 8 (b = 1500); 12 (b = 2000)	1
Slice thickness (mm)	3	3	3	3	3
Matrix size	384 × 384	384 × 384	384 × 384	90 × 90	160 × 140
Field of view	180 × 180	180 × 180	180 × 180	180 × 180	180 × 180
B values	n/a	n/a	n/a	50–800–1500–2000	n/a
Temporal resolution (s)	n/a	n/a	n/a	n/a	<15 (preferably 6)
Contrast media	n/a	n/a	n/a	n/a	Gadobutrol (0.1 mmol/kg)
1.5 T scanner					
Sequence	Sagittal	Coronal	Axial	Axial	Axial
	Fast recovery fast spin echo (FRFSE)			Echo planar imaging (EPI)	Gradient-echo
TE (ms)	108	146	146	73	1.76
TR (ms)	6700	6500	6400	3700	4.36
Number of averages	2	2	2	2 (b = 50); 6 (b = 800); 8 (b = 1500); 12 (b = 2000)	1
Slice thickness (mm)	3	3	3	3	3
M size	320 × 320	320 × 320	320 × 320	100 × 100	192 × 192
Field of view	200 × 200	200 × 200	200 × 200	200 × 200	260 × 260
B values	n/a	n/a	n/a	50–800–1500–2000	n/a
Temporal resolution (s)	n/a	n/a	n/a	n/a	<15 (preferably 6)
Contrast media	n/a	n/a	n/a	n/a	Gadobutrol (0.1 mmol/kg)

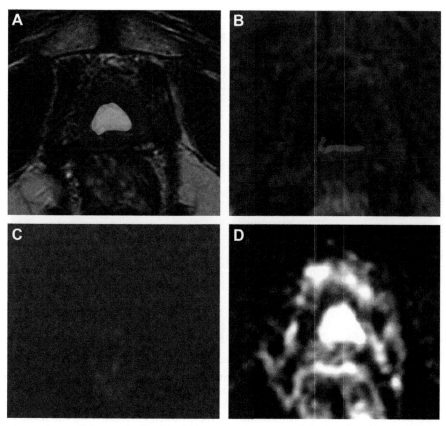

Fig. 1. Regular anatomy of the surgical bed in different MR sequences. (*A*) T2WI showing regular vesicourethral anastomosis with smooth borders (highlighted in light blue). (*B*) DCE sequence shows no focal or diffuse enhancement; highlighted in light yellow the enhancing urothelial mucosa. (*C*) No evidence of hyperintense signal in DWI or hypointense signal on (*D*) ADC map. ADC, apparent diffusion coefficient; DCE, dynamic contrast enhancement; DWI, diffusion-weighted imaging; T2WI, T2-weighted imaging.

assess appropriately the post-RT anatomy, the field of view should include the genitourinary diaphragm-prostate interface at the apex, and the bladder-prostate interface at the base.[27] More classical signs of pelvic irradiation, such as fatty replacement of the bone marrow, higher SI on T2WI of the bladder and rectal walls, the perirectal fascia, and the pelvic muscles, can be also identified.[6,17,28]

Examples of typical post-prostatectomy anatomy and post-radiation therapy changes are shown in **Figs. 1** and **2**, respectively.

Recurrence location

The most common site of local recurrence after RP, is the surgical bed, with additional common sites including the perianastomotic areas around the bladder neck or membranous urethra, the vesicorectal space, and the remnants of the seminal vesicles, when present.[29] After RT, the most common site of tumor recurrence is the location of the

original primary tumor, with disease developing elsewhere in only 4% to 9% of cases.[30–32]

Recurrence MR imaging semeiotics

In the post-surgical setting, local recurrence is typically observed as a soft tissue mass, with a lobulated morphology, located in the perianastomotic area, which appears slightly hyperintense on T2WI, shows early contrast enhancement on DCE imaging, and high signal on DWI matched by a low signal on the ADC map, when DWI/ADC is optimal in quality.[33] As a point of warning, recurrence in this setting needs to be differentiated from fibrosis, remnants of seminal vesicles, benign residual tissue, and blood products/surgical material.

After RT, local recurrence can manifest as an abnormality that resembles a mass, causing capsular bulging. This abnormality usually has slightly lower intensity on T2WI compared to the surrounding atrophic prostate tissue,[34] shows

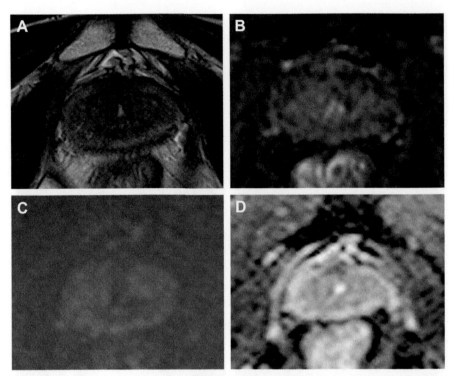

Fig. 2. Regular anatomy of the surgical bed in different MR sequences. (*A*) T2WI shows an atrophic prostate gland with a diffuse and homogenous hypointense signal. (*B*) DCE sequence with no focal nor diffuse enhancement. (*C*) No evidence of hyperintense signal in DWI or hypointense signal on (*D*) ADC map. ADC, apparent diffusion coefficient; DCE, dynamic contrast enhancement; DWI, diffusion-weighted imaging; T2WI, T2-weighted imaging.

hyperintense signal on DWI that matches an hypointense area on ADC, and early and focal hyper enhancement on DCE imaging, and may have similar imaging features and location to the dominant primary prostate tumor before RT. As a point of warning, due to reactive inflammation, glandular atrophy, and fibrosis, it can be more difficult to differentiate between the different zones of the prostate and to distinguish benign and malignant tissues.[27,35–40]

The Prostate Imaging for Local Recurrence Reporting Scoring System

The PI-RR is a scoring system designed to evaluate and report findings related to suspected local recurrence of PCa, after treatment with curative intent. The PI-RR scoring system is based on a combination of morphologic and functional imaging data and uses a 5-point scale to grade the likelihood of local recurrence, with higher scores indicating a higher likelihood of recurrence. The PI-RR scoring system includes evaluation of the treated prostate gland or prostate bed and

surrounding structures, including the seminal vesicles, lymph nodes, and pelvic bones.

Findings with a "very low" and "low" likelihood of recurrence are assigned scores of 1 and 2, respectively. If the presence of recurrence is "uncertain," a score of 3 is assigned. Scores of 4 and 5 are assigned for lesions with a "high" and "very high" likelihood of recurrence, respectively. Functional imaging findings are the basis of the reporting criteria. The size, location, and morphology/shape of the lesion are part of the anatomic criteria.

After RP, the location of relapsed tissue should be described using clock position with the vesicourethral anastomosis at the center, as per the PI-RR guidelines. To accurately identify local recurrence, it is important to interpret MR imaging with full review of the histopathology information from the prostatectomy or biopsy report, and from previous examinations, when available.[11,41] Per-sequence PI-RR categories after radical prostatectomy and radiation therapy are summarized in **Tables 2** and **3**, respectively.

Table 2
Per-sequence scoring categories following radical prostatectomy

Per-Sequence PI-RR Scoring after Radical Prostatectomy			
DCE—dominant sequence	**DWI**	**T2WI**	**Interpretation**
DCE 1: no enhancement at the surgical bed	DWI 1: no high SI on high b-value DWI and no low SI on the ADC map	T2W 1: Normal vesicourethral anastomosis/residual seminal vesicles	Very low likelihood of local recurrence
DCE 2: diffuse/ heterogeneous enhancement	DWI 2: diffuse moderate/ hyperintensity on high b-value DWI and/ or diffuse moderate hypointensity on the ADC map	T2W 2: thickened vesicourethral anastomosis/residual seminal vesicles or coarse scar in the seminal vesicle beds	Low likelihood of local recurrence
DCE 3: late phase focal/ mass-like enhancement	DWI 3: a focal hyperintense signal on high b-value DWI or a focal hypointense signal is on the ADC map, but not both	T2W 3: symmetric focal/ mass-like iso/hyper SI in the perianastomotic region/seminal vesicle bed	Equivocal case
DCE 4: focal/mass-like early enhancement not at the same site as the primary tumor, or when the tumor site is unknown	DWI 4: focal distinct hyperintensity on high b-value DWI and distinct hypointensity on the ADC map, not at the same location as the primary tumor, or the primary tumor site unknown	T2W 4: asymmetric focal/mass-like iso/ hyperintense SI in perianastomotic region/seminal vesicle bed, not at primary tumor site or when tumor location is unknown	High likelihood of local recurrence
DCE 5: focal/mass-like early enhancement at the same site as the primary tumor	DWI 5: focal distinct hyperintensity on high b-value DWI and distinct hypointensity on the ADC map, at the same site as the primary tumor	T2W 5: asymmetric focal or mass-like iso/ hyperintense SI in perianastomotic region/seminal vesicle bed on the same site as the primary tumor	Very high likelihood of local recurrence

Scoring after radical prostatectomy

T2-weighted imaging category Recurrent tumor tends to be slightly hyperintense on T2WI, which is also the same appearance as granulation tissue if the MR imaging is performed shortly after surgery. Although T2WI can provide useful information for locating recurrence, particularly when preoperative images are available, it is not included in the final assessment of PI-RADS scoring for post-RP patients.[42] When evaluating T2WI, 5 assessment categories are considered, depicted in **Table 2**.

Diffusion-weighted imaging category DWI has a lower sensitivity compared with DCE in identifying local recurrence. As for the primary tumor, local recurrence shows a high SI at high b value and low ADC values. However, after RP, it is difficult to achieve high-quality DWI due to the postoperative geometric distortions and presence of surgical clips causing artifacts. Nonetheless, DWI can still provide valuable information to help differentiate postoperative changes form residual tumor/local recurrence.[42]

The 5 assessment categories for DWI sequences are depicted in **Table 2**.

Dynamic contrast-enhanced category Although the diagnostic value of DCE-MR imaging is limited in naive patients, it plays a crucial role in identifying recurrent disease after RP. This is because the neoangiogenesis of recurrent tumors is characterized by disorganized and leaky blood vessels. Thus, early and focal enhancement, often with

Table 3
Per-sequence scoring categories following radiation therapy

Per-Sequence PI-RR Scoring after Radiation Therapy			
DCE—dominant sequence	**DWI—dominant sequence**	**T2WI**	**Interpretation**
DCE 1: no enhancement at the surgical bed	DWI 1: no high SI on high b-value DWI and no low SI on the ADC map	T2W 1: homogeneous signal intensity in the prostate	Very low likelihood of local recurrence
DCE 2: diffuse/ heterogeneous enhancement	DWI 2: diffuse moderate/ hyperintensity on high *b*-value DWI and/ or diffuse moderate hypointensity on the ADC map	T2W 2: linear/wedge-shaped, or diffuse hypointense areas, or BPH nodules	Low likelihood of local recurrence
DCE 3: late phase focal/ mass-like enhancement	DWI 3: a focal hyperintense signal on high *b*-value DWI or a focal hypointense signal is on the ADC map, but not both	T2W 3: patterns that do not fit in other categories	Equivocal case
DCE 4: focal/mass-like early enhancement not at the same site as the primary tumor, or when the tumor site is unknown	DWI 4: focal distinct hyperintensity on high b-value DWI and distinct hypointensity on the ADC map, not at the same location as the primary tumor, or the primary tumor site unknown	T2W 4: mild, focal, or mass-like areas of low SI not at the site of the primary tumor or when tumor location is unknown	High likelihood of local recurrence
DCE 5: focal/mass-like early enhancement at the same site as the primary tumor	DWI 5: focal distinct hyperintensity on high b-value DWI and distinct hypointensity on the ADC map, at the same site as the primary tumor	T2W 5: distinct circumscribed areas of hypointensity on the same side as the primary tumor	Very high likelihood of local recurrence

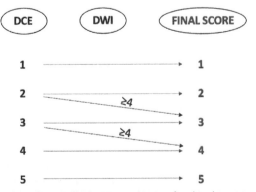

Fig. 3. Risk assessment categories after radical prostatectomy for local recurrence. DCE, dynamic contrast enhancement; DWI, diffusion-weighted imaging.

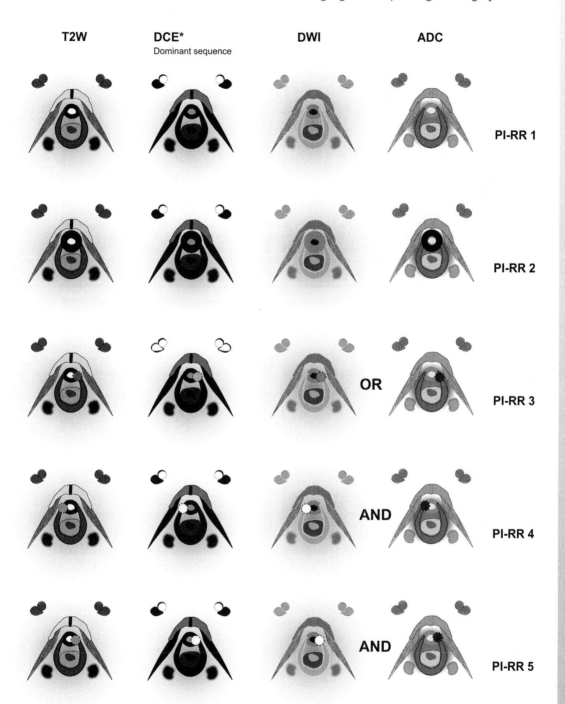

Fig. 4. A visual representation illustrating the various categories for assessing prostate cancer recurrence after radical prostatectomy (PI-RR).

contrast wash-out, is highly suspicious for local recurrence.[43] The kinetics of enhancement can help differentiate recurrence from postoperative changes, including residual glandular tissue, granulation tissue, and fibrosis. After RP, MR imaging should be performed at least 3 months later to avoid the presence of granulation tissue, which could be wrongly interpreted as residual tumor. As for fibrosis, it shows late and progressive enhancement, and normal residual tissue does

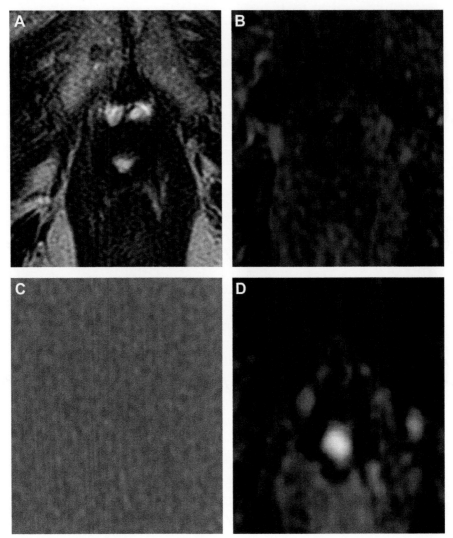

Fig. 5. Patient with pre-treatment PSA of 4.5 ng/mL who underwent radical prostatectomy; Gleason score 7 (3 + 4), pT2a N0. Twelve months after surgery PSA level is 0.04 ng/mL. (*A*) T2WI shows regular vesicourethral anastomosis with smooth borders with no evidence of focal lesions. (*B*) No focal or diffuse enhancement on DCE. No evidence of hyperintense signal on (*C*) DWI nor hypointense signal on (*D*) ADC map. This was scored as PI-RR 1. ADC, apparent diffusion coefficient; DCE, dynamic contrast enhancement; DWI, diffusion-weighted imaging; T2WI, T2-weighted imaging.

not show early enhancement.[44] The 5 assessment categories for DCE imaging are depicted in **Table 2**.

Final Prostate Imaging for local Recurrence Reporting assessment score after radical prostatectomy After surgery, DCE is the dominant sequence used for risk assessment of local recurrence, although the final score is based on the risk category of both DCE and DWI sequences. The DWI score can modify the overall risk assessment

when it is equal to or greater than 4, upgrading the final score from 2 to 3 and from 3 to 4, as illustrated in **Figs. 3** and **4**. Additionally, when discrepancies exist between the DWI and DCE sequences, T2WI may be employed to localize any recurrence. Examples of PI-RR scoring after RP are provided in **Figs. 5–9**.

Scoring after radiotherapy
T2-weighted imaging category Although T2WI provides detailed anatomic information, it has

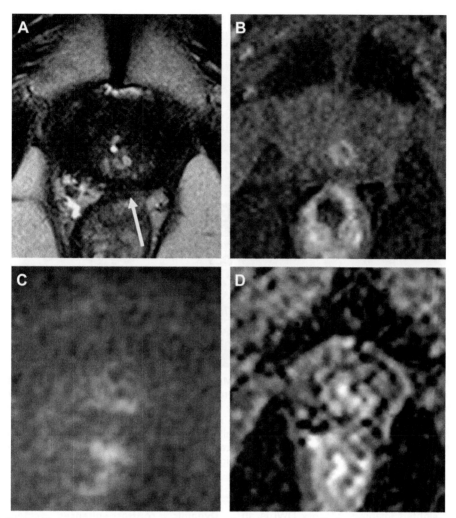

Fig. 6. Patient with pre-treatment PSA of 6.2 ng/mL who underwent radical prostatectomy; Gleason score 7 (4 + 3), pT2c N0. The PSA trend shows a slight increase, with the initial PSA level (t0) was 0.18 ng/mL, and the latest PSA level of 0.23 ng/mL. (*A*) T2WI shows benign prostatic hyperplasia glandular residue at 4 to 8 O' clock. (*B*) Focal enhancement of residual BPH on DCE. A slight hyperintensity on (*C*) DWI, with no hypointensity on (*D*) ADC map. This was scored as PI-RR 2. ADC, apparent diffusion coefficient; DCE, dynamic contrast enhancement; DWI, diffusion-weighted imaging; T2WI, T2-weighted imaging.

limited use in evaluating local recurrence. It can, however, be valuable in identifying BPH nodules and for comparing anatomic findings before and after treatment. T2WI after radiotherapy reveals several changes, such as glandular hypointensity in areas indicating tissue scarring and hyperintense signal abnormalities indicating fibrosis. This makes it difficult to distinguish between benign and malignant tissue. Additionally, post-treatment inflammation and swelling of the prostate gland can cause high SI areas on T2WI. Low-dose-rate (LDR) brachytherapy results in small ellipsoid signal voids from the radioactive seeds dispersed throughout the gland. Tissue changes are comparable to those seen in external beam radiation therapy (EBRT). In the case of local recurrence after EBRT, there may be a mass-like abnormality causing capsular bulging and slightly hypointense compared to treated prostatic tissue. However, focal SI changes on T2WI do not always indicate recurrence and other factors should be considered as the site of primary tumor. The evaluation categories considered for T2W images are depicted in Table 3.

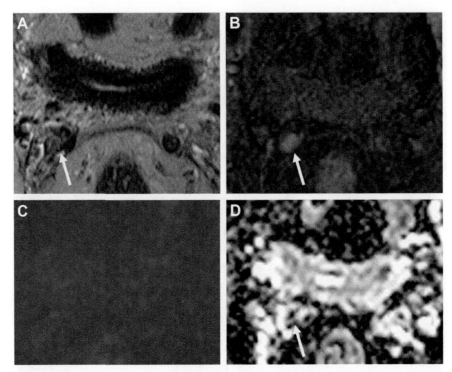

Fig. 7. Patient who underwent radical prostatectomy in March 2022; Gleason score 8 (4 + 4), tumor located in the mid-apex right peripheral zone, pT3bN1. Patient experienced PSA persistence–PSA level (t0) was 0.93 ng/mL. (*A*) The T2WI morphology shows a focal isointense mass-like lesion in the bed of the right seminal vesicles. (*B*) DCE demonstrates focal late enhancement in the bed of the right seminal vesicles. DWI (*C*)/ADC (*D*) reveals no evidence of distinct hyperintensity in DWI, but there is a mild focal hypointensity in the ADC map. The overall PI-RR score is 3 that requires a follow-up MR imaging scan in 3 months. ADC, apparent diffusion coefficient; DCE, dynamic contrast enhancement; DWI, diffusion-weighted imaging; T2WI, T2-weighted imaging.

Diffusion-weighted imaging category DWI is an essential sequence in the assessment of RT response; however, proper timing, awareness of potential artifacts, and proper technique selection are crucial to ensure the accuracy of the imaging interpretation. The early inflammatory effect of RT can mimic the high ADC values seen in benign tissue. Studies have shown that DWI is reliable when MR imaging is performed at least 6 weeks post-RT, which is considered the optimal time point. The quality of DWI sequences can also be affected by the presence of metals, and thus, it is imperative to assess the impact of marker placement on image quality. Susceptibility artifacts do not occur after high-dose-rate brachytherapy since no permanent seeds are implanted. The SI of local recurrence after RT is similar to that of the primary tumor; thus, suspicion of local recurrence can be raised by high signal intensity on DWI sequences and a corresponding low SI on the ADC map.[45] The 5 assessment categories for DWI sequences are similar to those after radical prostatectomy and are depicted in **Table 3**.

Dynamic contrast-enhanced category Early radiation-induced changes may increase vessel permeability, potentially leading to tumor flare. However, successful radiotherapy typically results in fibrosis and decreased blood flow and permeability. Therefore, to avoid mistaking granular inflammatory tissue and fibrosis for recurrent or residual tumor, MR imaging should be performed at least 3 months after treatment. Focal and early enhancement against a nonenhancing or late-enhancing background is suggestive for tumor recurrence.

The 5 assessment categories for DCE imaging are depicted in **Table 3**.

Final Prostate Imaging for local Recurrence Reporting assessment score after radiation therapy The final risk assessment after RT is determined by combining the scores from both DWI and DCE sequences, shown in **Figs. 10** and **11**. The final evaluation begins with the sequence between DWI and DCE with the highest score. If the areas of diffusion restriction and enhancement match, PI-RR 4 will

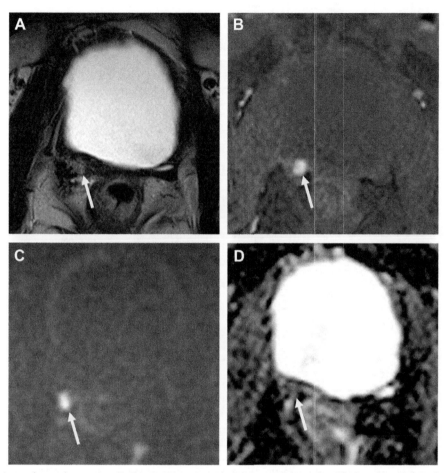

Fig. 8. Patient who underwent radical prostatectomy; Gleason score 8 (4 + 4), with the tumor located in the mid-apex on the left, pT2cN0. The PSA at the time of MR imaging was 0.15 ng/mL. (A) T2WI shows a focal hyperintense mass-like lesion on the right seminal vesicle bed. (B) DCE reveals early focal enhancement. (C) DWI reveals a focal hyperintensity. (D) ADC map shows a focal hypointense signal. The overall PI-RR score was 4. ADC, apparent diffusion coefficient; DCE, dynamic contrast enhancement; DWI, diffusion-weighted imaging; T2WI, T2-weighted imaging.

be upgraded to PI-RR 5. However, in cases where the location of the lesion differs between DWI and DCE sequences, T2WI can be useful in providing morphologic information. Examples of PI-RR scoring after RT are provided in **Figs. 12–16**.

Pitfalls and Differential Diagnosis

After radical prostatectomy

Residual glandular tissue and benign prostatic hyperplasia As previously mentioned, the timing of MR imaging after RP is crucial because several normal tissues can resemble a local recurrence. Residual glandular tissue may appear slightly hyperintense on T2WI and hypervascular on DCE images due to inflammatory changes. However, as with pre-treatment imaging, DWI remains the

dominant sequence for accurately diagnosing such cases. Regarding BPH nodules, the use of T2WI sequences can aid in their diagnosis, particularly if pre-treatment MR imaging is also available.[42,46]

Seminal vesicles and seminal colliculus The appearance of seminal vesicles on T2WI can differ based on the amount of fluid present at the time of imaging. Typically, the outer fibromuscular layer and the convoluted inner walls show low SI, whereas the fluid within the ducts appears as high SI, giving the seminal vesicles a distinctive "grape-like" shape. However, in some cases, they may become fibrotic and exhibit low SI on T2WI. To avoid mistaking these remnants for a local recurrence at the site of the seminal vesicles, it is

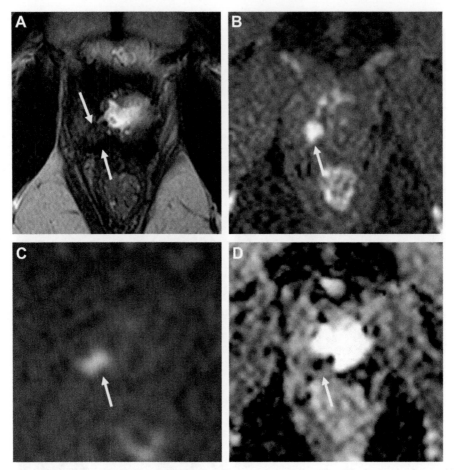

Fig. 9. Patient who underwent radical prostatectomy; Gleason score 7 (4 + 3), with the tumor located in the peripheral zone at mid-apex on the right, pT2cN0. The PSA at the time of MR imaging was 0.22 ng/mL. (*A*) T2WI shows a focal mildly hyperintense mass-like lesion on the right side of the vesicourethral anastomosis at 7 to 9 O' clock. (*B*) DCE shows early focal enhancement. (*C*) DWI a focal hyperintensity. (*D*) ADC reveals correspondent focal hypointensity. The overall PI-RR score was 5. ADC, apparent diffusion coefficient; DCE, dynamic contrast enhancement; DWI, diffusion-weighted imaging; T2WI, T2-weighted imaging.

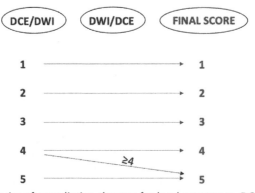

Fig. 10. Risk assessment categories after radiation therapy for local recurrence. DCE, dynamic contrast enhancement; DWI, diffusion-weighted imaging.

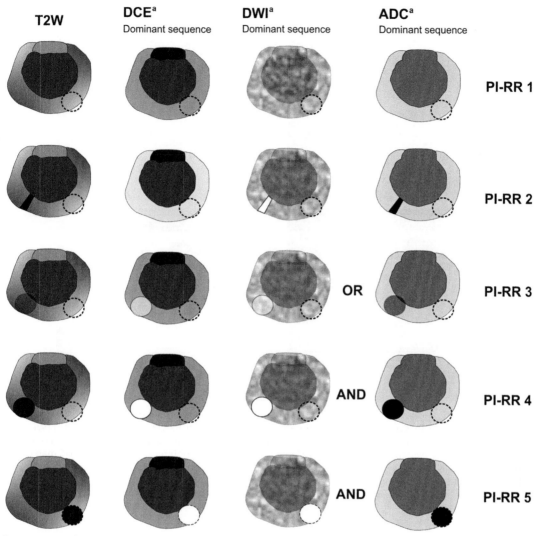

Fig. 11. A visual representation illustrating the various categories for assessing prostate cancer recurrence after radiation therapy (PI-RR). The primary tumor location is indicated by dashed lines, whereas the filled circles depict the location of the recurrence. [a] Dominant sequence.

important to carefully analyze DCE and DWI images. Local recurrence shows early enhancement, whereas fibrotic tissue demonstrates late enhancement, aiding in the differential diagnosis.[47]

The verumontanum, also known as the seminal colliculus, is a round bump located on the urethral crest within the back wall of the middle prostatic urethra. The prostatic utricle opens into it in the middle, and the 2 ejaculatory ducts open just after the utricle. Following RP, the seminal colliculus may occasionally persist and appear hyperintense on T2WI if hypertrophied or inflamed, with enhancement seen on DCE. However, it can be differentiated from a local recurrence as it does not show high SI on DWI.[42]

Inflammatory tissue and fibrosis Inflammatory granulation tissue can be detected on the surgical bed, particularly at the peri-anastomotic site, shortly after surgery. This tissue appears as hypointense on T2WI and may exhibit early enhancement due to its high vascular permeability. ADC map can help differentiate granular tissue from neoplastic tissue, as inflammatory tissue has a high SI on both DWI and ADC map. However, it is crucial to wait at least 3 months after surgery before performing an MR to avoid this pitfall.[23] Conversely, fibrosis or scar tissue is a finding that appears later at the surgical bed; the kinetics of enhancement can aid the differential diagnosis with local recurrence.[23]

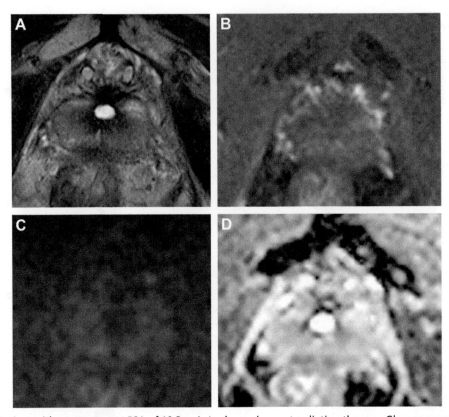

Fig. 12. Patient with pre-treatment PSA of 10.2 ng/mL who underwent radiation therapy; Gleason score 8 (4 + 4), pT2b N0. MR imaging scan is performed 12 months after radiation therapy, PSA level is 0.5 ng/mL. (*A*) T2WI shows a prostate gland with a diffuse and homogenous hypointense signal. (*B*) DCE sequence shows no focal or diffuse early enhancement. No evidence of hyperintense signal in (*C*) DWI or a hypointense signal in (*D*) ADC map can be appreciated. This was scored as PI-RR 1. ADC, apparent diffusion coefficient; DCE, dynamic contrast enhancement; DWI, diffusion-weighted imaging; T2WI, T2-weighted imaging.

Sealed off and conspicuous venous plexus At times, a distinct sealed-off venous plexus near the vesico-urethral anastomosis may appear as a mass-like tissue with high SI on T2WI. However, there is no post-contrast enhancement observed, which can aid in making the correct diagnosis. It can be challenging to differentiate between the prominent periprostatic venous plexus and recurrent tumors based solely on DCE imaging. In these cases, DWI is important to exclude the presence of tumorous tissue.[43] Examples of pitfalls after radical prostatectomy are shown in **Fig. 17.**

After radiation therapy
Inflammatory changes In the initial stage of RT, inflammation can cause a rise in blood flow and volume, resulting in potentially inaccurate interpretation of DCE images. However, high SI in ADC map helps the diagnosis of benign tissue. Hence, it is important to avoid performing MR imaging during or immediately after RT (**Fig. 18**).[18,46]

Anatomic distortion and fibrosis Radiation therapy may cause irregularities in the capsular profile, which can make it difficult to assess extracapsular extension of recurrence. Additionally, RT can lead to scarring and tissue distortion within the gland. These changes may resemble a local recurrence, particularly if with pseudonodular shape. These areas of glandular asymmetry do not appear hyperintense on DWI sequences and show late enhancement. It is essential to consider the primary tumor location as local recurrence after radiation therapy occurs at the site of the primary tumor and behaves similarly to the primary tumor in all sequences.[18,48]

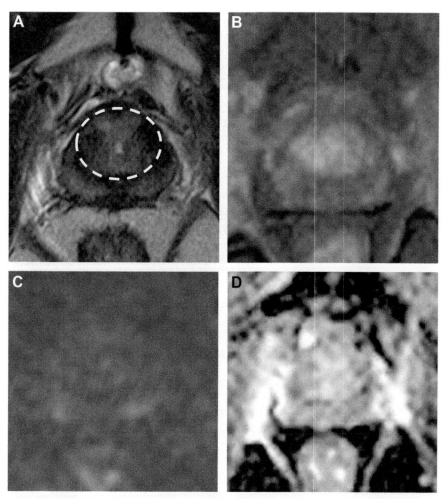

Fig. 13. Patient who underwent radiation therapy; Gleason score, 7 (3 + 4), pT2b N0. PSA level at the time of MR imaging was also 1.2 ng/mL. (*A*) T2WI: The prostate gland appears homogeneously hypointense. (*B*) DCE: There is diffuse enhancement in the transitional zone. (*C*) No significant hyperintensity on DWI. (*D*) Diffuse hypointense signal in the gland on ADC. This was scored as PI-RR 2. ADC, apparent diffusion coefficient; DCE, dynamic contrast enhancement; DWI, diffusion-weighted imaging; T2WI, T2-weighted imaging.

EVIDENCE ON PROSTATE IMAGING FOR LOCAL RECURRENCE REPORTING SCORING SYSTEM

After the introduction of PI-RR system in 2021, few studies have evaluated its performance in identifying local recurrence and its inter-reader agreement. A retrospective observational study by Pecoraro and colleagues[49] evaluated the performance of PI-RR for detecting local recurrence in patients with biochemical recurrence (BCR) after RT and RP. Four radiologists independently assigned a PI-RR score after analyzing 100 MR imaging scans. The study showed that in patients who underwent RT and RP, the area under the receiver operating

characteristic curve for local recurrence ranged from 0.77 to 0.92 and 0.80 to 0.88, respectively. The inter-reader agreement was optimal (interclass correlation coefficient of 0.87). The study assessed for the first time the diagnostic performance of PI-RR and optimal reproducibility. Also, Ciaccarese and colleagues[50] conducted a retrospective study to evaluate PI-RR score's diagnostic accuracy and interobserver variability compared with histopathological data. PI-RR scoring was compared with PET/CT findings. The study found that PI-RR score had an accuracy of 68.4% and excellent inter-reader agreement (k = 0.884). Compared with choline-PET/CT and PSMA-PET/CT, PI-RR score showed a higher detection rate (69.6% vs 19.6%

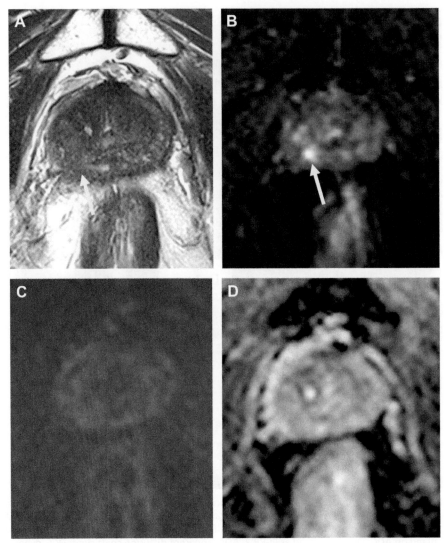

Fig. 14. Patient who underwent radiation therapy; Gleason score 7 (3 + 4), pT2b N0. PSA level at the time of MR imaging was 1.4 ng/mL. (*A*) T2WI: The prostate gland appears homogeneously hypointense. (*B*) DCE: There is a focal late enhancement in the peripheral zone on the right. (*C*) No focal distinct hyperintensity on DWI. (*D*) No focal hyperintense signal in ADC map. This was scored as PI-RR 3. ADC, apparent diffusion coefficient; DCE, dynamic contrast enhancement; DWI, diffusion-weighted imaging; T2WI, T2-weighted imaging.

and 59.1% vs 22.7%, respectively). In recent retrospective observational study, Bergalio and colleagues[51] evaluated the reproducibility of the PI-RR scoring system among readers with different expertise. Two radiologists and one radiology resident served as readers evaluating a total of 67 MR imagings. PI-RR resulted to have a diagnostic accuracy range of 75% to 80%. When using a binary evaluation (PI-RR ≥ 3 as positive MR imaging), the interreader agreement showed a correlation coefficient (k) of 0.74. The findings of this study confirmed the diagnostic accuracy of MR imaging and the promising reproducibility among readers with varying

levels of experience. Finally, Park and colleagues[52] showed how a PI-RR score of 4 and 5 on postprostatectomy MR imaging was associated with adverse clinicopathologic characteristics and could predict biochemical recurrence at 1 year.

CLINICAL IMPLICATIONS

Lack of a standardized pathway to determine local recurrence after radiation therapy/radical prostatectomy leads to delaying salvage therapy in many patients.

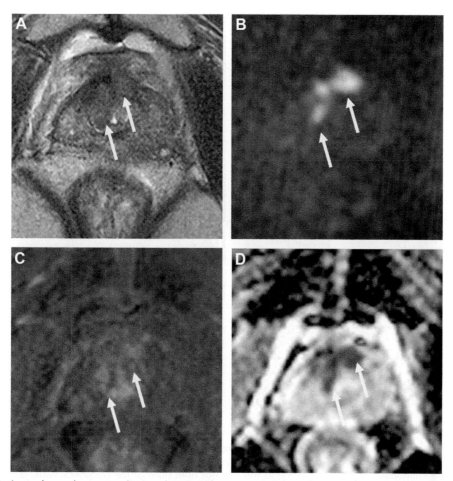

Fig. 15. Patient who underwent radiation therapy; Gleason score 8 (4 + 4), pT2c N0. The PSA level at the time of MR imaging was 2.4 ng/mL. (*A*) T2WI: multiple pseudo-nodular hypointense lesions in the anterior transitional zone. (*B*) Focal late enhancement on DCE. (*C*) Focal distinct hyperintensity on DWI. (*D*) Correspondent hypointensity of the signal on ADC map. This was scored as PI-RR 4 as the side of the primary lesion was not known and it did not match early enhancement on DCE. ADC, apparent diffusion coefficient; DCE, dynamic contrast enhancement; DWI, diffusion-weighted imaging; T2WI, T2-weighted imaging.

Various studies have demonstrated that delaying sRT can be a controversial decision, as it may increase the risk of disease progression and reduce the effectiveness of treatment. Early initiation of sRT after PSA failure is associated with better outcomes, including improved cancer-specific survival and overall survival, compared with delayed initiation. Also delaying sRT can increase the risk of distant metastasis and reduce the chances of achieving a durable PSA response.[46,53,54] Recently, Panebianco and Turkbey[41] proposed a personalized diagnostic pathway for patients with PCa who have undergone whole-gland treatment, based on European Association of Urology BCR risk groups (depicted in **Table 4**), incorporating the PI-RR scoring. They focus on the importance of a standardized diagnostic approach in case of biochemical recurrence to reduce overtreatment in the first place, but also to avoid delaying salvage therapy, increase the overall survival rate, and eventually lower related expenses. A standardized diagnostic approach for patients with rising PSA is essential to achieve an accurate diagnosis with optimal timing. The diagnostic pathway needs to be a personalized process that takes into account various factors, including pre- and post-treatment risk factors, and equipment availability.

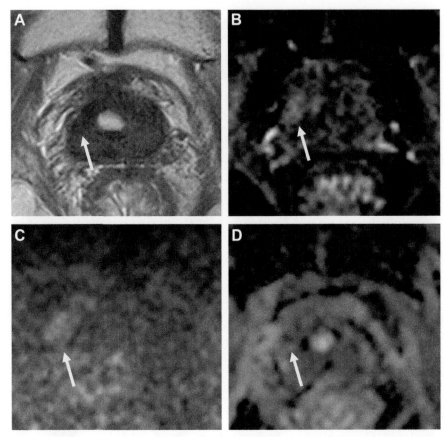

Fig. 16. Patient who underwent radiation therapy; Gleason score 8 (4 + 4), the primary tumor was located at the right mid-apex in the peripheral zone, pT2c N0. PSA level at the time of MR imaging was 3.1 ng/mL. (*A*) T2WI showed a pseudo-nodular hypointense lesion at the anterior right horn of the peripheral zone. (*B*) Focal early enhancement on DCE. (*C*) Focal hyperintensity on DWI. (*D*) Correspondent hypointensity on the ADC map. This was scored as PI-RR 5 as the local relapse is on the same side of the primary tumor and DWI and DCE alteration location matches. ADC, apparent diffusion coefficient; DCE, dynamic contrast enhancement; DWI, diffusion-weighted imaging; T2WI, T2-weighted imaging.

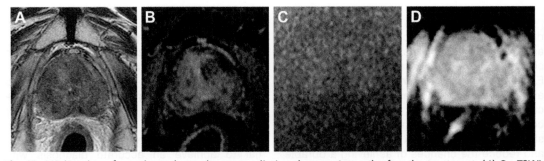

Fig. 17. MR imaging of a patient who underwent radiation therapy, 1 month after the treatment. (*A*) On T2WI the prostate gland shows a heterogeneous signal. (*B*) DCE shows diffuse whole gland enhancement. (*C*) No focal significant hyperintensity on DWI. (*D*) No focal hypointensity on ADC map. This is a case example of post-radiotherapy inflammation which highlights the importance of the right timing of imaging after treatment. ADC, apparent diffusion coefficient; DCE, dynamic contrast enhancement; DWI, diffusion-weighted imaging; T2WI, T2-weighted imaging.

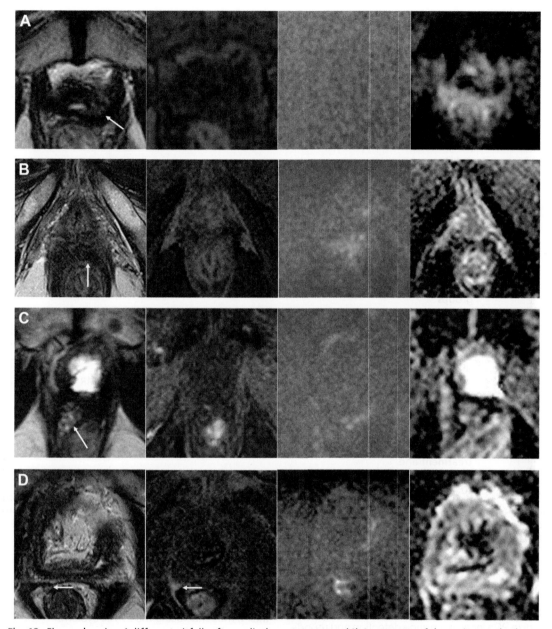

Fig. 18. Figure showing 4 different pitfalls after radical prostatectomy. (*A*) Asymmetry of the vesico-urethral anastomosis (3–6 O' clock), with no functional MR pattern compatible with recurrent tissue. (*B*) Fibrotic sling at the vesico-urethral anastomosis (4–6 O' clock). (*C*) Right seminal vesicle remnant with no functional MR pattern compatible with recurrent tissue. (*D*) A small hypointense tissue is seen on T2WI image, which shows focal enhancement on DCE without hyperintensity in DWI nor hypointensity on ADC map. This is a case example of a prominent vessel. T2WI, T2-weighted imaging; DWI, diffusion-weighted imaging; ADC, apparent diffusion coefficient; DCE, dynamic contrast enhancement.

Communication and collaboration among different specialties can lead to effective decision-making and improved patient outcomes. Therefore, a risk-adapted strategy for addressing recurrent PCa should be pursued in clinical practice, using a standardized diagnostic approach and multidisciplinary teamwork. This approach can have a significant clinical impact on patient management and outcomes.

Table 4
Tailored diagnostic pathways for patients experiencing biochemical recurrence after whole-gland prostate cancer therapies, proposed by Panebianco and Turkbey.[41]

Pathway	Patient Group	First-Line Imaging Modality	Imaging Result	Next Steps
1	Low-risk pre-treatment and post-treatment prognostic risk groups	MR imaging and PI-RR	Negative Positive (PI-RR 3–5)	PSA monitoring Targeted biopsy and/or salvage therapy
2	Intermediate-risk pre-treatment and low-risk post-treatment risk groups	MR imaging and PI-RR	Negative Positive (PI-RR 3–5)	PSMA-PET/CT Targeted biopsy and/or salvage therapy
3	High-risk pre-treatment and low-risk post-treatment risk groups	MR imaging and PI-RR	Negative	PSMA-PET/CT
	Low-risk pre-treatment and high-risk post-treatment risk groups		Positive (PI-RR 3–5)	Salvage therapy
4	Intermediate-risk pre-treatment and high-risk post-treatment risk groups	PSMA-PET/CT	Negative	Pelvis MR imaging and/or whole-body MR imaging
	High-risk pre-treatment and high-risk post-treatment risk groups		Positive	Salvage therapy

Abbreviations: PI-RR, Prostate Imaging for Recurrence Reporting; PSA, Prostate Specific Antigen; PSMA-PET/CT, Prostate Specific Antigen - Positron Emission Tomography/Computed Tomography.

SUMMARY

PI-RR is a scoring system developed to standardize PCa local recurrence detection and reporting after whole-gland therapies with curative intent, using the same MR imaging acquisition protocol described in PI-RADS guidelines. PI-RR is a tool that can be used to differentiate local recurrence from residual tissue, granulation tissue, sealed off and conspicuous venous plexus and fibrosis after surgery and radiation therapy, and has shown promising results in early validation studies. MR imaging and PI-RR can be of aid to direct patient care in men experiencing biochemical recurrence to a risk-based therapeutic planning, especially for those at low risk of developing bone or visceral metastasis. Currently, albeit MR imaging is widely used in clinical practice, its widespread use for recurrence detection is limited due to narrow expertise; therefore, radiologists might improve their confidence using the PI-RR system.

CLINICS CARE POINTS

- The MRI protocol after radical prostatectomy and radiation therapy follows PI-RADS version 2.1 guidelines, which include T2-weighted imaging (T2WI, Dynamic Contrast Enhancement (DCE) imaging, and Diffusion Weighted Imaging (DWI).

- After radical prostatectomy, DCE is the main sequence for assessing the risk of local recurrence.

- The risk assessment after radiation therapy is established by combining scores from both DWI and DCE sequences.
- Local recurrence occurs mostly on the site of primary tumor, pre- treatment mpMRI can help.

DISCLOSURE

The authors have nothing to disclose.

REFERENCES

1. Simon NI, Parker C, Hope TA, et al. Best approaches and updates for prostate cancer biochemical recurrence. Am Soc Clin Oncol Educ Book 2022;42:352–9.
2. Van den Broeck T, van den Bergh RCN, Briers E, et al. Biochemical recurrence in prostate cancer: the european association of urology prostate cancer guidelines panel recommendations. Eur Urol Focus 2020;6(2):231–4.
3. Jambor I, Falagario U, Ratnani P, et al. Prediction of biochemical recurrence in prostate cancer patients who underwent prostatectomy using routine clinical prostate multiparametric MRI and decipher genomic score. J Magn Reson Imaging 2020;51(4):1075–85.
4. Picchio M, Mapelli P, Panebianco V, et al. Imaging biomarkers in prostate cancer: role of PET/CT and MRI. Eur J Nucl Med Mol Imaging 2015;42(4):644–55.
5. Panebianco V, Sciarra A, Marcantonio A, et al. Conventional imaging and multiparametric magnetic resonance (MRI, MRS, DWI, MRP) in the diagnosis of prostate cancer. Q J Nucl Med Mol Imaging 2012;56(4):331–42.
6. Richenberg J, Løgager V, Panebianco V, et al. The primacy of multiparametric MRI in men with suspected prostate cancer. Eur Radiol 2019;29(12):6940–52.
7. De Visschere PJL, Standaert C, Fütterer JJ, et al. A systematic review on the role of imaging in early recurrent prostate cancer. Eur Urol Oncol 2019;2(1):47–76.
8. Barchetti F, Stagnitti A, Megna V, et al. Unenhanced whole-body MRI versus PET-CT for the detection of prostate cancer metastases after primary treatment. Eur Rev Med Pharmacol Sci 2016;20(18):3770–6.
9. Maurer T, Eiber M, Fanti S, et al. Imaging for prostate cancer recurrence. Eur Urol Focus 2016;2(2):139–50.
10. Barchetti F, Panebianco V. Multiparametric MRI for recurrent prostate cancer post radical prostatectomy and postradiation therapy. BioMed Res Int 2014;2014:1–23.
11. Panebianco V, Villeirs G, Weinreb JC, et al. Prostate magnetic resonance imaging for local recurrence reporting (pi-rr): international consensus -based guidelines on multiparametric magnetic resonance imaging for prostate cancer recurrence after radiation therapy and radical prostatectomy. Eur Urol Oncol 2021;4(6):868–76.
12. Schaeffer E, Srinivas S, Antonarakis ES, et al. NCCN Guidelines Insights: Prostate Cancer, Version 1.2021: Featured Updates to the NCCN Guidelines. J Natl Compr Canc Netw 2021;19(2):134–43.
13. Crocerossa F, Marchioni M, Novara G, et al. Detection rate of prostate specific membrane antigen tracers for positron emission tomography/computerized tomography in prostate cancer biochemical recurrence: a systematic review and network meta-analysis. J Urol 2021;205(2):356–69.
14. Trabulsi EJ, Rumble RB, Jadvar H, et al. Optimum imaging strategies for advanced prostate cancer: ASCO guideline. J Clin Oncol 2020;38(17):1963–96.
15. Turkbey B, Rosenkrantz AB, Haider MA, et al. Prostate imaging reporting and data system version 2.1: 2019 update of prostate imaging reporting and data system version 2. Eur Urol 2019;76(3):340–51.
16. Artibani W, Cacciamani G. Is the choice between clips and no clips or cautery and no cautery still a dilemma in robot-assisted radical prostatectomy? Eur Urol Open Sci 2022;44:76–7.
17. Vargas HA, Wassberg C, Akin O, et al. MR imaging of treated prostate cancer. Radiology 2012;262(1):26–42.
18. Haider MA, Chung P, Sweet J, et al. Dynamic contrast-enhanced magnetic resonance imaging for localization of recurrent prostate cancer after external beam radiotherapy. Int J Radiat Oncol 2008;70(2):425–30.
19. Engels RRM, Israël B, Padhani AR, et al. Multiparametric magnetic resonance imaging for the detection of clinically significant prostate cancer: what urologists need to know. part 1: acquisition. Eur Urol 2019. https://doi.org/10.1016/j.eururo.2019.09.021. S0302283819307419.
20. Prabhakar S, Schieda N. Patient preparation for prostate MRI: A scoping review. Eur J Radiol 2023;162:110758.
21. Lopes Dias J, Lucas R, Magalhães Pina J, et al. Post-treated prostate cancer: normal findings and signs of local relapse on multiparametric magnetic resonance imaging. Abdom Imaging 2015;40(7):2814–38.
22. Allen SD, Thompson A, Sohaib SA. The normal post-surgical anatomy of the male pelvis following radical prostatectomy as assessed by magnetic resonance imaging. Eur Radiol 2008;18(6):1281–91.
23. Sella T, Schwartz LH, Swindle PW, et al. Suspected local recurrence after radical prostatectomy: endorectal coil MR imaging. Radiology 2004;231(2):379–85.

24. Potretzke TA, Froemming AT, Gupta RT. Post-treatment prostate MRI. Abdom Radiol 2020;45(7): 2184–97.

25. Mertan FV, Greer MD, Borofsky S, et al. Multiparametric magnetic resonance imaging of recurrent prostate cancer. Top Magn Reson Imaging 2016; 25(3):139–47.

26. Asuncion A, Walker PM, Bertaut A, et al. Prediction of prostate cancer recurrence after radiation therapy using multiparametric magnetic resonance imaging and spectroscopy: assessment of prognostic factors on pretreatment imaging. Quant Imaging Med Surg 2022;12(12):5309–25.

27. Patel P, Mathew MS, Trilisky I, et al. Multiparametric MR imaging of the prostate after treatment of prostate cancer. Radiographics 2018;38(2):437–49.

28. Gaur S, Turkbey B. Prostate MR imaging for post-treatment evaluation and recurrence. Radiol Clin North Am 2018;56(2):263–75.

29. Cirillo S, Petracchini M, Scotti L, et al. Endorectal magnetic resonance imaging at 1.5 Tesla to assess local recurrence following radical prostatectomy using T2-weighted and contrast-enhanced imaging. Eur Radiol 2009;19(3):761–9.

30. Patel P, Oto A. Magnetic resonance imaging of the prostate, including pre- and postinterventions. Semin Interv Radiol 2016;33(03):186–95.

31. Arrayeh E, Westphalen AC, Kurhanewicz J, et al. Does local recurrence of prostate cancer after radiation therapy occur at the site of primary tumor? Results of a longitudinal MRI and MRSI study. Int J Radiat Oncol Biol Phys 2012;82(5): e787–93.

32. Jalloh M, Leapman MS, Cowan JE, et al. Patterns of Local Failure following Radiation Therapy for Prostate Cancer. J Urol 2015;194(4):977–82.

33. Faiella E, Santucci D, Vertulli D, et al. The role of multiparametric mri in the diagnosis of local recurrence after radical prostatectomy and before salvage radiotherapy. Actas Urol Esp Engl Ed 2022;46(7): 397–406.

34. McCammack KC, Raman SS, Margolis DJ. Imaging of local recurrence in prostate cancer. Future Oncol Lond Engl 2016;12(21):2401–15.

35. Sugimura K, Carrington BM, Quivey JM, et al. Post-irradiation changes in the pelvis: assessment with MR imaging. Radiology 1990;175(3):805–13.

36. Chan TW, Kressel HY. Prostate and seminal vesicles after irradiation: MR appearance. J Magn Reson Imaging JMRI 1991;1(5):503–11.

37. Maurer T, Eiber M, Fanti S, et al. Imaging for prostate cancer recurrence. Eur Urol Focus 2016;2(2): 139–50.

38. Sciarra A, Panebianco V, Ciccariello M, et al. Magnetic resonance spectroscopic imaging ([1] H-MRSI) and dynamic contrast-enhanced magnetic resonance (DCE-MRI): pattern changes from inflammation to prostate cancer. Cancer Invest 2010;28(4):424–32.

39. Serinelli S, Panebianco V, Martino M, et al. Accuracy of MRI skeletal age estimation for subjects 12–19. Potential use for subjects of unknown age. Int J Legal Med 2015;129(3):609–17.

40. Del Giudice F, Pecoraro M, Vargas HA, et al. Systematic review and meta-analysis of vesical imaging-reporting and data system (VI-RADS) inter-observer reliability: an added value for muscle invasive bladder cancer detection. Cancers 2020; 12(10). https://doi.org/10.3390/cancers12102994.

41. Panebianco V, Turkbey B. Magnetic resonance imaging for prostate cancer recurrence: it's time for precision diagnostic with Prostate Imaging for Recurrence Reporting (PI-RR) score. Eur Radiol 2022;33(2):748–51.

42. Panebianco V, Barchetti F, Barentsz J, et al. Pitfalls in Interpreting mp-MRI of the prostate: a pictorial review with pathologic correlation. Insights Imaging 2015;6(6):611–30.

43. Renard-Penna R, Zhang-Yin J, Montagne S, et al. Targeting local recurrence after surgery with MRI imaging for prostate cancer in the setting of salvage radiation therapy. Front Oncol 2022;12: 775387.

44. Myers RP, Cahill DR, Devine RM, et al. Anatomy of radical prostatectomy as defined by magnetic resonance imaging. J Urol 1998;159(6):2148–58.

45. Song I, Kim CK, Park BK, et al. Assessment of response to radiotherapy for prostate cancer: value of diffusion-weighted MRI at 3 T. Am J Roentgenol 2010;194(6):W477–82.

46. Panebianco V, Giganti F, Kitzing YX, et al. An update of pitfalls in prostate mpMRI: a practical approach through the lens of PI-RADS v. 2 guidelines. Insights Imaging 2018;9(1):87–101.

47. Sella T, Schwartz LH, Hricak H. Retained seminal vesicles after radical prostatectomy: frequency, MRI characteristics, and clinical relevance. Am J Roentgenol 2006;186(2):539–46.

48. Pucar D, Hricak H, Shukla-Dave A, et al. Clinically significant prostate cancer local recurrence after radiation therapy occurs at the site of primary tumor: magnetic resonance imaging and step-section pathology evidence. Int J Radiat Oncol 2007;69(1): 62–9.

49. Pecoraro M, Turkbey B, Purysko AS, et al. Diagnostic accuracy and observer agreement of the mri prostate imaging for recurrence reporting assessment score. Radiology 2022;304(2): 342–50.

50. Ciccarese F, Corcioni B, Bianchi L, et al. Clinical application of the new prostate imaging for recurrence reporting (PI-RR) score proposed to evaluate the local recurrence of prostate cancer after radical prostatectomy. Cancers 2022;14(19):4725.

51. Bergaglio C, Giasotto V, Marcenaro M, et al. The role of mpMRI in the assessment of prostate cancer recurrence using the PI-RR system: diagnostic accuracy and interobserver agreement in readers with different expertise. Diagnostics 2023;13(3):387.

52. Park MY, Park KJ, Kim MH, et al. Focal nodular enhancement on DCE MRI of the prostatectomy bed: radiologic-pathologic correlations and prognostic value. Eur Radiol 2023;33(4):2985–94.

53. Bottke D, Bartkowiak D, Siegmann A, et al. Effect of early salvage radiotherapy at PSA < 0.5 ng/ml and impact of post-SRT PSA nadir in post-prostatectomy recurrent prostate cancer. Prostate Cancer Prostatic Dis 2019;22(2):344–9.

54. Tilki D, Chen MH, Wu J, et al. Prostate-specific antigen level at the time of salvage therapy after radical prostatectomy for prostate cancer and the risk of death. J Clin Oncol 2023;22:02489.

Prostate-Specific Membrane Antigen PET/ Computed Tomography
Pearls and Pitfalls

Larissa Bastos Costa, MD[a,b], Renata Moreira, MD[c],
Priscilla Romano Gaspar, MD[d], Felipe de Galiza Barbosa, MD[a,b],*

KEYWORDS

• PSMA-PET • Prostate cancer • Pitfalls • Molecular imaging

KEY POINTS

• Prostate-specific membrane antigen PET (PSMA-PET) is the most accurate imaging method for prostate cancer assessment.
• PSMA-PET outperforms conventional imaging (computed tomography and bone scan) for detecting prostate cancer nodal and bone metastases.
• PSMA-PET can have benign pitfalls and detect atypical disease spread; therefore, it is fundamental to understand its peculiarities in prostate cancer.

INTRODUCTION

Accurate staging and management of prostate cancer are crucial for optimal patient outcomes. Conventional imaging modalities, such as computed tomography (CT) and bone scans (BSs), have limitations in detecting small lesions and accurately assessing disease extent.[1,2] However, recent advancements in molecular imaging have led to the emergence of prostate-specific membrane antigen positron emission tomography (PSMA-PET) as an improved tool in prostate cancer imaging.

PSMA, a transmembrane protein highly expressed in prostate cancer cells, serves as a target for molecular imaging. PSMA-PET uses radiotracers labeled with PSMA-targeting ligands, which bind to PSMA and emit positron emissions that are detected by PET scanners.[3,4] This imaging technique provides enhanced sensitivity and specificity compared with conventional imaging, enabling the detection of primary prostate cancer, lymph node staging, and evaluation of distant metastases. Furthermore, PSMA-PET has shown promise in the assessment of treatment response and guiding salvage therapy decisions.[5]

Despite the remarkable advancements and growing use of PSMA-PET, there are several pearls and pitfalls associated with this imaging modality. This review article aims to explore the principles of PSMA-PET, discuss its clinical applications in prostate cancer, highlight its advantages and pearls, address its limitations and pitfalls, examine current guidelines and recommendations, and shed light on the future directions of PSMA-PET on prostate cancer management.

[a] Radiology and Nuclear Medicine Department, Hospital Sirio Libanes, Rua Adma Jafet 91, São Paulo, Brazil; [b] Radiology and Nuclear Medicine Department, Americas Group, Rua Tupi 535, São Paulo, Brazil; [c] Radiology and Nuclear Medicine Department, Casa de Saúde São José, R. Macedo Sobrinho, 21 - Humaitá, Rio de Janeiro 22271-080, Brazil; [d] Nuclear Medicine Department, Hospital Vitória (Americas Group) and Hospital de Força Aérea do Galeão, Avenida Jorge Curry 550, Rio de Janeiro, Brazil
* Corresponding author. Departamento de Medicina Nuclear - Hospital Sirio Libanes, Rua Adma Jafet 115 - CEP: 01308-050.
E-mail address: felipegaliza@gmail.com

Radiol Clin N Am 62 (2024) 161–175
https://doi.org/10.1016/j.rcl.2023.07.002
0033-8389/24/© 2023 Elsevier Inc. All rights reserved.

PRINCIPLES OF PROSTATE-SPECIFIC MEMBRANE ANTIGEN PET IMAGING

Radiopharmaceuticals Used in Prostate-Specific Membrane Antigen PET Imaging (PSMA Agents)

PSMA is a transmembrane glycoprotein enzyme on the cell surface of normal prostate tissue that it is overexpressed in prostate cancer.[3,6–9]

Some PSMA-PET agents are labeled with 68 Ga, whereas others are labeled with 18F. 68 Ga has a shorter half-life (68 minutes) and higher positron energies resulting in slightly blurrier images compared with 18F with a 110-minute half-life and lower positron energies. 68Ga-PSMA-HBED-CC (also known as 68Ga-PSMA-11 or sometimes simply as 68Ga-PSMA) is the most widely used radioligand in clinical practice.[10]

18F-labeled PSMA-targeted PET imaging agents (eg, 18F-DCFBC, 18F-DCFPyL, and 18F-PSMA-1007), due to their favorable physical properties, have higher production capacity and improved imaging characteristics.[11,12]

18F-fluciclovine (anti-1-amino-3-18F-fluorocyclobutane-1-carboxylic acid [18F-FACBC]) is a synthetic nonmetabolized leucine amino acid analog that demonstrates high uptake in tissues that produce proteins or process amino acids. Amino acid transporter systems are upregulated in many carcinomas, including prostate cancer. This radiotracer is FDA approved currently for biochemical recurrence (BCR) assessment, however, has lower sensitivity compared with PSMA-radioligands. In a head-to-head comparison, 68Ga-PSMA-11 PET/CT outperformed 18F-fluciclovine, by detecting positive findings in 50% (5 out of 10) of patients who had a negative 18F-fluciclovine scan, and by detecting additional lesions in 20% of the patients who were positive with both scans.[13] The role of 18F-FACBC for prostate cancer diagnosis and workup is unclear presently, although it could be considered an alternative to PSMA radioligands in prostate cancer (PCa) with low PSMA expression.

Mechanism of Prostate-Specific Membrane Antigen Targeting and Uptake

PSMA transmembrane conformational structure enables it to exhibit an internalization functionality by means of endosomal complexes, which is a highly attractive feature for targeted diagnostic and therapeutic approaches, especially with radiopharmaceuticals.[6–8,14,15] PSMA expression occurs in normal epithelial prostate cells and is highly upregulated in PCa cells according to the biological aggressiveness of the disease, generally becoming more intense in high Gleason score, castration-resistant, and metastatic tumors.

Prostate-Specific Membrane Antigen Physiologic Uptake

Physiologic high-intensity activity is seen in the lacrimal, parotid, and submandibular glands. The precise mechanism of uptake remains uncertain but probably reflects a combination of nonspecific excretion and PSMA expression in these tissues. As with radioiodine, PSMA can be secreted in saliva, which may result in oropharyngeal, laryngeal, or esophageal uptake. High-intensity uptake may also be seen in the small bowel, primarily in the duodenum, where PSMA expression may facilitate absorption of dietary folates. Moderate-intensity uptake is seen in the liver and spleen.[3]

For [68 Ga]Ga-PSMA-11 and [18F]DCFPyL, high uptake is noted in the cortex of the kidneys, parotid and submandibular salivary glands, and duodenum. Moderate median uptake is noted in the spleen, liver, and lacrimal glands.[6–8] In comparison to [68 Ga]Ga-PSMA-11, the uptake of [18F]PSMA-1007 is higher in the liver, gallbladder, pancreas (due to predominant hepatobiliary excretion) and lower in the kidneys, bladder, and lacrimal glands.[16] Low urinary excretion of 18F-PSMA-1007 might be advantageous for delineation of local recurrence or pelvic lymph node metastases (**Fig. 1**).[12]

One limitation of both [68 Ga]Ga-PSMA-11 and [18F]DCFPyL is their increased urinary excretion in the ureters and the bladder, which limits the detection of local recurrence in the prostate bed.[16] Several techniques, including administration of furosemide, delayed imaging, and use of intravenous contrast material in a delayed urographic phase, can be helpful in differentiating physiologic urinary activity from pathologic uptake.[3]

Imaging Protocols and Techniques Used in Prostate-Specific Membrane Antigen PET Imaging

Tracer activity used should be reported in MBq, whether fixed 333 MBq for [18F]DCFPyL or patient-specific 1.8 to 2.2 MBq/kg for [68 Ga]Ga-PSMA-11 and 4 MBq/kg for [18F]PSMA-1007.[16]

For [68 Ga]Ga-PSMA-11 and [18F]DCFPyL, imaging is performed approximately 45 to 75 minutes after radiotracer administration, and for [18F]PSMA-1007, imaging is performed approximately 60 to 120 minutes after radiotracer administration. The standard acquisition should be from the vertex to the midthigh, with an acquisition time of 3 to 4 minutes per bed position.[6–8,16,17] A diagnostic CT scan with or without contrast media is performed.[17] The patient should be well hydrated and should void immediately before the scan.[3,9]

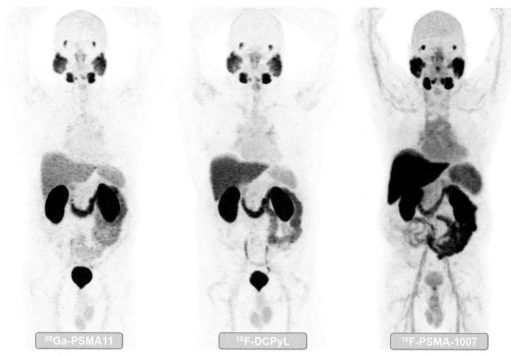

68Ga-PSMA11   18F-DCPyL   18F-PSMA-1007

Fig. 1. Normal biodistribution of the most common radiopharmaceuticals used in PSMA-PET imaging.

Additional PET imaging acquisition (early and delayed) has been studied, and the diagnostic benefits are controversial.[18]

Pitfalls and Limitations of Prostate-Specific Membrane Antigen PET Imaging

False-positive findings and potential causes

Despite PSMA-PET high specificity as an imaging tool, imaging readers must be aware of a variety of physiologic and other pathologic processes that can express PSMA, including normal nonprostatic epithelial cells, inflammation/infection, nonprostatic neoplastic cells, and nonprostatic tumor-associated neovasculature (endothelial expression),[19] and result in an interpretative error. Most of the nonprostate processes have a low intensity of tracer uptake or are nonfocal, in contrast to the focal and usually intense uptake associated with PCa lesions.[3]

Bone-related conditions

Most common pitfalls are healing bone fractures and degenerative bone changes.[20,21] [18F] PSMA-1007 has been described as having more unspecific benign bone uptake compared with [68 Ga]Ga-PSMA-11.[16,20,21] Another very common finding on PSMA-PET imaging is a single mild tracer uptake in the ribs (**Fig. 2**). The most prevalent pitfalls are described in the following (**Table 1**).

Ganglia of the sympathetic trunk

Radiotracer uptake by ganglia of the sympathetic trunk can be confused with lymph node metastasis. Lymph nodes are the second most common site of metastasis in patients with prostate cancer. Ganglia can be distinguished from lymph node metastases based on location (most prevalent: celiac, stellate, and sacral ganglia), low level of tracer uptake, and configuration (comma-shaped).[12,22] Conversely, lymph node metastases show significantly more intense uptake, and demonstrate a nodular configuration.[22]

Prostate-specific membrane antigen PET in other malignancies

PSMA expression has been described in various other tumor types, and it is mainly related to the expression in the tumor neovasculature rather than in the tumor cells themselves. High-intensity tracer uptake is seen in several malignant tumor types, including clear cell renal carcinoma,[16,23] salivary gland ductal carcinoma, glioblastoma multiforme, hepatocellular carcinoma, and gastric and pancreatic cancers.[1,19] Lower intensity uptake may be observed in a wide range of tumors.[19] Nevertheless, very-high intensity uptake is most frequently seen in prostate cancer, and the other tumor types can usually be differentiated by different patterns of spread and correlative anatomic appearances. Identification of synchronous PSMA-expressing

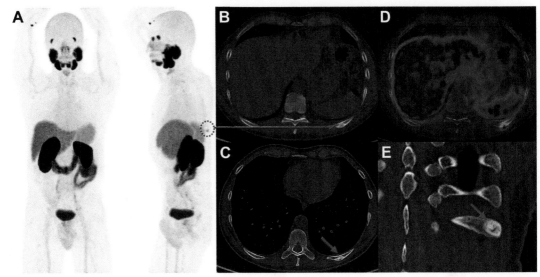

Fig. 2. MIP images from 68Ga-PSMA-PET (*A*) and axial (*B, C*), coronal (*E*) CT, and PET/CT (*D*) show a single focus of faint radiotracer uptake (*dashed circle* on *A*) in a typical fibrous osseous defect of the third right rib (*red arrow* on *B, C,* and *E*).

Table 1
Spectrum of reported benign bone pathologies with prostate-specific membrane antigen-uptake PET imaging that can mimic prostate cancer metastases

Bone		
	PSMA Expression	Notes
Osteodegenerative changes	Low-to-moderate	Osteodegenerative changes are very common among patients with PCa but only very few of them may present mild PSMA uptake, especially in the spine. The clue for diagnosis is the typical morphologic appearance of articular narrowing with sclerosis and osteophytosis[19]
Fracture Fibrous cortical defect	Low-to-moderate Low-to-moderate	Single mild tracer uptake in the ribs; it is usually not related to PCa and does not require further investigation because the dedicated CT from PET/CT is often sufficient for a confident diagnosis. Fibrous cortical defect can seem as a lucent area with sclerotic rim. In few unclear cases, a dedicated CT with a bone filter should offer a better morphologic correlation[19]
Paget disease	Diffuse low-to-moderate and heterogeneous uptake delineating the cortex of pelvic bones	Typical morphologic changes, such as diffuse sclerosis, thickened cortex, bone expansion, and coarsened trabeculae. Close anatomic correlation usually enables these entities to be characterized with confidence
Hemangioma	Low-to-moderate	Thickened bone trabeculae (salt and pepper)

malignancies has been reported to be very uncommon (0.7%).[3,24]

False-negative findings and potential challenges

Although most pitfalls represent false-positive findings, some factors may induce false-negative findings as well. Up to 5% of prostate adenocarcinomas do not express PSMA. Furthermore, aggressive forms of primary neuroendocrine PCa or neuroendocrine dedifferentiation in metastatic castration-resistant PCa (mCRPC) may show a reduced PSMA expression.[16] 18F-FDG-PET/CT can have a role for the disease assessment in such scenarios.[12]

Technical considerations and limitations, availability limitations

Lesion evaluation can be challenging in specific situations, and practitioners should use a combination of aspects: (1) molecular (ie, uptake intensity and extension), (2) morphologic (ie, based on the CT/MR imaging findings [9] [10]), and (3) biological/clinical (ie, does it fit with known PCa staging, predicted spread, and/or prostate-specific antigen [PSA] values?).[19]

When findings are equivocal, a contrast-enhanced CT within the PET/CT study may be requested or subsequent evaluation by dedicated MR imaging may be suggested to aid in clarification. Sometimes, however, differentiation to a secondary malignancy is difficult, and a biopsy is required for the diagnosis.[19]

CLINICAL APPLICATIONS OF PROSTATE-SPECIFIC MEMBRANE ANTIGEN PET

Detection and Primary Staging of Prostate Cancer

Imaging initial staging of prostate cancer for decades has been done with bone scintigraphy and abdominal CT scan depending on the risk for metastatic disease. Low-risk tumor patients (ISUP 1 and 2) usually do not have indication for systemic imaging staging, due to its very low probability of metastatic disease. However, intermediate-risk and high-risk patients should undergo imaging workup to determine the locoregional nodal (N) and distant metastasis (M) staging. More recent with the incorporation of multiparametric magnetic resonance (mpMR) of the prostate in early stages of PCa screening and diagnosis, it is also recommended and feasible to assess the local (T) staging, which can increase the accuracy of clinical nomograms to assess the probability of extraprostatic extension (EPE) and consequently customize treatment

approach (nerve sparing, surgical margins, and so forth).[25]

Currently for T of PCa, mpMR imaging has the highest spatial resolution and offers a more accurate assessment compared with CT. For such reason PSMA-PET/CT has a limited role for this purpose because the CT component is not accurate for EPE risk stratification. A straight comparison between mpMR imaging and PSMA-PET/CT demonstrated that both methods had comparable intraprostatic tumor detection; however, mpMR imaging was superior to assess extracapsular extension (ECE) and seminal vesicle invasion.[26] The majority of prostate cancer has PSMA expression (95%) on PET, and there is a good correlation of uptake intensity (measured by standard uptake value [SUV]) and histology grading (Gleason/ISUP). More aggressive tumors (Gleason score > 7) tend to have higher uptake (SUV >10).[27] This information can be helpful to decide treatment plan in a scenario where there is a discrepancy between clinical information and biopsy histology. Primary tumor PSMA-radioligand uptake also has a prognostic value, as cancers with higher SUVs tend to have earlier and higher rates of BCR,[28] which translates a relevant prognostic biomarker.

The main purpose of systemic staging is to determine extraprostatic disease to lymph nodes (N) and distant organ (M), fundamental for deciding patient management and therapy strategies. This is the additional role of PSMA-PET for PCa initial disease. The literature has increasing data supporting the superior accuracy to detect N and M compared with conventional (CT and BS). The proPSMA trial demonstrated that prospectively, with a higher accuracy (92% vs 65%), greater treatment influence, and fewer uncertain finding (7% vs 23%).[29] Such data led to the inclusion of PSMA-PET on the National Comprehensive Case Network (NCCN) guideline in 2021.[30]

PSMA-PET has a higher sensitivity and specificity compared with CT to detect nodal disease. The average sensitivity in the literature is around 50% to 60%.[27,29,31] The relatively low sensitivity is attributed to the limited detection of micrometastasis. Tumor deposits of less than 4 mm have lower detection rates, and their prevalence is not low in PCa.[32] Nevertheless, the specificity is very high (>90%), which leads to a high confidence in reducing the need for histology confirmation of findings, and consequently a reliable noninvasive test for staging (**Fig. 3**). Pelvic nodal disease detected on PSMA has prognostic implication that can change management. Nodal positive disease on PSMA-PET has a higher chance of not being cured with prostatectomy alone, more persistent disease, and correlates with early BCR,

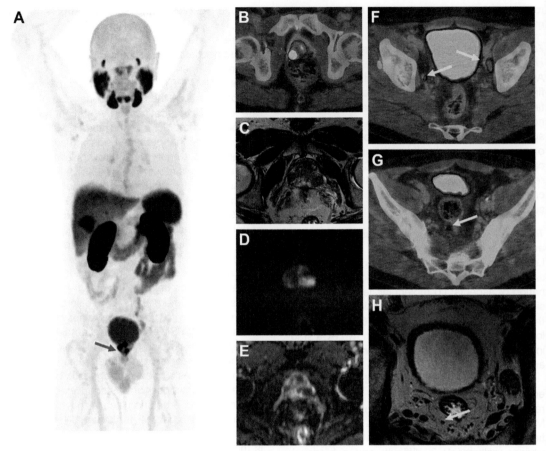

Fig. 3. (A–H) Initial staging of prostate cancer in a 58-year-old patient (PSA 150 ng/mL, Gleason 8/ISUP 4). MIP images from ^{68}Ga-PSMA-PET (A) and axial (B, F, G) PET/CT images show high radiotracer uptake in a right peripheral zone lesion—one of the multifocal lesions (red arrow on A and B), which correlates with the findings at MR images (C, D, and E). Also noted that one small mesorectal lymph node was considered negative at the MR images due to small size (yellow arrow on H) but positive on PET/CT images with moderate to high radiotracer uptake (yellow arrow on G). Bilateral positive external iliac nodes are also noted (yellow arrows on F).

despite the pathologic N status.[31] Moreover, PSMA detects sites of nodal spread that are not traditionally included on radical treatment (ie, prostatectomy or radiation therapy [RT]), such as in the mesorectal and perivesical regions.

Bone metastasis is the most prevalent site of distant metastasis in PCa. PSMA-PET has a higher sensitivity and specificity compared with BS, with less uncertain findings.[29] In the PROSTAGE trial, PSMA-PET had superior sensitivity for detection of bone metastasis compared all available whole-body (WB) imaging methods to stage high-risk PCa, including whole-body magnetic ressonance (WB-MR) and bone single photon emission computed tomography (SPECT)-CT scintigraphy.[33] All morphologic patterns of bone metastasis (ie, lytic, blastic, and medullary) can express PSMA, whereas BS has limited detection of nonsclerotic lesions (Fig. 4).[18]

There is an emerging role of PSMA-PET in the early PCa diagnosis. MpMR imaging is established as the imaging method that improves the detection of clinical significant PCa (csPCa) while reducing the detection of insignificant PCa that require no treatment. Still a nonnegligible number of csPCa are not detected by mpMR imaging. Early retrospective data demonstrated a higher detection rate of intraprostatic tumor foci by PSMA-PET compared with MR, and recently prospective data in an early diagnostic scenario demonstrated PSMA-PET added value to mpMR imaging in detecting csPCa. PSMA-PET combined with mpMR imaging increased negative predictive value to 91% (MR alone—72%) and also increased sensitivity to 97% (MR alone—83%).[34] There are prostate regions where tumor detection can be challenging for mpMR imaging (eg, very distal close to pelvic floor, anterior fibromuscular stroma,

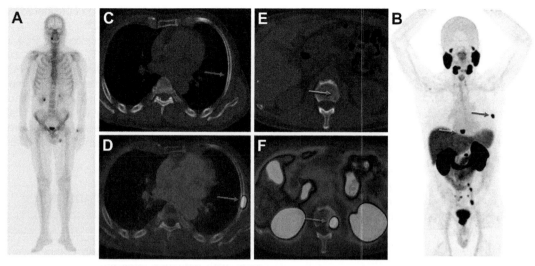

Fig. 4. Initial staging of prostate cancer in a 66-year-old patient (PSA 18 ng/mL, Gleason 8/ISUP 4). Bone scintigraphy was considered negative (*A*). MIP images from ^{68}Ga-PSMA-PET (*B*) and axial (*C–F*) PET/CT images show high radiotracer uptake in a sclerotic lesion in a left rib (*red arrow on B, C and D*) and a lytic lesion on left lateral half of D5 (*red arrow on B, E and F*).

periurethral, and central zone),[35] and perhaps PSMA-PET can help overcome this limitation (**Fig. 5**). Data on how to implement PSMA-PET in this setting is lacking but patients with earlier negative biopsy and mpMR imaging who have persistent clinical suspicious for PCa (eg, persistently elevated or increasing PSA), may benefit from the high sensitivity of PSMA-PET for PCa detection.[36] There are ongoing trials to determine the real role of PSMA-PET combined with mpMR in the early PCa detection scenario.

Assessment of Biochemical Recurrence

PCa recurrence is a frequent concern for patients after radical prostatectomy (RP) or RT. Studies show that between 25% and 55% of patients will experience an increase in PSA levels after those treatments.[37] PCa BCR is characterized by a PSA level greater than 0.2 ng/mL (0.2 µg/L) in 2 consecutive measurements following RP, when the PSA level is equal to or greater than 2.0 ng/mL above the lowest recorded value after RT (nadir).[38]

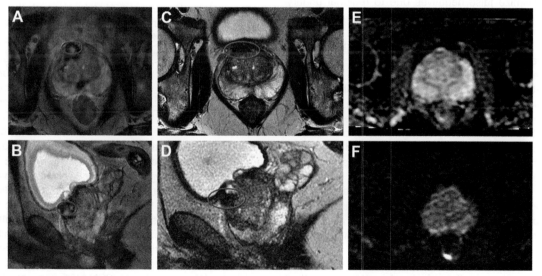

Fig. 5. A 57-year-old patient (PSA 9.8 ng/mL) with 2 prior negative transrectal ultrasound-guided systematic prostate biopsies. Axial (*A*) and sagittal (*B*) images from ^{68}Ga-PSMA-PET/MR show moderate radiotracer uptake in an ill-defined anterior fibromuscular stroma lesion (*red circle on A–D*) without restricted diffusion (*E* and *F*).

Although high levels of PSA usually appear before a detectable lesion is found on conventional imaging, PSMA-PET shows substantially higher detection rates than those reported for conventional imaging modalities, and at lower PSA levels, with higher sensitivity and specificity in this scenario.[18] PSMA-PET presents a detection rate of 38% for PSA levels less than 0.5 ng/mL; 57% for 0.5 to less than 1.0 ng/mL; 84% for 1.0 to less than 2.0 ng/mL, 86% for 2.0 to less than 5.0 ng/mL, and 97% for 5.0 ng/mL or greater.[31]

Abdominopelvic lymph nodes are the predominant site of metastasis, occurring in around 50% of cases, whereas local recurrence and bone metastases occur in approximately 35% of the cases.[17] The prevalence and site of recurrence vary depending on the chosen curative-intent treatment, either RT or RP.

LOCAL RECURRENCE AFTER RADICAL PROSTATECTOMY

Typical sites—The most frequent sites of local recurrence after surgery are the vesicourethral anastomosis (~62% of cases), the lateral surgical margins or remnant ducti deferentia (~25% of cases) and the retrovesical region, topography of rectoprostatic/Denonvilliers fascia (8%–21% of cases).[39]

Most vesicourethral anastomosis positive cases on PSMA-PET do not exhibit tomographic findings, relying solely on the criteria of a mild-to-moderate focal radiotracer uptake within the fibrotic tissue (**Fig. 6**).[17] Administering diuretics before or after PET image acquisition can help minimize false negatives due to regional urinary radiotracer activity and enhance the accuracy of the examination.[40]

Atypical sites—The emergence of PSMA-PET has redefined several anatomic concepts regarding how PCa behaves and spreads.[41] Atypical metastatic sites (ie, penile urethra, bladder wall, and rectum) that were previously difficult to detect can now be characterized using PSMA-PET, thereby aiding in the choice of new therapeutic approaches, and reducing the chance of subjecting patients to inappropriate treatments.

Although penile urethral metastatic deposits secondary to PCa are rarely documented in the literature, the available reports indicate an association with an aggressive disease progression and unfavorable prognosis, particularly those originating from ductal tumors.[42,43] Urethral metastases typically occur through direct involvement with a prostate bed lesion. The morphologic appearance (wall thickening) is indistinguishable from that of urothelial cancer, which should be considered as the primary differential diagnosis.[43]

Another rare site for local recurrence of PCa is the rectum. Before PSMA-PET, this diagnosis was typically made in metastatic patients (mPC) with poor survival outcomes and significant symptoms. The morphologic features include an anterior mass or irregular wall thickening, with annular wall infiltration, potentially accompanied by stricture. The degree of PSMA uptake can vary alongside these manifestations.[44]

LOCAL RECURRENCE AFTER RADIATION THERAPY

Although there is limited literature on PSMA-PET in local BCR after RT, it is a relatively common scenario, with detection rates ranging from 10% to 60% in external beam radiation therapy (EBRT) and 7% to 35% in brachytherapy. The PSMA-PET detection rate is significantly higher in patients who underwent EBRT (~95%) compared with brachytherapy (~75%).[45,46]

Typical sites—Most reccurrences identified by PSMA-PET after RT are characterized by focal tracer uptake in the prostate or seminal vesicles, often at the same location as the primary lesion before treatment. Unlike after RP, urinary excretion does not appear to hamper the detection of local recurrence after RT.[46]

Atypical sites—There are no major differences from the atypical findings seen after RP. The bladder wall represents an uncommon site for local PCa recurrence, often located at a considerable distance from the bladder neck in contact with prostate. Some case reports suggest that upfront external beam RT may be preferred over brachytherapy to reduce the risk of viable malignant cell dislodgement into the bladder because the bladder neck is typically not included in the high-dose area.[47]

REGIONAL NODAL RECURRENCE

As previously mentioned, pelvic lymph nodes are the primary site of metastasis in patients with BCR, occurring in approximately 40% to 60% of cases.[17] The nodal status plays a crucial role in determining the appropriate therapeutic approach. Recent studies have demonstrated that PSMA-PET has a detectability limit of 5 mm for identifying positive lymph nodes. Although smaller positive lymph nodes may occasionally result in false negatives, PSMA-PET imaging sensibility still surpasses that of conventional methods.[48]

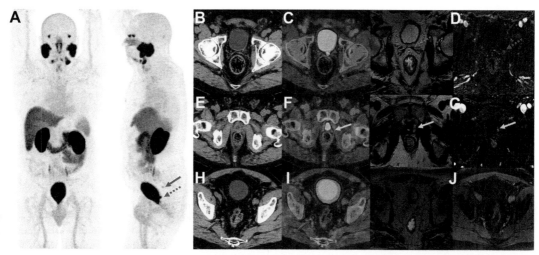

Fig. 6. Prostate cancer BCR (PSA 0.37 ng/mL) in a 67-year-old patient after RP for Gleason 9/ISUP 5 prostate cancer. *(A–J)* MIP images from ^{68}Ga-PSMA-PET *(A)* and axial *(A, B, C, E, F, H,* and *I)* CT and PET/CT images show high radiotracer uptake in the vesicourethral anastomosis *(yellow arrow* in *A* and *F)*, retrovesical space *(dashed red arrow* in *A, B* and *C)* and right internal iliac lymph node *(red arrow* in *A, H* and *I)*. Axial T2-weighted and dynamic contrast-enhanced MR images *(dashed red arrow* and *yellow arrow* in *A, D* and *G)* show mild early enhancement considered suspicious findings, not being able to characterize the pelvic lymph node *(J)*. Eiber M., Maurer T., Souvatzoglou M., et al. Evaluation of Hybrid 68Ga-PSMA Ligand PET/CT in 248 Patients with Biochemical Recurrence After Radical Prostatectomy. J Nucl Med 2015;56(5):668–74. © SNMM

Typical spread—Nodal involvement in PCa typically shows lateralization corresponding to the dominant side of the primary disease.[3]

Pelvic lymph nodes, particularly those in the obturator fossae, external iliac, and internal iliac regions, are the most commonly involved.[49] However, after RP followed by lymphadenectomy, the common iliac and retroperitoneal nodes (nonregional) become more frequently affected. This change in the lymph node distribution highlights the importance of thorough lymphadenectomy and the need to consider these nonregional nodes as potential sites of metastasis. Understanding this altered nodal pattern is crucial for accurate staging and treatment planning, including the consideration of adjuvant therapies targeting the nonregional nodes.[50]

Atypical spread—Pelvic lymph node dissection usually follows a standard template (external and internal iliac nodes and obturator nodes) or an extended template (standard template plus para-aortic and presacral nodes).[51] Therefore, the diagnosis of atypical nodal involvement sites (such as mesorectal and retroperitoneal nodes) is crucial for determining therapeutic/surgical planning.[51,52]

PSMA-PET imaging has revealed previously unnoticed mesorectal metastases in up to 15% of patients with prostate cancer. These metastases, often overlooked by conventional imaging methods due to their small size, can now be more accurately identified (**Fig. 7**).[53] These findings

highlight the importance of considering this region for treatment planning.[3,53] Isolated retroperitoneal lymph node involvement with sparing of the pelvic region is uncommon.[54]

One potential pitfall develops while interpreting mild tracer uptake on normal-sized inguinal, axillary, and mediastinal lymph nodes, which should be considered negative for metastasis, and possibly related to inflammatory scenarios.

Evaluation of Metastatic Disease

Approximately 65% of men with PSA failure after RP may develop metastatic disease within 10 years.[55] A retrospective study showed that 59% of mPC had bone involvement, 32% had limited lymph node metastases (mainly in pelvic nodes), and 6% had lung or liver metastases.[56] Distant lymph node metastases can occur in various locations, including mediastinal and cervical nodes.[57]

Typical sites—Bone is the most common site of PCa metastases[56,58] and although bone scintigraphy and CT are effective in detecting osteoblastic lesions, their ability to detect osteolytic and bone marrow metastases is limited (**Fig. 8**).[1,2] PSMA-PET reveals distinct expression patterns in different types of bone metastases (osteoblastic, osteolytic, and bone marrow). Higher PSMA uptake is observed in osteolytic and bone marrow lesions, suggesting a greater number of viable tumor

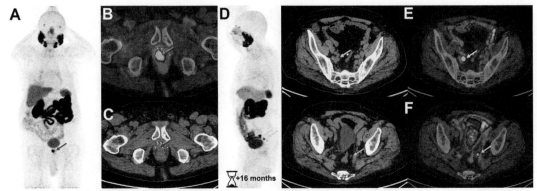

Fig. 7. Prostate cancer BCR (PSA 6.7 ng/mL) in an 84-year-old patient after brachytherapy. (A–C)[68]Ga-PSMA-PET (A), CT (B), and PET/CT (C) images show exclusive prostate gland recurrence with intense tracer accumulation in the right peripheral zone (arrow in A–C). MR imaging examination (not shown) was considered negative. Patient underwent SBRT. After 16 months, the patient presented with new BCR (PSA 8.4 ng/mL). (D–F) ^{68}Ga-PSMA-PET/CT (E and F) images show intense tracer accumulation in a right internal iliac (yellow arrow in E) and mesorectal lymph node (green arrow in D and F).

cells and increased malignancy.[59] Moreover, osteolytic lesions may exhibit rapid tumor growth, elevated PSMA expression, and enhanced neovascularization.

In advanced stages of prostate cancer, lung, and liver lesions frequently emerge as additional sites of distant recurrence, often coexisting with bone metastases.[58,60]

Atypical sites—Rare metastatic sites, affecting less than 5% of patients, can manifest in any

organ, including the brain and meninges, thyroid gland, adrenal glands, peritoneum, gastrointestinal tract (stomach and intestine), and urinary tract (ureter, urethra, and kidney).[58,61–64]

Oligometastatic vs Polymetastatic—Over time, patients with PCa can develop castration-sensitive distant metastases, which may eventually progress to castration-resistant disease that continues to grow despite anti-androgen deprivation therapy (ADT).

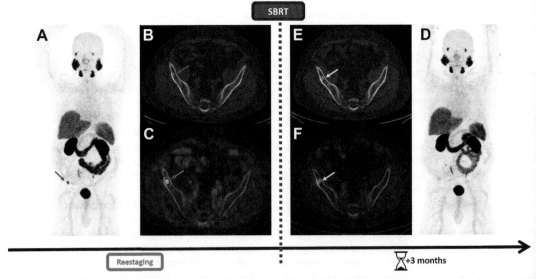

Fig. 8. Therapeutic response assessment after SBRT of a single metastatic bone lesion in the right ilium in a 72-year-old patient with prostate cancer (PSA 186 ng/mL, Gleason score 9) treated with RT 21 years before. Coronal MIP PET (A), transverse CT (B), and transverse PET/CT (C) images before treatment show an intense PSMA uptake in a sclerotic lesion (red arrow A-C). After SBRT (D–F), the lesion became more sclerotic and showed lower radiotracer uptake (yellow arrow D-F).

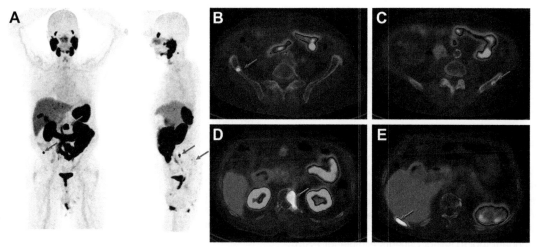

Fig. 9. Prostate cancer restaging in a patient with rising PSA (3.9 ng/mL) scheduled for RT of prostatic bed recurrence and SBRT of two metastatic bone lesions. Besides identifying the local recurrence, PSMA-PET/CT detected at least 6 additional bone lesions (*red arrows A-E*) missed on BS. Because of the additional sites of disease detected, the patient management was changed to systemic therapy.

Furthermore, they can present with either oligometastatic or polymetastatic disease. Oligometastases is a term used to describe a state between localized and disseminated disease, in which fewer than 3 to 5 metastatic lesions are present.[65] Metastasis-directed therapy (MDT), such as stereotactic body radiation therapy (SBRT) and pelvic salvage lymph node dissection surgery, has been found to improve clinical outcomes in patients with oligometases.[18] In addition, it is established that early curative MDT can delay ADT initiation and minimize toxicities, providing effective disease control (**Fig. 9**).[65,66]

In this setting, PSMA-PET enhances accuracy in detecting and distinguishing nodal, bone, visceral, and mixed oligometastatic PCa recurrence compared with conventional imaging. This enables early identification of oligometastatic disease and facilitates targeted treatments because CT and BS may underestimate the number of lesions due to their limited sensitivity.[18,67]

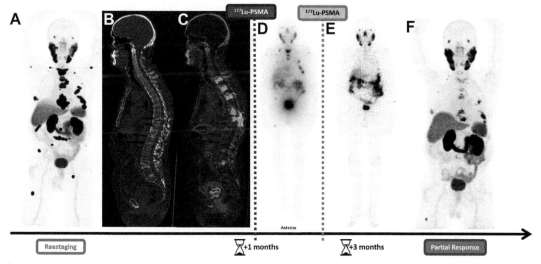

Fig. 10. Restaging of a mCRPC (PSA 186 ng/mL) in an 86-year-old patient after RT, ADT, and 223Ra radionuclide therapy. MIP (*A*), sagittal CT reconstruction (*B*), and fused PSMA-PET/CT images (*C*) show multifocal osseous metastases. The patient underwent 2 cycles of ^{177}Lu-PSMA radionuclide therapy. Posttreatment whole-body scans (*D* and *E*) and ^{68}Ga-PSMA-PET MIP (*F*) images show persistent but decreased radiotracer uptake by the metastatic lesions, compatible partial response to treatment.

Up to 20% of patients with advanced PCa will progress while receiving ADT, a disease status known as mCRPC, which has a poor prognosis and impaired quality of life.[68] Available therapeutic modalities for mCRPC include second-generation ADT, chemotherapy, immunotherapy, and radionuclide therapy. PSMA-PET can be a reliable baseline parameter for future systemic response assessment or as a theranostic selector for radionuclide PSMA-based therapy.[67,69]

The principle of any targeted therapy infers that the target structure is abundantly expressed from tumor cells, and PSMA-based therapy is no different. Unfortunately, PCa is characterized by high genetic and phenotypic heterogeneity, especially in the late-stage setting.[70] Therefore, PSMA-PET is an important tool to select patients eligible for PSMA-based therapy (ie, 177Lutetium-PSMA; Fig. 10).

There is no consensus on what should be considered an adequate tumor uptake at one of the PSMA-ligand PET agents for patient selection. There is, however, evidence that SUVs of the related pretreatment PSMA-PET/CT correlate with tumor absorbed dose and consequently a higher level of biochemical response.[71] According to previous studies, it is suggested that adequate tumor uptake should be at least higher than the liver.[72,73] Tumor uptake greater than 1.5 to 2-fold liver background for 68Ga-PSMA-11 and tumor uptake is greater than salivary gland uptake for 18F-PSMA-1007 seems to be a valuable threshold.[74]

Many imaging criteria have been proposed to assess the therapeutic response of metastatic PCa. For PSMA-PET, Fanti and colleagues[75] proposed a response assessment criteria, the PSMA-PET Progression criteria, which has some similarities with the PET Response Criteria in Solid Tumors[76] and considered clinical and laboratory data besides imaging to define progression. This criteria still needs further validation in clinical trials.

One of the uncertainties regarding PSMA-PET concerns the effect of ADT on imaging. Short-term ADT may increase PSMA expression (flare phenomenon),[77–79] whereas long-term ADT probably has the opposite effect.[80] Long-term ADT induces apoptosis of androgen-sensitive cells, causing a reduction in tumor volume and a subsequent decrease in PSA levels and PSMA uptake. However, one-third of patients undergoing long-term ADT still had visible lesions at PSMA-PET, despite complete biochemical remission. In this context, PSMA-PET-positive lesions correlate with PCa cell clones that became castration resistant.[81] There is no ideal time point for PSMA-PET response assessment during ADT; it is recommended at least a 3-month interval to avoid misinterpretation.

SUMMARY

PSMA-PET has emerged as a valuable tool in the management of PCa, providing clinicians with enhanced capabilities in accurate staging and treatment planning. The advantages of PSMA-PET compared with conventional imaging include its improved detection sensitivity and specificity and high-resolution imaging capabilities. These advancements have contributed to improved patient outcomes.

However, it is essential to acknowledge the limitations and pitfalls of PSMA-PET. False-positive and false-negative findings, technical challenges, and cost and availability issues pose challenges in its widespread adoption.

Current guidelines and recommendations recognize the value of PSMA-PET in clinical practice, and evidence supporting its integration continues to grow. The future of PSMA-PET holds great promise, with ongoing research focusing on optimizing imaging techniques, radiotracer development, and further validating its prognostic implications.

CLINICS CARE POINTS

- Recognizing the differences between the PSMA tracers and their features, as well as the main pitfalls, is fundamental to the interpretation of the examination.
- The CT component and the tracer uptake pattern evaluation are essential in differentiating PSMA-PET pitfalls from metastases.
- PSMA-PET is superior to CT and bone scintigraphy and can change management in staging and BCR.

DISCLOSURE

All authors disclose not having any commercial or financial conflicts of interest and any funding sources.

REFERENCES

1. Lange MB, Nielsen ML, Andersen JD, et al. Diagnostic accuracy of imaging methods for the diagnosis of skeletal malignancies: A retrospective analysis against a pathology-proven reference. Eur J Radiol 2016;85(1):61–7.
2. Evangelista L, Panunzio A, Polverosi R, et al. Early bone marrow metastasis detection: the additional value of FDG-PET/CT vs. CT imaging. Biomed Pharmacother 2012;66(6):448–53.

3. Hofman MS, Hicks RJ, Maurer T, et al. Prostate-specific Membrane Antigen PET: Clinical Utility in Prostate Cancer, Normal Patterns, Pearls, and Pitfalls. Radiographics 2018;38(1):200–17.

4. Eder M, Schäfer M, Bauder-Wüst U, et al. 68Ga-complex lipophilicity and the targeting property of a urea-based PSMA inhibitor for PET imaging. Bioconjug Chem 2012;23(4):688–97.

5. Barbosa FG, Queiroz MA, Ferraro DA, et al. Prostate-specific Membrane Antigen PET: Therapy Response Assessment in Metastatic Prostate Cancer. Radiographics 2020;40(5):1412–30.

6. O'Keefe DS, Bacich DJ, Huang SS, et al. A Perspective on the Evolving Story of PSMA Biology, PSMA-Based Imaging, and Endoradiotherapeutic Strategies. J Nucl Med 2018;59(7):1007–13.

7. Carter RE, Feldman AR, Coyle JT. Prostate-specific membrane antigen is a hydrolase with substrate and pharmacologic characteristics of a neuropeptidase. Proc Natl Acad Sci U S A 1996;93(2):749–53.

8. Pfob CH, Ziegler S, Graner FP, et al. Biodistribution and radiation dosimetry of (68)Ga-PSMA HBED CC-a PSMA specific probe for PET imaging of prostate cancer. Eur J Nucl Med Mol Imaging 2016; 43(11):1962–70.

9. Pomykala KL, Farolfi A, Hadaschik B, et al. Molecular Imaging for Primary Staging of Prostate Cancer. Semin Nucl Med 2019;49(4):271–9.

10. Basu S, Alavi A. PET-based molecular imaging in evolving personalized management design, an issue of PET clinics (The Clinics: Internal Medicine Book 11). E-Book. Elsevier Health Sciences; 2016.

11. Sanchez-Crespo A. Comparison of Gallium-68 and Fluorine-18 imaging characteristics in positron emission tomography. Appl Radiat Isot 2013;76:55–62.

12. Sheikhbahaei S, Werner RA, Solnes LB, et al. Prostate-Specific Membrane Antigen (PSMA)-Targeted PET Imaging of Prostate Cancer: An Update on Important Pitfalls. Semin Nucl Med 2019;49(4):255–70.

13. Mena E, Lindenberg LM, Choyke PL. New Targets for PET Molecular Imaging of Prostate Cancer. Semin Nucl Med 2019;49(4):326–36.

14. Rajasekaran SA, Anilkumar G, Oshima E, et al. A novel cytoplasmic tail MXXXL motif mediates the internalization of prostate-specific membrane antigen. Mol Biol Cell 2003;14(12):4835–45.

15. Liu H, Rajasekaran AK, Moy P, et al. Constitutive and antibody-induced internalization of prostate-specific membrane antigen. Cancer Res 1998;58(18):4055–60.

16. Ceci F, Oprea-Lager DE, Emmett L, et al. E-PSMA: the EANM standardized reporting guidelines v1.0 for PSMA-PET. Eur J Nucl Med Mol Imaging 2021; 48(5):1626–38.

17. Eiber M, Maurer T, Souvatzoglou M, et al. Evaluation of Hybrid 68Ga-PSMA Ligand PET/CT in 248 Patients with Biochemical Recurrence After Radical Prostatectomy. J Nucl Med 2015;56(5):668–74.

18. Barbosa FG, Queiroz MA, Nunes RF, et al. Revisiting Prostate Cancer Recurrence with PSMA PET: Atlas of Typical and Atypical Patterns of Spread. Radiographics 2019;39(1):186–212.

19. de Galiza Barbosa F, Queiroz MA, Nunes RF, et al. Nonprostatic diseases on PSMA PET imaging: a spectrum of benign and malignant findings. Cancer Imaging 2020;20(1):23.

20. Uprimny C, Kroiss AS, Decristoforo C, et al. Early dynamic imaging in Ga- PSMA-11 PET/CT allows discrimination of urinary bladder activity and prostate cancer lesions. Eur J Nucl Med Mol Imaging 2017;44(5):765–75.

21. Panagiotidis E, Paschali A, Giannoula E, et al. Rib Fractures Mimicking Bone Metastases in 18F-PSMA-1007 PET/CT for Prostate Cancer. Clin Nucl Med 2019;44(1):e46–8.

22. Rischpler C, Beck TI, Okamoto S, et al. Ga-PSMA-HBED-CC Uptake in Cervical, Celiac, and Sacral Ganglia as an Important Pitfall in Prostate Cancer PET Imaging. J Nucl Med 2018;59(9):1406–11.

23. Blute ML, Chang SL. Renal cancer: old and new paradigms, an issue of urologic clinics: Volume 50-2, 1st Edition. E-Book. Elsevier Health Sciences; 2023.

24. Osman MM, Iravani A, Hicks RJ, et al. Detection of Synchronous Primary Malignancies with Ga-Labeled Prostate-Specific Membrane Antigen PET/CT in Patients with Prostate Cancer: Frequency in 764 Patients. J Nucl Med 2017;58(12):1938–42.

25. Mehralivand S, Shih JH, Harmon S, et al. A Grading System for the Assessment of Risk of Extraprostatic Extension of Prostate Cancer at Multiparametric MRI. Radiology 2019;290(3):709–19.

26. Sonni I, Felker ER, Lenis AT, et al. Head-to-Head Comparison of 68Ga-PSMA-11 PET/CT and mpMRI with a Histopathology Gold Standard in the Detection, Intraprostatic Localization, and Determination of Local Extension of Primary Prostate Cancer: Results from a Prospective Single-Center Imaging Trial. J Nucl Med 2022;63(6):847–54.

27. Yaxley JW, Raveenthiran S, Nouhaud F-X, et al. Risk of metastatic disease on 68 gallium-prostate-specific membrane antigen positron emission tomography/computed tomography scan for primary staging of 1253 men at the diagnosis of prostate cancer. BJU Int 2019;124(3):401–7.

28. Roberts MJ, Morton A, Papa N, et al. Primary tumour PSMA intensity is an independent prognostic biomarker for biochemical recurrence-free survival following radical prostatectomy. Eur J Nucl Med Mol Imaging 2022;49(9):3289–94.

29. Hofman MS, Lawrentschuk N, Francis RJ, et al. Prostate-specific membrane antigen PET-CT in patients with high-risk prostate cancer before curative-intent surgery or radiotherapy (proPSMA): a prospective, randomised, multicentre study. Lancet 2020;395(10231):1208–16.

30. Schaeffer E, Srinivas S, Antonarakis ES, et al. NCCN Guidelines Insights: Prostate Cancer, Version 1.2021. J Natl Compr Canc Netw 2021;19(2):134–43.

31. Fendler WP, Calais J, Eiber M, et al. Assessment of 68Ga-PSMA-11 PET Accuracy in Localizing Recurrent Prostate Cancer: A Prospective Single-Arm Clinical Trial. JAMA Oncol 2019;5(6):856–63.

32. van Leeuwen PJ, Emmett L, Ho B, et al. Prospective evaluation of 68Gallium-prostate-specific membrane antigen positron emission tomography/computed tomography for preoperative lymph node staging in prostate cancer. BJU Int 2017;119(2):209–15.

33. Anttinen M, Ettala O, Malaspina S, et al. A Prospective Comparison of 18F-prostate-specific Membrane Antigen-1007 Positron Emission Tomography Computed Tomography, Whole-body 1.5 T Magnetic Resonance Imaging with Diffusion-weighted Imaging, and Single-photon Emission Computed Tomography/Computed Tomography with Traditional Imaging in Primary Distant Metastasis Staging of Prostate Cancer (PROSTAGE). Eur Urol Oncol 2021; 4(4):635–44.

34. Emmett L, Buteau J, Papa N, et al. The Additive Diagnostic Value of Prostate-specific Membrane Antigen Positron Emission Tomography Computed Tomography to Multiparametric Magnetic Resonance Imaging Triage in the Diagnosis of Prostate Cancer (PRIMARY): A Prospective Multicentre Study. Eur Urol 2021;80(6):682–9.

35. Rosenkrantz AB, Verma S, Turkbey B. Prostate cancer: top places where tumors hide on multiparametric MRI. AJR Am J Roentgenol 2015;204(4):W449–56.

36. Lopci E, Saita A, Lazzeri M, et al. 68Ga-PSMA Positron Emission Tomography/Computerized Tomography for Primary Diagnosis of Prostate Cancer in Men with Contraindications to or Negative Multiparametric Magnetic Resonance Imaging: A Prospective Observational Study. J Urol 2018;200(1):95–103.

37. Sanda MG, Cadeddu JA, Kirkby E, et al. Clinically Localized Prostate Cancer: AUA/ASTRO/SUO Guideline. Part II: Recommended Approaches and Details of Specific Care Options. J Urol 2018; 199(4):990–7.

38. Freedland SJ, Rumble RB, Finelli A, et al. Adjuvant and salvage radiotherapy after prostatectomy: American Society of Clinical Oncology clinical practice guideline endorsement. J Clin Oncol 2014; 32(34):3892–8.

39. Sella T, Schwartz LH, Swindle PW, et al. Suspected local recurrence after radical prostatectomy: endorectal coil MR imaging. Radiology 2004;231(2):379–85.

40. Fendler WP, Eiber M, Beheshti M, et al. PSMA PET/CT: joint EANM procedure guideline/SNMMI procedure standard for prostate cancer imaging 2.0. Eur J Nucl Med Mol Imaging 2023;50(5):1466–86.

41. Dureja S, Thakral P, Pant V, et al. Rare Sites of Metastases in Prostate Cancer Detected on Ga-68 PSMA PET/CT Scan-A Case Series. Indian J Nucl Med 2017;32(1):13–5.

42. Mary Mansbridge Margaret, Strahan Andrew, Parker Jonathon, et al. PSMA-PET/CT-avid metastatic prostate cancer to the penis. BMJ Case Rep 2020;13(3):e233522.

43. Ellis CL, Epstein JI. Metastatic prostate adenocarcinoma to the penis: a series of 29 cases with predilection for ductal adenocarcinoma. Am J Surg Pathol 2015;39(1):67–74.

44. Bowrey DJ, Otter MI, Billings PJ. Rectal infiltration by prostatic adenocarcinoma: report on six patients and review of the literature. Ann R Coll Surg Engl 2003;85(6):382–5.

45. Hruby G, Eade T, Kneebone A, et al. Delineating biochemical failure with Ga-PSMA-PET following definitive external beam radiation treatment for prostate cancer. Radiother Oncol 2017;122(1):99–102.

46. Einspieler I, Rauscher I, Düwel C, et al. Detection Efficacy of Hybrid Ga-PSMA Ligand PET/CT in Prostate Cancer Patients with Biochemical Recurrence After Primary Radiation Therapy Defined by Phoenix Criteria. J Nucl Med 2017;58(7):1081–7.

47. Raleigh DR, Hsu I-C, Braunstein S, et al. Bladder wall recurrence of prostate cancer after high-dose-rate brachytherapy. Brachytherapy 2015;14(2): 185–8.

48. Hövels AM, Heesakkers RAM, Adang EM, et al. The diagnostic accuracy of CT and MRI in the staging of pelvic lymph nodes in patients with prostate cancer: a meta-analysis. Clin Radiol 2008;63(4):387–95.

49. Buyyounouski MK, Choyke PL, McKenney JK, et al. Prostate cancer - major changes in the American Joint Committee on Cancer eighth edition cancer staging manual. CA Cancer J Clin 2017;67(3): 245–53.

50. Briganti A, Suardi N, Capogrosso P, et al. Lymphatic spread of nodal metastases in high-risk prostate cancer: The ascending pathway from the pelvis to the retroperitoneum. Prostate 2012;72(2):186–92.

51. Osmonov DK, Aksenov AV, Trick D, et al. Cancer-specific and overall survival in patients with recurrent prostate cancer who underwent salvage extended pelvic lymph node dissection. BMC Urol 2016;16(1):56.

52. Osmonov DK, Aksenov AV, Boller A, et al. Extended salvage pelvic lymph node dissection in patients with recurrent prostate cancer. Extended Salvage Pelvic Lymph Nodes Dissection in Patients with Recurrent Prostate Cance. Adv Urol 2014. https://doi.org/10.1155/2014/321619.

53. Hijazi S, Meller B, Leitsmann C, et al. See the unseen: Mesorectal lymph node metastases in prostate cancer. Prostate 2016;76(8):776–80.

54. Griffin N, Burke C, Grant LA. Common primary tumours of the abdomen and pelvis and their patterns of tumour spread as seen on multi-detector

computed tomography. Insights Imaging 2011;2(3): 205–14.

55. Pound CR, Partin AW, Eisenberger MA, et al. Natural history of progression after PSA elevation following radical prostatectomy. JAMA 1999;281(17):1591–7.

56. Yossepowitch O, Bianco FJ Jr, Eggener SE, et al. The natural history of noncastrate metastatic prostate cancer after radical prostatectomy. Eur Urol 2007;51(4):940–7 [discussion: 947–8].

57. Saitoh H, Hida M, Shimbo T, et al. Metastatic patterns of prostatic cancer. Correlation between sites and number of organs involved. Cancer 1984; 54(12):3078–84.

58. Gandaglia G, Abdollah F, Schiffmann J, et al. Distribution of metastatic sites in patients with prostate cancer: A population-based analysis. Prostate 2014;74(2):210–6.

59. Janssen J-C, Woythal N, Meißner S, et al. [Ga] PSMA-HBED-CC Uptake in Osteolytic, Osteoblastic, and Bone Marrow Metastases of Prostate Cancer Patients. Mol Imaging Biol 2017;19(6):933–43.

60. Große Hokamp N, Kobe C, Linzenich E, et al. Solitary PSMA-Positive Pulmonary Metastasis in Biochemical Relapse of Prostate Cancer. Clin Nucl Med 2017;42(5):406–7.

61. Chakraborty PS, Kumar R, Tripathi M, et al. Detection of brain metastasis with 68Ga-labeled PSMA ligand PET/CT: a novel radiotracer for imaging of prostate carcinoma. Clin Nucl Med 2015;40(4):328–9.

62. Chan M, Hsiao E, Turner J. Cerebellar Metastases From Prostate Cancer on 68Ga-PSMA PET/CT. Clin Nucl Med 2017;42(3):193–4.

63. Weiberg D, Radner H, Derlin T, et al. Early Detection of Bilateral Testicular Metastases From Prostatic Adenocarcinoma Using 68Ga-PSMA Ligand PET/ CT. Clin Nucl Med 2017;42(7):563–4.

64. Serfling S, Luther A, Kosmala A, et al. Epididymal Metastasis of Prostate Cancer Detected With 68Ga-PSMA-PET/CT. Clin Nucl Med 2016;41(10):792–3.

65. Tosoian JJ, Gorin MA, Ross AE, et al. Oligometastatic prostate cancer: definitions, clinical outcomes, and treatment considerations. Nat Rev Urol 2017; 14(1):15–25.

66. Ost P, Reynders D, Decaestecker K, et al. Surveillance or Metastasis-Directed Therapy for Oligometastatic Prostate Cancer Recurrence: A Prospective, Randomized, Multicenter Phase II Trial. J Clin Oncol 2018;36(5):446–53.

67. Ballas LK, de Castro Abreu AL, Quinn DI. What Medical, Urologic, and Radiation Oncologists Want from Molecular Imaging of Prostate Cancer. J Nucl Med 2016;57(Suppl 3). 6S – 12S.

68. Scher HI, Fizazi K, Saad F, et al. Increased survival with enzalutamide in prostate cancer after chemotherapy. N Engl J Med 2012;367(13):1187–97.

69. Rauscher I, Maurer T, Fendler WP, et al. 68)Ga-PSMA ligand PET/CT in patients with prostate

cancer: How we review and report. Cancer Imaging 2016;16(1):14.

70. Burchardt T, Burchardt M, Chen MW, et al. Transdifferentiation of prostate cancer cells to a neuroendocrine cell phenotype in vitro and in vivo. J Urol 1999; 162(5):1800–5.

71. Violet J, Jackson P, Ferdinandus J, et al. Dosimetry of Lu-PSMA-617 in Metastatic Castration-Resistant Prostate Cancer: Correlations Between Pretherapeutic Imaging and Whole-Body Tumor Dosimetry with Treatment Outcomes. J Nucl Med 2019;60(4):517–23.

72. Kratochwil C, Fendler WP, Eiber M, et al. EANM procedure guidelines for radionuclide therapy with Lu-labelled PSMA-ligands (Lu-PSMA-RLT). Eur J Nucl Med Mol Imaging 2019;46(12):2536–44.

73. Hofman MS, Violet J, Hicks RJ, et al. [Lu]-PSMA-617 radionuclide treatment in patients with metastatic castration-resistant prostate cancer (LuPSMA trial): a single-centre, single-arm, phase 2 study. Lancet Oncol 2018;19(6):825–33.

74. Giesel FL, Hadaschik B, Cardinale J, et al. F-18 labelled PSMA-1007: biodistribution, radiation dosimetry and histopathological validation of tumor lesions in prostate cancer patients. Eur J Nucl Med Mol Imaging 2017;44(4):678–88.

75. Fanti S, Hadaschik B, Herrmann K. Proposal for Systemic-Therapy Response-Assessment Criteria at the Time of PSMA PET/CT Imaging: The PSMA PET Progression Criteria. J Nucl Med 2020;61(5): 678–82.

76. O JH, Lodge MA, Wahl RL. Practical PERCIST: A Simplified Guide to PET Response Criteria in Solid Tumors 1.0. Radiology 2016;280(2):576–84.

77. Evans MJ, Smith-Jones PM, Wongvipat J, et al. Noninvasive measurement of androgen receptor signaling with a positron-emitting radiopharmaceutical that targets prostate-specific membrane antigen. Proc Natl Acad Sci U S A 2011;108(23):9578–82.

78. Meller B, Bremmer F, Sahlmann CO, et al. Alterations in androgen deprivation enhanced prostate-specific membrane antigen (PSMA) expression in prostate cancer cells as a target for diagnostics and therapy. EJNMMI Res 2015;5(1):66.

79. Emmett L, Yin C, Crumbaker M, et al. Rapid Modulation of PSMA Expression by Androgen Deprivation: Serial Ga-PSMA-11 PET in Men with Hormone-Sensitive and Castrate-Resistant Prostate Cancer Commencing Androgen Blockade. J Nucl Med 2019;60(7):950–4.

80. Afshar-Oromieh A, Debus N, Uhrig M, et al. Impact of long-term androgen deprivation therapy on PSMA ligand PET/CT in patients with castration-sensitive prostate cancer. Eur J Nucl Med Mol Imaging 2018;45(12):2045–54.

81. Ware RE, Williams S, Hicks RJ. Molecular Imaging of Recurrent and Metastatic Prostate Cancer. Semin Nucl Med 2019;49(4):280–93.

Prostate-Specific Membrane Antigen-Ligand Therapy
What the Radiologist Needs to Know

Steven P. Rowe, MD, PhD[a],*, Mohammad S. Sadaghiani, MD[a],
Andrei Gafita, MD[a], Sara Sheikhbahaei, MD, MPH[a],
Martin G. Pomper, MD, PhD[a], Jeffrey Young, BS, CNMT[b], Avery Spitz, RN[c],
Rudolf A. Werner, MD[d], Jorge D. Oldan, MD[e], Lilja B. Solnes, MD, MBA[a]

KEYWORDS

- PRLT • Prostate cancer • Radioligand therapy • Theranostics • Endoradiotherapy

KEY POINTS

- Prostate-specific membrane antigen (PSMA)-targeted radioligand therapy (PRLT) is a novel and effective therapy for men with metastatic, castration-resistant prostate cancer.
- The pivotal trial for approval of the first PRLT in the U.S. was called VISION and demonstrated improvements in progression-free and overall survival when PSMA RLT was added to standard-of-care.
- Successful implementation of a PRLT clinic requires key personnel, necessary infrastructure, and collaborative decision-making and management of patients.

INTRODUCTION

Diagnostic imaging with new targeted positron emission tomography (PET) radiotracers, in combination with analogous small-molecule theranostic agents/radioligand therapies (RLT), have revitalized the field of nuclear medicine in recent years.[1] Pre-eminent among those classes of agents are compounds that target the prostate-specific membrane antigen (PSMA),[2] a transmembrane, type II glycoprotein that is highly expressed on the vast majority of prostate cancer (PCa) epithelial cells[3] and the neovascular endothelial cells of non-prostate cancers.[4]

In men with metastatic, castration-resistant prostate cancer (mCRPC), PSMA-targeted RLT (PRLT) has been shown to be an effective and well-tolerated therapeutic approach.[5] In the United States, a pivotal, phase III clinical trial (the VISION trial[6]) has led to the regulatory approval of the first PRLT agent, ^{177}Lu-PSMA-617 (tradename, Pluvicto). However, questions remain regarding the use of PRLT in terms of managing toxicities, understanding which patients will respond and to what extent they will respond, how to deploy PRLT in the clinic, how best to support patient access, and how we, as a field, can best scale our impact to meet the considerable demand,[7] among others.

[a] The Russell H. Morgan Department of Radiology and Radiological Science, Johns Hopkins University School of Medicine, 601 North Caroline Street, Baltimore, MD 21287, USA; [b] Johns Hopkins Hospital, 600 North Wolfe Street, Baltimore, MD 21287, USA; [c] Sidney Kimmell Comprehensive Cancer Center, Johns Hopkins University School of Medicine, 401 North Broadway Street, Baltimore, MD 21231, USA; [d] Department of Nuclear Medicine, University Hospital Würzburg Oberdürrbacherstraße 6, 97080 Würzburg, Germany; [e] Department of Radiology, University of North Carolina, 101 Manning Drive, Chapel Hill, NC 27514, USA
* Corresponding author. The Russell H. Morgan Department of Radiology and Radiological Science, Johns Hopkins University School of Medicine, 600 North Wolfe Street, Baltimore, MD 21287.
E-mail address: srowe8@jhmi.edu

Radiol Clin N Am 62 (2024) 177–187
https://doi.org/10.1016/j.rcl.2023.07.003
0033-8389/24/© 2023 Elsevier Inc. All rights reserved.

In this article, we will answer a number of those questions. Specifically, we aim to provide information on the underlying efficacy and toxicities associated with PRLT, describe the key personnel and infrastructure necessary to set up a successful PRLT clinic, discuss challenging cases and situations that providers should be aware of, and proffer potential future directions for this rapidly evolving field.

KEY CLINICAL STUDIES ON PROSTATE-SPECIFIC MEMBRANE ANTIGEN RADIOLIGAND THERAPY

Prior to 2021, the vast majority of work carried out with PRLT was composed of single-center retrospective and prospective studies that were highly heterogeneous in their methodologies.[5] Nonetheless, a meta-analysis of 24 of those studies demonstrated their overall efficacy in patients with mCRPC, with a pooled proportion of 0.71 (95% confidence interval [CI] [0.66, 0.75]) with any decrease in serum prostate-specific antigen (PSA) level after treatment with either ^{177}Lu-PSMA-617 or the similar agent ^{177}Lu-PSMA-I&T. The pooled proportion of patients with an objective biochemical response to either of those agents, defined as a PSA drop ≥50%, was 0.41 (95% CI [0.36, 0.47]).

In the vast majority of cases, toxicities from PRLT with ^{177}Lu-labeled agents are low-grade, self-limited, and generally tolerable for patients.[5] A meta-analysis of the toxicities from these agents found that the estimated proportion of patients who would have any-grade anemia was 0.28 (95% CI [0.17, 0.42]), any-grade fatigue was 0.25 [95% CI (0.16, 0.37)], any-grade leukopenia was 0.28 (95% CI [0.22, 0.35]), and any-grade nephropathy was 0.13 [95% CI (0.07, 0.24)].[5] Grade 3 or 4 toxicities were distinctly uncommon, with anemia occurring most frequently with an estimated proportion of 0.08 (95% CI [0.05, 0.12]).[5]

In the VISION trial, 831 patients with mCRPC who were previously treated with at least one androgen-receptor-pathway inhibitor and one or two taxane regimens with positive ^{68}Ga-PSMA-11 scans were randomized 2:1 to receive either ^{177}Lu-PSMA-617 or standard of care. After 20.9 months of median follow-up, there was significantly higher radiographic progression-free survival (median, 8.7 versus 3.4 months, hazard ratio 0.4, 99.2% CI 0.29–0.57) and overall survival (median 15.3 vs 11.3 months, hazard ratio 0.62 95% CI 0.52 to 0.74) in patients who had received ^{177}Lu-PSMA-617. All key secondary endpoints (overall response rate, disease control rate, time to symptomatic skeletal event, progression-free survival, percentage of patients achieving a PSA response, and proportion of patients achieving at least an 80% decrease in PSA) favored ^{177}Lu-PSMA-617; incidence of adverse events of grade 3 or above was higher (52.7% vs 38.0%), though the quality of life was not affected.[6]

In the TheraP trial, a total of 183 patients with mCRPC with positive ^{68}Ga-PSMA-11 scans (and no discordant FDG-positive/PSMA-negative lesions) for whom cabazitaxel was considered an appropriate next step were randomized 1:1 to either cabazitaxel or ^{177}Lu-PSMA-617. PSA responses were more frequent among men in the ^{177}Lu-PSMA-617 group [66% vs 37% by intention to treat, difference of 29% (95% CI 16–42%) and 66% versus 44% by treatment, difference of 23% (95% CI 9–37%)]. Grade 3-4 adverse events were less frequent (33% vs 53%) and no deaths were attributed to treatment with ^{177}Lu-PSMA-617, although progression-free survival was not significantly different and overall survival data is forthcoming.[8]

While an endpoint such as overall survival is how we should judge prospectively designed clinical trials, on a practical level, we should also be able to determine whether individual patients are responding to therapy without waiting to see how their disease ultimately manifests. In regard to PSMA expression and response assessment, the patterns on follow-up PET scans can be confusing.[9,10] However, with directly cytotoxic therapy such as PRLT, the response-assessment patterns on the scan should be straightforward, as has generally been proposed by in standardized frameworks such as PSMA PET progression (PPP)[11] and Response Evaluation Criteria in PSMA-PET/Computed Tomography (RECIP) version 1.0.[12] As the name would suggest, PPP focuses on defining progression of disease with three different criteria; (I) the appearance of two or more new PSMA-positive distant lesions, (II) the appearance of one new PSMA-positive lesion with consistent clinical or laboratory data, and (III) at least 30% increase in size or uptake in one or more lesions with consistent clinical or laboratory data, and recommended confirmation by biopsy or correlative imaging within 3 months of PSMA-PET as may be warranted (criteria II, III).[11] RECIP and PPP criteria are summarized in **Table 1**.

A number of recent studies suggested that early response assessment based on the determination of total viable tumor burden on PSMA PET/CT (considering volume and PSMA density of all metastases) can independently predict survival in patients with mCRPC who received PSMA-targeted RLT.[12,13] RECIP has specifically been validated to show that patients with RECIP progressive disease (RECIP-PD, defined as ≥20% increase in the

Table 1
RECIP 1.0 and PPP criteria for response evaluation during PRLT

Criteria	Definition
RECIP 1.0	
PD	Total tumor volume increase $\geq$ 20% and new lesions
PR	Total tumor volume decrease $\geq$ 30% without new lesions
CR	Absence of any PSMA-uptake on PET
SD	all other
PPP	
PD	a. Volume increase of any metastasis $\geq$ 30% and consistent clinical/lab Or b. Two or more new PSMA-positive lesions Or c. one new PSMA-positive lesion and consistent clinical/lab data
Non-PD	All other

Abbreviations: CR, complete remission; PD, progressive disease; PPP, PSMA PET progression; PR, partial remission; RECIP, response evaluation criteria in PSMA-imaging; SD, stable disease.

volume of PSMA-avid tumor and the appearance of new lesions) have shorter overall survival than patients with RECIP partial response (RECIP-PR, defined as $\geq$30% decrease in the volume of PSMA-avid tumor and no new lesions) or patients with RECIP stable disease (RECIP-SD, ie, any disease state other than RECIP-PD or RECIP-PR).[12] Preliminarily, RECIP 1.0 appears to offer the best prognostication among the currently proposed criteria.[14] Future prospective studies are warranted to determine the optimal timing of PSMA imaging after PRLT and further explore and validate its role as a therapeutic response biomarker.

Note that existing response-assessment criteria such as RECIP and PPP are predicated upon the ready availability of PSMA-targeted PET. Many clinical trials may continue to use traditional response assessment (such as changes in the diameters of soft-tissue lesions[15] or the appearance of new lesions on bone scan[16]), although such criteria may miss early progression that is visible with PSMA imaging.[17] Cross-sectional imaging readers could potentially encounter the typical changes seen with responding PCa, such as increased sclerosis in bone lesions and decreased sizes of lymph nodes. However, the routine use of

PSMA-targeted PET for response assessment in patients undergoing PRLT will hopefully come to be more commonplace.

PERSONNEL AND INFRASTRUCTURE

Based on the VISION trial protocol, it is typical for patients to have treatment plans that call for 6 doses of 7.4 MBq (200 mCi) spaced at 8-week intervals.[6] A typical infusion session that includes IV hydration will take approximately 2 hours. Therefore, any theranostics center that plans to do PRLT should allocate the appropriate space for the number of infusion rooms that may meet their local demand.[7] Dosimetry can be acquired based on the γ-ray emission from lutetium-177 and the use of single-photon emission computed tomography and/or planar imaging,[18] although the exact role of dosimetry in routine clinical practice is unclear.

There are a number of key personnel who are necessary for effective running of a PRLT theranostics center (**Fig. 1**). The first person a patient is likely to interface with is a nurse navigator. The nurse navigator performs an initial intake screen of the patient, undertakes a medical chart review of labs, and helps to obtain any available internal or external PSMA PET images. This helps to consolidate information and allow the nuclear medicine physician to identify patients that are good candidates for therapy (**Box 1**). The patient then comes to the clinic to discuss PET scan results and go over the therapy plan, including the review of potential toxicities, benefits vs risks of treatment, and the scheduling of follow-up procedures. The nurse navigator also coordinates labs before each therapy and at chosen intervals for follow-up. Education and coordination are the key components of the nurse navigator's responsibilities. This includes ensuring patient follow-up blood count monitoring, imaging, and check-ins with the medical oncology team. This multidisciplinary approach provides continuity of care with the medical oncologist and minimizes stress for the patient. A background in oncology can help to assist with the triage of toxicities, such as fatigue, nausea, nutrition/hydration status, and low blood count review and management during the treatment period. The nurse navigator also assists with education about radiation safety precautions for both the patient and their family.

One or more specialized nuclear medicine technologists are vital to a successful, safe, and efficient theranostics center. The therapy technologist needs to come from a solid foundation of nuclear medicine, with an emphasis on detail and patient care. Patients with PRLT lie in a grey area

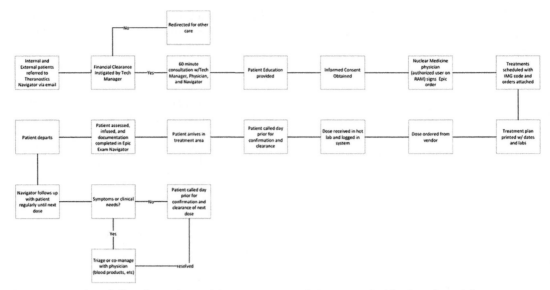

Fig. 1. Proposed work-flow for patients with prostate cancer being treated with PSMA-ligand therapy.

Box 1

Summary of selected criteria currently utilized in clinical practice for selecting patients for PRLT

Imaging Inclusion Criteria

- PSMA uptake at least as high as the liver in at least one metastatic lesion
- No lymph node lesions ≥2.5 cm in diameter with PSMA uptake less than liver
- No solid organ metastases ≥1.0 cm in diameter with PSMA uptake less than liver
- No bone metastases with soft tissue portion ≥1.0 cm in diameter with PSMA uptake less than liver

Clinical Inclusion Criteria

- Progressing metastatic castration-resistant prostate cancer after treatment with at least one targeted anti-androgen and one taxane-based chemotherapy
- Eastern Cooperative Oncology Group score of 0, 1, or 2
- Adequate organ and bone marrow function. Special consideration must be given to patients with extensive bone marrow infiltration by prostate cancer who have baseline cytopenias

Credit Line: Data from Sartor O, de Bono J, Chi KN, et al. Lutetium-177-PSMA-617 for Metastatic Castration-Resistant Prostate Cancer. N Engl J Med. 2021;385(12):1091-103."

---

between radiology and oncology, where the role of the technologist is to provide a service and not just perform an examination.

As is often the case in medicine, a part of the successful technologist's role is a checklist that covers key aspects of the therapy session. Important pre-infusion steps include, but are not limited to: confirming that patients are not experiencing any issues or concerns prior to the start of the infusion and establishing that labs have been performed within the past 7 days and are within acceptable ranges (eg, glomerular filtration rate, creatinine, blood urea nitrogen, hemoglobin, platelets, white-blood-cell count, absolute neutrophil count, and alkaline phosphatase).

Day of treatment preparation is key for the successful and safe administration of PRLT. Ensure infusion rooms and bathrooms are properly set up to minimize radioactive contamination surrounding the treatment area. All infusion rooms should be set up with appropriate safety equipment, including radiation shields around the patients and infusion set ups. Follow proper hot lab preparation for therapy radioisotope, inspect vial, confirm the amount of radioactivity with an appropriate dose calibrator, use tongs when handling to minimize radiation exposure, aseptic technique, and disposal of unused product and waste according to your hospital and/or state guidelines. **Fig. 2** includes photographs of one of the infusion rooms at Johns Hopkins.

A proper written directive signed by the covering nuclear medicine physician or radiologist and a timeout taken by the treatment team prior to beginning the infusion are important considerations on

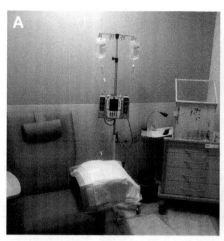 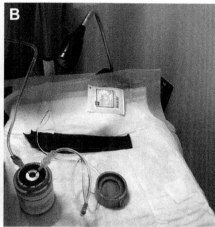

Fig. 2. (*A, B*) Representative photographs of an infusion set-up. (*A*) The overall set-up, with the infusion chair on the left, an IV stand and the infusion pump in the middle, and the vial containing the therapeutic dose on the right, behind a shield. (*B*) A close-up picture of the vial containing the therapeutic dose and the associated apparatus for "vial method" infusion of the agent.

the day of therapy. A peripheral IV should be placed and hydration started 30 minutes prior to the infusion of PRLT. This will help ensure patency and to minimize the risk of extravasation prior to the administration of therapy. PRLT should be administered according to locally developed departmental guidelines. Optional vital signs can be collected 15 minutes before administration, as well as 30 minutes and 60 minutes following administration. A review of radiation safety instructions, as well as general precautions to follow upon discharge, should be performed prior to the discharge of the patient. Treatment rooms and bathrooms should be surveyed for any contamination. All radioactive waste material should be disposed of in accordance with institutional/state guidelines.

A nuclear medicine physician or nuclear radiologist who is trained in the supervision of the administration of parenteral radioactive therapies should be available on-site during infusion and should be ready to address any medical issues that arise during the infusion process. That physician, or one of his/her colleagues, should meet with the patient prior to the day of infusion to discuss multiple issues, including the data that justify the use of PRLT, expectations regarding efficacy and toxicities, plans for follow-up, and radiation precautions. It is also the responsibility of the physician to review the PSMA PET scan, to ensure that the patient is appropriate for treatment, and the baseline laboratory values to confirm it would be safe to treat the patient. In our clinical practices, we typically hew to the "VISION criteria" for PSMA PET in which at least one metastatic lesion must have uptake above liver background and no lesions (lymph nodes ≥ 2.5 cm in short axis, visceral metastases

≥1.0 cm in short axis, or bone lesions with soft-tissue component ≥ 1.0 cm) have uptake at or below liver background.[6] Regarding laboratory values, patients should have glomerular filtration rates ≥30 mL/min and adequate bone marrow reserve, with preferences for platelets >100,000/μL and hemoglobin >9 g/dL.[6] Of course, all treatment decisions should ultimately be made in a multi-disciplinary fashion with input from members of the care team and at the discretion of the treating physician.

CASE AND SITUATION EXAMPLES

Despite pivotal clinical trials that have established the safety and efficacy of PRLT, and an understanding of the personnel and infrastructure needed for the safe administration of such agents, difficult cases still arise and there is a great deal we, as a field, still need to learn. The following situational examples are from our clinical practice and highlight some of the common cases in which decision-making must be undertaken in a PRLT theranostic clinic.

Fig. 3 demonstrates a patient with widespread metastatic disease with high avidity. The patient has both high disease burden but also discrete lesions, suggesting that he may respond to therapy while also not suffering unnecessary bone marrow toxicity. Indeed, the patient had an objective biochemical response with a PSA drop of more than 50% following the completion of 6 doses of ^{177}Lu-PSMA-617 therapy.

However, other patients with high uptake in their tumors may still have disease that is refractory with PRLT for reasons that remain obscure.

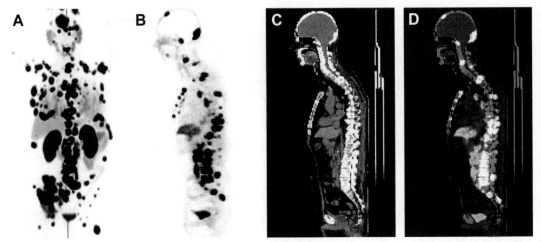

Fig. 3. 64-year-old man with widespread mCRPC. (*A*) Anterior, maximum intensity projection (MIP) image of a ^{18}F-DCFPyL PET scan, with (*B*) lateral PET, (*C*) lateral CT, and (*D*) lateral PET/CT images demonstrating widespread, radiotracer-avid lesions. Given that his tumors were very avid and that he did not have significant hemodynamic abnormalities based on same-day laboratory evaluation, we elected to treat the patient. His skeletal pain resolved and PSA went from 2,684 ng/dL to 918 ng/dL, an objective biochemical response.

Fig. 4 is an example of a patient with high baseline uptake who had such refractory disease, as was apparent on the follow-up scan with a rising PSA. The ability to identify such patients early in the treatment course will be imperative to avoid futile therapy with PRLT.

In our collective clinical experience, the timing of PSMA-targeted PET is also important for patient selection. **Fig. 5** demonstrates a patient whose baseline PET (prior to the initiation of chemotherapy) showed high uptake in relatively limited lymph node and bone-metastatic disease. Following progression on chemotherapy, his repeat PET scan showed new metastatic lesions with uptake below liver. Two cycles of PRLT did not demonstrate any evidence of response, demonstrating the importance of high uptake in lesions at the start of PRLT.

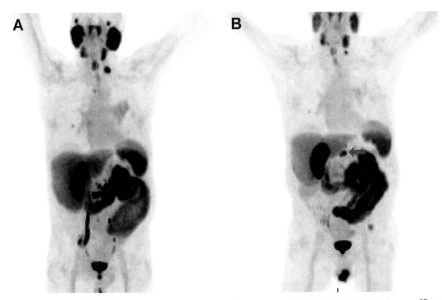

Fig. 4. 73-year-old man with bone metastatic PCa. (*A*) Baseline MIP and (*B*) follow-up MIP from a ^{18}F-DCFPyL PET. The patient underwent six cycles of PRLT but had a rising PSA at the end of therapy (from 4.2 ng/mL prior to therapy to 5.3 ng/mL after therapy) and was found to have new lesions on follow-up PSMA-targeted PET [including a new T12 lesion denoted by the *arrow* in (*B*)].

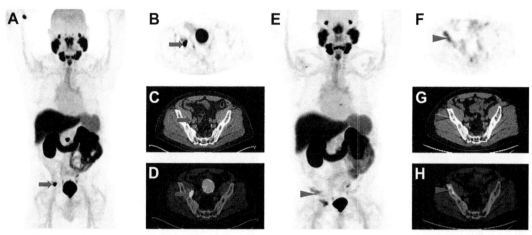

Fig. 5. 68-year-old man with mCRPC who was imaged prior to starting chemotherapy (A-D). (A) Maximum intensity projection image, (B) axial PET, (C) axial CT, and (D) axial PET/CT images demonstrating intense uptake in nodal (*arrows*) and bone metastatic disease. The patient subsequently progressed after chemotherapy (PSA from 4.8 ng/mL to 19.8 ng/mL) and was re-imaged prior to starting PRLT (E–H). Although the progressive lesions are apparent on the second PSMA scan (*arrowheads*), and have relatively low uptake (less than liver), the patient still elected to undergo PRLT. After two rounds of PRLT, his PSA continued to rise and was 24.8 ng/mL at the time of this writing.

Lastly, Fig. 6 is an example of a patient who should only be treated with PRLT with caution. The diffusely infiltrative nature of his bone metastases with relatively low uptake (although above liver) suggests this patient may have more hematologic toxicity than meaningful response to therapy. At the discretion of the nuclear medicine physician, such patients can be treated with

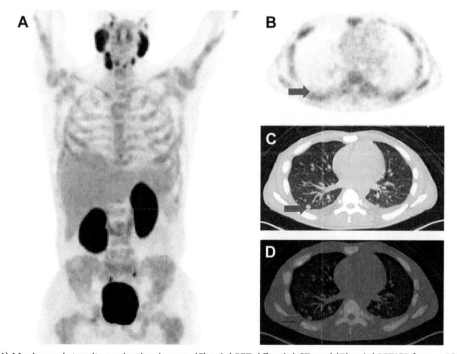

Fig. 6. (A) Maximum intensity projection image, (B) axial PET, (C) axial CT, and (D) axial PET/CT from a 52-year-old man with aggressive mCRPC that had diffusely infiltrated his bone marrow and led to numerous lung metastases (*arrows, B–D*). Given the uptake above the liver in the diffuse bone metastases and the small size of the lung nodules, the patient was started on PRLT. However, he continued to have rapidly progressive disease and passed away soon after the first cycle of PRLT.

PRLT, although they should be counseled that their pattern of disease could portend a poor response to therapy. Unfortunately, this patient passed away from multiple factors after only receiving one dose of PRLT.

FUTURE DIRECTIONS

To date, there are two common lutetium-177-labeled PSMA radiopharmaceuticals used in the clinic worldwide, and those are ^{177}Lu-PSMA-617 and ^{177}Lu-PSMA-I&T.[5,19] Of note, the underlying chemical structures vary among those radiopharmaceuticals.[19] While the urea-binding motif of the two target molecules is identical, the chelators have inherent differences, with ^{177}Lu-PSMA-617 being linked to a DOTA and ^{177}Lu-PSMA-I&T to a DOTAGA chelator.[19] Nonetheless, those dissimilarities have not led to outcome differences, as a recent matched-pair analysis yielded comparable survival for both agents.[19]

Head-to-head comparisons of outcome prediction with those two radiopharmaceuticals are, however, lacking, as predictive biomarker studies have typically included only one of these PSMA-targeted agents. Nonetheless, those studies provided virtually identical clinical biomarkers for identifying high-risk individuals. For instance, using ^{177}Lu-PSMA-617, Ferdinandus, and colleagues and Rahbar and coworkers reported that alkaline phosphatase (AP) and lactate dehydrogenase (LDH) as independent outcome predictors.[20,21] Grubmüller and colleagues,[22] however, provided evidence that C-reactive protein (CRP) may be suitable for predicting progressive disease. Ahmadzadehfar, and colleagues[23] further investigated survival predictors and demonstrated that liver-functional parameters including albumin, aspartate aminotransferase (AST) and the presence of hepatic tumor burden are also tightly linked to outcome. Beyond those laboratory-based values, recent efforts have also focused on advanced analysis of pretherapeutic PSMA-targeted PET/CT. Among others, Seifert and colleagues[24] have shown that for patients planned for treatment with ^{177}Lu-PSMA-617, PSMA-avid tumor volume and total-lesion quotient, defined as PSMA tumor burden divided by mean standardized uptake value, may serve as a negative prognosticator for survival.

Relative to ^{177}Lu-PSMA-617, such outcome prediction studies using ^{177}Lu-PSMA-I&T have been uncommon. Hartrampf, and colleagues[25] described 92 men with PC, showing that CRP, LDH, AST, and time since diagnosis were linked to overall survival. A recent study included 301 patients being treated with ^{177}Lu-PSMA-I&T and also reported on pretherapeutic prognosticators, such as AP, LDH, PSA levels, and preceding chemotherapeutic protocols along with the presence of hepatic metastases.[26] Of note, that study also investigated the use of post-therapeutic scintigraphy and demonstrated that patients responding to therapy on those scans also have favorable outcomes, including progression-free and overall survival.[26]

Taken together, regardless of which radiotracer is used for PSMA-directed RLT, easily obtainable laboratory values reflecting hepatic function or established parameters of response such as LDH (most likely reflecting tumor cell destruction) may also be helpful to identify patients at increased risk for therapeutic failure. Recent efforts, however, have turned towards more detailed analyses of pretherapeutic imaging. For instance, Moazemi, and colleagues investigated mathematically extracted features (radiomics) from PSMA-targeted PET using ^{68}Ga-labeled radiopharmaceuticals and those image-based items may also serve as prognostic factors.[27,28] However, radiomics with PET must be viewed with caution, as a recent prospective study provided evidence that those radiomics features have a low test-retest reproducibility.[29]

Conventional parameters, such as SUV, have provided robust repeatability and thus, may be better suited for outcome prediction in patients scheduled for PSMA-targeted radioligand therapy.[30] The plethora of parameters for outcome prediction in the context of ^{177}Lu-labeled therapy may pose a challenge for the referring urologist or treating nuclear medicine expert. As such, Gafita and colleagues[31] recently demonstrated that normograms weighing those parameters may further refine outcome prediction, which has been also validated in an external setting. Further efforts have also included artificial intelligence applications,[28,32] which allows for faster and more reliable identification of patients responding to therapy.

Recently, a prospective study investigated DNA damage response markers in peripheral blood lymphocytes to test whether individual radiosensitivity may also serve as an outcome predictor. As established markers of cellular DNA damage response, decreasing peripheral lymphocytic baseline γ-H2AX and 53BP1 foci were linked to less favorable outcome.[33] This suggests an impending important role for genomics in identifying novel biomarkers for treatment response with PRLT.

It is likely that all PCa will eventually develop resistance to currently approved PRLT, which may arise through loss of PSMA expression, selection for those cells with intact and/or superior DNA-repair machinery, dose-limiting toxicities, or other mechanisms. For a subset of patients, specifically those that have become resistant to ^{177}Lu-based PRLT but whose tumors maintain PSMA expression, the use of agents labeled with radionuclides that decay by α-particle emission may be appropriate. At the current time, such compounds are not regulatory approved. Some of the initial responses to therapy have been encouraging,[34] although toxicities have proven difficult to alleviate.[35] In the end, the proper balance between efficacy and toxicities may come down to ligand design and the proper selection of radionuclide.[36]

Particularly as it may be possible to improve the efficacy of PRLT, it is expected that available agents will be utilized earlier in the course of the disease (eg, in men with hormone-sensitive metastatic disease) and in combination with other agents (eg, immunotherapies).[37] As long as adequate PSMA expression is confirmed by PET, PRLT is likely to be effective in those contexts. However, significant unanswered questions remain, such as [1] will combination therapies lead to additive or synergistic therapeutic benefit and/or additive or synergistic toxicities; and [2] if PRLT is used early in the course of disease, what options will be left for men who have progressed on androgen-targeted therapies and taxane-based chemotherapy?

As a final thought regarding the future direction of PRLT, we would be remiss in not mentioning the potential role of artificial intelligence (AI). AI will undoubtedly impact every aspect of radiology.[38] In regard to PSMA PET, AI has already demonstrated the ability to find and characterize lesions,[39] which indicates that it may be able to automatically place patients into actionable categories. Indeed, AI is capable of synthesizing imaging and clinical data to attempt to identify those patients that will benefit from PRLT.[28] The combination of new molecular imaging targets and scaffolds with the power of AI will drive the wider adoption of theranostics, including PRLT.[40]

SUMMARY

In an era in which more and more patients with PCa are treated with multiple agents in the up-front metastatic setting, orthogonal therapies that leverage new targets via novel mechanisms are necessary. PRLT is one such approach, whereby the near-universal expression of PSMA is used to deliver cytotoxic levels of radiation to the PCa cells. This approach requires specialized personnel and careful selection of patients to optimize efficacy while limiting toxicity. Although PRLT with ^{177}Lu-labeled

agents is already an accepted standard-of-care for men with mCRPC who have previously been treated with chemotherapy, there remains a tremendous amount to learn. Eventually, new therapeutic agents will coalesce with improved nomograms and patient-selection algorithms, as well as AI, to maximally benefit patients.

CLINICS CARE POINTS

- Prostate-specific membrane antigen (PSMA)-based imaging and therapy have altered the clinical approach to men with prostate cancer.

- PSMA radioligand therapy (PRLT) is an effective and well-tolerated standard-of-care for the treatment of men with castration-resistant, metastatic prostate cancer in the post-chemotherapy setting.

- It is expected that PRLT will soon move into pre-chemotherapy and hormone-sensitive settings. In combination with new ligand structures, combination therapies, and advanced imaging biomarker development, PRLT will become an increasingly important part of the management of prostate cancer.

CONFLICT OF INTEREST

M.G. Pomper is a coinventor on a US patent covering ^{18}F-DCFPyL and as such is entitled to a portion of any licensing fees and royalties generated by this technology. This arrangement has been reviewed and approved by Johns Hopkins University in accordance with its conflict of interest policies. S.P. Rowe is a consultant for Progenics Pharmaceuticals Inc., United States, a wholly owned subsidiary of Lantheus Pharmaceuticals, Inc. and the licensee of ^{18}F-DCFPyL. M.G. Pomper and S.P. Rowe have received research funding from Progenics Pharmaceuticals. All other authors declare that there is no relevant conflict of interest.

REFERENCES

1. Rowe SP, Pomper MG. Molecular imaging in oncology: current impact and future directions. CA Cancer J Clin 2022;72(4):333–52.

2. Rowe SP, Gorin MA, Pomper MG. Imaging of prostate-specific membrane antigen with small-molecule PET radiotracers: from the bench to advanced clinical applications. Annu Rev Med 2019;70:461–77.

3. Wright GL Jr, Haley C, Beckett ML, et al. Expression of prostate-specific membrane antigen in normal,

benign, and malignant prostate tissues. Urol Oncol 1995;1(1):18–28.

4. Chang SS, O'Keefe DS, Bacich DJ, et al. Prostate-specific membrane antigen is produced in tumor-associated neovasculature. Clin Cancer Res 1999; 5(10):2674–81.

5. Sadaghiani MS, Sheikhbahaei S, Werner RA, et al. A systematic review and meta-analysis of the effectiveness and toxicities of lutetium-177-labeled prostate-specific membrane antigen-targeted radioligand therapy in metastatic castration-resistant prostate cancer. Eur Urol 2021;80(1):82–94.

6. Sartor O, de Bono J, Chi KN, et al. Lutetium-177-PSMA-617 for metastatic castration-resistant prostate cancer. N Engl J Med 2021;385(12):1091–103.

7. Czernin J, Calais J. How many theranostics centers will we need in the United States? J Nucl Med 2022; 63(6):805–6.

8. Hofman MS, Emmett L, Sandhu S, et al. [(177)Lu]Lu-PSMA-617 versus cabazitaxel in patients with metastatic castration-resistant prostate cancer (TheraP): a randomised, open-label, phase 2 trial. Lancet 2021;397(10276):797–804.

9. Hope TA, Truillet C, Ehman EC, et al. 68Ga-PSMA-11 PET imaging of response to androgen receptor inhibition: first human experience. J Nucl Med 2017; 58(1):81–4.

10. Zukotynski KA, Emmenegger U, Hotte S, et al. Prospective, single-arm trial evaluating changes in uptake patterns on prostate-specific membrane antigen-targeted (18)F-DCFPyL PET/CT in patients with castration-resistant prostate cancer starting abiraterone or enzalutamide. J Nucl Med 2021; 62(10):1430–7.

11. Fanti S, Hadaschik B, Herrmann K. Proposal for systemic-therapy response-assessment criteria at the time of PSMA PET/CT imaging: the PSMA PET progression criteria. J Nucl Med 2020;61(5):678–82.

12. Gafita A, Rauscher I, Weber M, et al. Novel framework for treatment response evaluation using PSMA PET/CT in patients with metastatic castration-resistant prostate cancer (RECIP 1.0): an international multicenter study. J Nucl Med 2022;63(11):1651–8.

13. Rosar F, Wenner F, Khreish F, et al. Early molecular imaging response assessment based on determination of total viable tumor burden in [(68)Ga]Ga-PSMA-11 PET/CT independently predicts overall survival in [(177)Lu]Lu-PSMA-617 radioligand therapy. Eur J Nucl Med Mol Imaging 2022;49(5):1584–94.

14. Gafita A, Rauscher I, Fendler WP, et al. Measuring response in metastatic castration-resistant prostate cancer using PSMA PET/CT: comparison of RECIST 1.1, aPCWG3, aPERCIST, PPP, and RECIP 1.0 criteria. Eur J Nucl Med Mol Imaging 2022;49(12): 4271–81.

15. Eisenhauer EA, Therasse P, Bogaerts J, et al. New response evaluation criteria in solid tumours: revised RECIST guideline (version 1.1). Eur J Cancer 2009; 45(2):228–47.

16. Scher HI, Morris MJ, Stadler WM, et al. Trial design and objectives for castration-resistant prostate cancer: updated recommendations from the prostate cancer clinical trials working group 3. J Clin Oncol 2016;34(12):1402–18.

17. Markowski MC, Velho PI, Eisenberger MA, et al. Detection of early progression with (18)F-DCFPyL PET/CT in men with metastatic castration-resistant prostate cancer receiving bipolar androgen therapy. J Nucl Med 2021;62(9):1270–3.

18. Schuchardt C, Zhang J, Kulkarni HR, et al. Prostate-specific membrane antigen radioligand therapy using (177)Lu-PSMA I&T and (177)Lu-PSMA-617 in patients with metastatic castration-resistant prostate cancer: comparison of safety, biodistribution, and dosimetry. J Nucl Med 2022;63(8):1199–207.

19. Hartrampf PE, Weinzierl FX, Buck AK, et al. Matched-pair analysis of [(177)Lu]Lu-PSMA I&T and [(177)Lu]Lu-PSMA-617 in patients with metastatic castration-resistant prostate cancer. Eur J Nucl Med Mol Imaging 2022;49(9):3269–76.

20. Rahbar K, Boegemann M, Yordanova A, et al. PSMA targeted radioligandtherapy in metastatic castration resistant prostate cancer after chemotherapy, abiraterone and/or enzalutamide. A retrospective analysis of overall survival. Eur J Nucl Med Mol Imaging 2018;45(1):12–9.

21. Ferdinandus J, Violet J, Sandhu S, et al. Prognostic biomarkers in men with metastatic castration-resistant prostate cancer receiving [177Lu]-PSMA-617. Eur J Nucl Med Mol Imaging 2020;47(10): 2322–7.

22. Grubmuller B, Senn D, Kramer G, et al. Response assessment using (68)Ga-PSMA ligand PET in patients undergoing (177)Lu-PSMA radioligand therapy for metastatic castration-resistant prostate cancer. Eur J Nucl Med Mol Imaging 2019;46(5):1063–72.

23. Ahmadzadehfar H, Schlolaut S, Fimmers R, et al. Predictors of overall survival in metastatic castration-resistant prostate cancer patients receiving [(177) Lu]Lu-PSMA-617 radioligand therapy. Oncotarget 2017;8(61):103108–16.

24. Seifert R, Kessel K, Schlack K, et al. PSMA PET total tumor volume predicts outcome of patients with advanced prostate cancer receiving [(177)Lu]Lu-PSMA-617 radioligand therapy in a bicentric analysis. Eur J Nucl Med Mol Imaging 2021;48(4): 1200–10.

25. Hartrampf PE, Seitz AK, Weinzierl FX, et al. Baseline clinical characteristics predict overall survival in patients undergoing radioligand therapy with [(177)Lu] Lu-PSMA I&T during long-term follow-up. Eur J Nucl Med Mol Imaging 2022;49(12):4262–70.

26. Karimzadeh A, Heck M, Tauber R, et al. ^{177}Lu-PSMA-I&T for Treatment of Metastatic Castration-

Resistant Prostate Cancer: Prognostic Value of Scintigraphic and Clinical Biomarkers. J Nucl Med 2023; 64(3):402–9.

27. Moazemi S, Erle A, Lutje S, et al. Estimating the potential of radiomics features and radiomics signature from pretherapeutic PSMA-PET-CT scans and clinical data for prediction of overall survival when treated with (177)Lu-PSMA. Diagnostics 2022; 11(2):186.

28. Moazemi S, Erle A, Khurshid Z, et al. Decision-support for treatment with (177)Lu-PSMA: machine learning predicts response with high accuracy based on PSMA-PET/CT and clinical parameters. Ann Transl Med 2021;9(9):818.

29. Werner RA, Habacha B, Lutje S, et al. Lack of repeatability of radiomic features derived from PET scans: Results from a (18) F-DCFPyL test-retest cohort. Prostate 2023;83(6):547–54.

30. Werner RA, Habacha B, Lutje S, et al. High SUVs have more robust repeatability in patients with metastatic prostate cancer: results from a prospective test-retest cohort imaged with (18)F-DCFPyL. Mol Imaging 2022;2022:7056983.

31. Gafita A, Calais J, Grogan TR, et al. Nomograms to predict outcomes after (177)Lu-PSMA therapy in men with metastatic castration-resistant prostate cancer: an international, multicentre, retrospective study. Lancet Oncol 2021;22(8):1115–25.

32. Xue S, Gafita A, Dong C, et al. Application of machine learning to pretherapeutically estimate dosimetry in men with advanced prostate cancer treated with (177)Lu-PSMA I&T therapy. Eur J Nucl Med Mol Imaging 2022;49(12):4064–72.

33. Widjaja L, Werner RA, Krischke E, et al. Individual radiosensitivity reflected by gamma-H2AX and 53BP1 foci predicts outcome in PSMA-targeted radioligand therapy. Eur J Nucl Med Mol Imaging 2023;50(2):602–12.

34. Kratochwil C, Bruchertseifer F, Giesel FL, et al. 225Ac-PSMA-617 for PSMA-Targeted alpha-Radiation Therapy of Metastatic Castration-Resistant Prostate Cancer. J Nucl Med 2016;57(12):1941–4.

35. Rathke H, Kratochwil C, Hohenberger R, et al. Initial clinical experience performing sialendoscopy for salivary gland protection in patients undergoing (225)Ac-PSMA-617 RLT. Eur J Nucl Med Mol Imaging 2019;46(1):139–47.

36. Mease RC, Kang CM, Kumar V, et al. An improved (211)At-Labeled Agent for PSMA-targeted alpha-therapy. J Nucl Med 2022;63(2):259–67.

37. Patell K, Kurian M, Garcia JA, et al. Lutetium-177 PSMA for the treatment of metastatic castrate resistant prostate cancer: a systematic review. Expert Rev Anticancer Ther 2023;23(7):731–44.

38. Soyer P, Fishman EK, Rowe SP, et al. Does artificial intelligence surpass the radiologist? Diagn Interv Imaging 2022;103(10):445–7.

39. Erle A, Moazemi S, Lutje S, et al. Evaluating a machine learning tool for the classification of pathological uptake in whole-body PSMA-PET-CT scans. Tomography 2021;7(3):301–12.

40. Rowe SP. Artificial intelligence in molecular imaging: at the crossroads of revolutions in medical diagnosis. Ann Transl Med 2021;9(9):817.

Prostate Cancer Diagnosis with Micro-ultrasound
What We Know now and New Horizons

Adriano Basso Dias, MD[a], Sangeet Ghai, MD[a],*

KEYWORDS

• Prostate cancer • Micro-ultrasound • Cancer detection

KEY POINTS

• Micro-Ultrasound (MicroUS) is a novel high-resolution 29-MHz ultrasound with ~three times greater resolution compared to conventional transrectal ultrasound, potentially improving accuracy of targeted prostate biopsy.
• A growing body of literature is available supporting the use of MicroUS with comparable accuracy to multiparametric MRI, for guidance of targeted prostate biopsy.
• The ongoing OPTIMUM randomized controlled trial will help to establish the role of MicroUS in the diagnostic algorithm for the detection of clinically significant prostate cancer.

INTRODUCTION

Prostate cancer (PCa) is the most common non-cutaneous cancer diagnosed in men worldwide, accounting for 15% of the total new cancer cases in the male population and responsible for 375,000 deaths in 2020.[1] Population screening using prostate-specific antigen (PSA) and digital rectal examination is recommended by the NCCN, EAU and other clinical guidelines.[2,3] Over the past decade, the use of multiparametric magnetic resonance imaging (mpMRI) for the diagnosis of PCa has exponentially increased, with increased utilization in the PCa diagnosis pathway. Multiple level one evidence studies, including PRECISION, 4M, MRI-FIRST, PRECISE, and PROMIS, have confirmed MRI-targeted biopsy as being not inferior to (possible superiority) TRUS-guided systematic biopsies for clinically significant (cs) PCa detection with fewer core biopsies and substantially less insignificant PCa diagnosed[4–8] These studies have resulted in widespread acceptance of mpMRI prior to biopsy and inclusion of this method in most clinical guidelines.[2,3] Although

mpMRI has improved detection rates, there are issues related to MRI cost, access, interpretation, fusion biopsy expertise and variability in scan quality.[9] Additionally, many patients within this population will have relative contraindications to mpMRI such as implanted devices, claustrophobia and impaired renal function.

More recently, high frequency Micro-Ultrasound (MicroUS) has emerged as a promising imaging technology for PCa diagnosis.[10] The most recent edition of the NCCN,[3] EAU[2] and AFU[11] guidelines mention the novel MicroUS imaging modality for the detection of PCa citing recent studies.[12–17] This modality has the potential to add value to mpMRI, in addition to easy access and a cost-effective tool for diagnosis of PCa, with the capability to improve sensitivity and negative predictive value (NPV) for csPCa, mainly due to its capacity of visualizing and targeting under real-time lesions suspicious for PCa.[18] The purpose of this review is to provide the reader an overview of the role of micro-US for diagnosis of PCa, discussing its diagnostic performance, technical considerations and limitations.

a Joint Department of Medical Imaging, University Medical Imaging Toronto, University Health Network–Mount Sinai Hospital–Women's College Hospital, University of Toronto, 585 University Avenue, 1PMB-298, Toronto, ON M5G 2N2, Canada
* Corresponding author.
E-mail address: sangeet.ghai@uhn.ca

Radiol Clin N Am 62 (2024) 189–197
https://doi.org/10.1016/j.rcl.2023.06.014
0033-8389/24/© 2023 Elsevier Inc. All rights reserved.

HIGH RESOLUTION MICRO-ULTRASOUND
Overview

MicroUS is a novel imaging technique, developed by Exact Imaging (Toronto, Ontario, Canada), which has received regulatory approval in the European Union (CE Mark), the United States (FDA), and Canada (Health Canada medical device license) for visualization and biopsy of the prostate. MicroUS operates at frequencies of 29 MHz and allows for a roughly fourfold higher crystal density along the transducer (512 vs 128 crystals). The resolution of MicroUS is 70 microns, which is the diameter of a typical prostatic duct, as opposed to 200 microns or more of TRUS, which provides a threefold improvement in special resolution compared to conventional frequency TRUS.[18–20] The high resolution of the MicroUS system permits the visualization of the ductal anatomy and cellular density, resulting in a more detailed view of the prostate anatomy (Fig. 1). As a consequence, MicroUS has emerged as a promising new imaging device for targeted biopsy, with the potential to improve sensitivity for csPCa, due to its ability of visualizing and targeting under real-time lesions suspicious for PCa.[18] The first generation of MicroUS technology, the ExactVu 29 MHz system, was originally assessed in a pilot study in 2013 on a radical

prostatectomy series.[10] Second generation high resolution MicroUS was released in 2017 and included additional advances in image quality and ergonomics, including redesign of the side fire transducer, which presents similar circumference (64 mm) as most of the TRUS transducers (58–74 mm),[21] and has been usually well tolerated by patients. For instance, in Klotz and colleagues,[12] a total of 1040 MicroUS procedures were performed with no drop-out for tolerability of the probe.

Prostate Risk Identification using Micro-Ulltrasound Grading System

In 2016, "Prostate Risk Identification using Micro-Ulltrasound" (PRI-MUS) grading system was proposed and validated to assess the risk of PCa for targeted biopsy with the MicroUS platform (Table 1).[22] The PRI-MUS scale ranges from 1 to 5, where a lesion ranked as a 1 implies a low risk for cancer while a lesion ranked as a 5 visualize a high risk for cancer. In contrast to PI-RADS (for mpMRI), PRI-MUS protocol is designed to take advantage of the real-time nature of ultrasound to be applied live during real-time TRUS biopsy. However, it refers to suspicious areas only in the peripheral zone of the prostate and the present version does not include a scoring system for the transition zone. Conversely, PI-RADS assesses lesions in the entire prostate gland. MicroUS paired with the PRI-MUS protocol can be used to inform biopsy decisions, guide prostate biopsy and aid in the detection of suspicious prostatic lesions in the same way as mpMRI. Furthermore, it also provides real-time visualization during the biopsy rather than requiring MRI/US fusion for targeting suspicious sites identified on mpMRI.

Technique

MicroUS-guided prostate biopsy can be performed by a transrectal or transperineal approach. Biopsy preparation and potential complications are similar to those related with TRUS-guided biopsy. Overall, recommendations concerning antibiotic prophylaxis, bowel preparation, anticoagulation withdrawal, and anesthesia delivery should follow the same local urologic guidelines.

The prostate is scanned in the parasagittal plane with MicroUS, since its high-resolution probe corresponds to a linear transducer. The first step of the study usually consists in measuring the prostate volume. For this assessment, initially a sweep is completed, which generates an axial view (Fig. 2A), and is used for the calculation of the maximum transverse diameter of the prostate. Subsequently, the midline sagittal plane is used for the measurement of the anteroposterior and

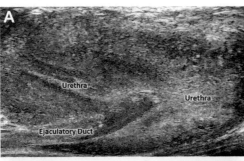
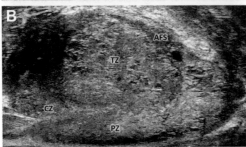

Fig. 1. Prostate MicroUS using a 29-MHz transducer showing the main anatomic landmarks of the prostate (sagittal plane). Midline view (A) showing clearly the urethra and ejaculatory duct. Paramedian view (B) demonstrating the four prostate zones: AFS, TZ, CZ and PZ. AFS, anterior fibromuscular stroma; CZ, central zone; PZ, peripheral zone; TZ, transition zone.

Table 1
PRI-MUS risk table

PRI-MUS Risk Score	Cancer Risk	Findings
1	Very Low	Small regular ducts, "Swiss cheese" with no other heterogeneity or bright echoes
2	Some	Hyperechoic with or without ductal patches (possible ectatic glands or cysts)
3	Indeterminate	Mild heterogeneity or bright echoes in hyperechoic tissue
4	Significant	Heterogeneous cauliflower/smudgy/mottled appearance or bright echoes (possible comedonecrosis)
5	Very High	Irregular shadowing (originating in prostate, not prostate border) or mixed echo lesions, or irregular prostate and/or peripheral zone border

craniocaudal diameters (**Fig. 2**B), which allows the estimation of the prostate volume. The second stage of the procedure consists in scanning carefully the entire prostate to depict morphologic abnormalities and lesions according to PRI-MUS score.

Systematic biopsy is performed in the sagittal plane similar to conventional TRUS-guided biopsies. If MRI has been performed prior to biopsy, the prostate is initially assessed for visibility of MRI lesions and for additional areas based on PRI-MUS scoring system for the peripheral zone. For MRI lesions visible on MicroUS, visually directed real-time targeted biopsy (**Fig. 3**) is performed rather than requiring use of additional software fusion with conventional TRUS and thereby provides for accurate targeting.[13]

Multiparametric Magnetic Resonance Imaging/Micro-Ultrasound Fusion

The first commercial MicroUS device (ExactVu, Exact Imaging, Markham Canada) also includes the ability to perform mpMRI/microUS fusion (FusionVu). It has been shown that TRUS visibility of prostatic lesions facilitates targeted biopsy.[23] The capacity to visualize the abnormal tissue in the real-time on MicroUS may therefore improve the accuracy of mpMRI-targeted biopsy by obviating the need to rely upon elastic or rigid deformation calculations and frequent corrections for patient movement or capsule marking errors. MicroUS/MRI fusion (FusionVu) biopsies are performed using software platforms to combine the MRI data to the US for targeted biopsies if they are not visible on MicroUS imaging (**Fig. 4**). The software aligns the tumor boundary identified on MRI as an overlay on the real-time Micro-US image to enable a direct targeted biopsy.[13] This tool is especially useful for suspicious lesions in the anterior transition zone of the gland that may not be visible on MicroUS in real-time for biopsy.

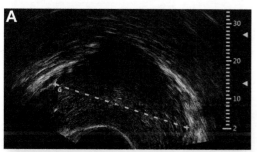
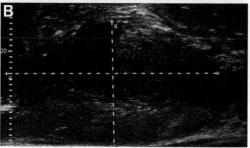

Fig. 2. Prostate volume calculation with MicroUS. Firstly, a sweep is performed with the probe and that generates an axial view (A) which is used for the measurement of the maximum transverse diameter of the prostate. Subsequently, the midline sagittal plane (B) is used for the calculation of the anteroposterior and craniocaudal diameters.

Diagnostic Performance

MicroUS presents three times greater resolution as compared with conventional TRUS resolution, potentially resulting in improvement in accuracy of targeted prostate biopsy.[24] For example, a multicenter randomized controlled trial, previously showed that MicroUS is more sensitive than conventional TRUS in detecting PCa.[25]

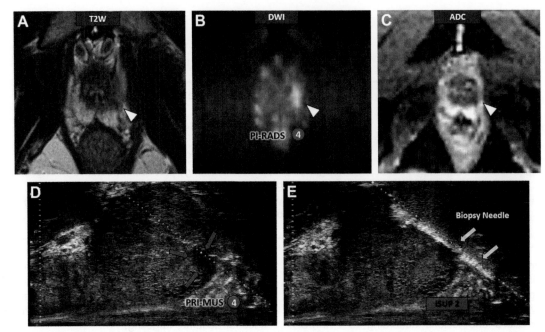

Fig. 3. Images in a 60-year-old man with prostate-specific antigen level of 4.5 ng/mL. Multiparametric MRI scans (axial T2-weighted image [A], diffusion-weighted image [B and ADC map [C]) show a PI-RADS 4 lesion in the left apex peripheral zone (*arrowheads*). MicroUS scan (D) shows the corresponding index lesion with smudgy pattern (PRI-MUS 4) (red *arrows*). Targeted biopsy revealed grade group 2 disease (E). PI-RADS, Prostate Imaging Reporting and Data System; PRI-MUS, Prostate Risk Identification Using Micro-Ultrasound.

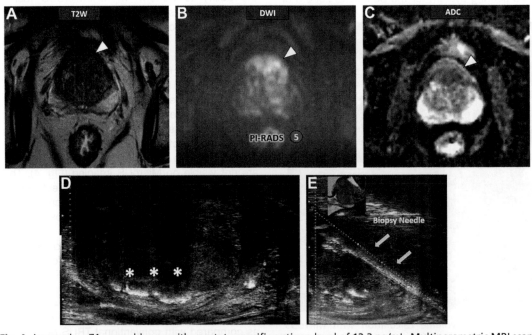

Fig. 4. Images in a 71-year-old man with prostate-specific antigen level of 12.3 ng/mL. Multiparametric MRI scans (T2-weighted [A], diffusion-weighted imaging [B] and ADC map [C] show a 2-cm PI-RADS 5 lesion (*arrowheads*) in the anterior transition zone. (C) MicroUS scan (D) failed to detect the site of the tumor, due to shadowing from calcification in corpora amylacea (*asterisks*), limiting the assessment of anterior gland. Targeted MicroUS/MRI fusion (FusionVu) (E) biopsies (using software platforms to integrate the MRI and ultrasound data) revealed grade group 2 disease. PI-RADS, Prostate Imaging Reporting and Data System.

More recently, multiple studies have also shown that the sensitivity of MicroUs is comparable to that of mpMRI for PCa detection (**Fig. 5**). The first study comparing MicroUS and mpMRI was published in 2018 by Eure and colleagues,[26] and showed that MicroUS could potentially be as sensitive to csPCa as mpMRI in the active surveillance cohort. This feasibility study had many limitations including small sample size, however it demonstrated that blinding between the two modalities was possible and that a within-patient comparison was feasible. Subsequently, multiple studies highlighting the similarities of csPCa detection rates between mpMRI and microUS have been published since 2019.[13]

In 2020, Socarras and colleagues performed a single center prospective trial where 194 patients first underwent microUS targeted biopsy while the operator was blinded to the mpMRI results.[27] While multiple studies have demonstrated the benefit of adding mpMRI to systematic biopsies for the detection of csPCa,[28] Socarras and colleagues showed additional benefit of adding MicroUS to mpMRI and systematic mapping, owing to its potential to detect csPCa that may be invisible on mpMRI. MicroUS detected 11% additional cancers not detected by MRI or systematic biopsy in their

study. Likewise, Lughezzani and colleagues assessed diagnosis of csPCa with MicroUS in a cohort of 320 patients with a positive MRI (PI-RADS ≥3).[29] This study showed a 2.6% improvement in csPCa detection by adding MicroUS targets to that of MRI targets and systematic biopsy. Furthermore, they concluded that these two modalities (MicroUS and MRI) appear to provide complementary information that could be combined to maximize the detection of csPCa. This may additionally have implications for patients being considered for focal therapy.

In 2021, Klotz and colleagues published the first multi-center prospective registry trial (11 institutions; 1040 patients) to compare the diagnostic performance of mpMRI targeted biopsy to microUS targeted biopsy.[12] Any man with an indication for prostate biopsy (elevated PSA or abnormal DRE) was included in the study. The authors concluded that MicroUS had comparable or higher sensitivity for csPCa compared to mpMRI. In this study, MicroUS and mpMRI sensitivity were 94% versus 90%, respectively (*P* = .03), and negative predictive value (NPV) for the two modalities was 85% versus 77%, respectively. An important limitation of this study was the methodological differences between sites. For example, 7 of the 11 sites were unblinded

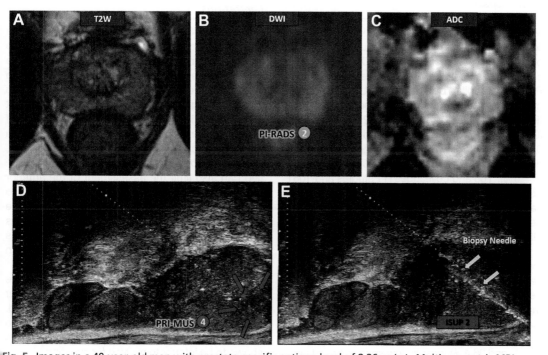

Fig. 5. Images in a 49-year-old man with prostate-specific antigen level of 8.26 ng/mL. Multiparametric MRI scans (T2-weighted [*A*], diffusion-weighted imaging [*B*] and ADC map [*C*] did not show any suspicious lesion (PI-RADS 2). MicroUS scan (*D*) showed a 6mm-hypoechoic lesion with smudgy pattern (PRI-MUS 4) in the left midgland peripheral zone (red *arrows*). Targeted biopsy revealed grade group 2 disease (*E*). PI-RADS, Prostate Imaging Reporting and Data System; PRI-MUS, Prostate Risk Identification Using Micro-Ultrasound.

to the mpMRI before using microUS; however, the results between blinded and unblinded groups were similar.

In 2022, Ghai and colleagues[15] and Hofbauer and colleagues[16] compared detection rate of csPCa using microUS targeted biopsy and mpMRI targeted biopsy. In Hofbauer and colleagues's multi-center prospective study, microUS found 73% of csPCa cases and mpMRI found 76%. MicroUS was non-inferior to mpMRI (P = .023) for detecting csPCa on biopsy. In Ghai and colleagues's single-center prospective trial, of the 94 men biopsied, mpMRI targeted biopsy found csPCa (GG $\geq$ 2) in 37 (39%) of the men and microUS found csPCa in 33 (35%) of the men. This study showed that the two modalities had comparable detection rates, nevertheless MicroUS would not have permitted avoidance of biopsy in as many cases as mpMRI. Interestingly, the detection of high-risk pathologic features (intraductal carcinoma and cribriform subtypes) was nearly equal between modalities. The combination of the two modalities, mpMRI targeted and microUS guided biopsy, allowed the detection of csPCa in 39 (40%) of the men in the trial. This study in particular suggests the potential added benefit of using mpMRI combined with microUS and reinforced that there was no value in adding systematic biopsies to mpMRI and microUS targeted biopsies.

Two recent metanalyses have also compared MicroUS and mpMRI for PCa detection. In Sountoulides and colleagues[17] study (13 studies and 1125 patients), the detection rate of csPCa and insignificant PCa, as well as the overall detection rate of PCa were similar between MicroUS-guided and mpMRI-targeted prostate biopsy. The pooled detection ratio for Grade group (GG) $\geq$ 2 PCa was 1.05 (95% CI 0.93–1.19, I^2 = 0%), and 0.94 (95% CI 0.73–1.22, I^2 = 0%) for GG1 PCa. The overall detection ratio for PCa was 0.99 (95% CI 0.89–1.11, I^2 = 0%). You and colleagues (11 studies and 1081 patients)[30] also concluded that there was no significant difference between MicroUS and mpMRI in the detection of csPCa, showing an odds ratio of 1.01 (95% CI: 0.83–1.22, P = .92) for csPCa detection.

In 2023, Avolio and colleagues[31] assessed the performance of MicroUS for predicting csPCa in patients with a persistent clinical suspicion of PCa despite negative mpMRI. The authors concluded that MicroUS may represent an effective tool for the diagnosis of csPCa in men with negative mpMRI, providing high sensitivity and NPV (respectively, 97.1% and 96.4%), despite low specificity and positive predictive value (29.7% and 34.0%, respectively).

Overall, available evidence has demonstrated that MicroUS detection rates for csPCa diagnosis are comparable to the detection rates of mpMRI guided biopsy procedures. The conclusions presented are uniform and include three studies providing level 1a evidence (per the OCEBM criteria for diagnostics tests)[32]; however, scarce randomized controlled trial data is available and some of the studies mentioned in this review have limitations with risk of bias. The OPTIMUM trial (ClinicalTrials.gov Identifier: NCT05220501) will address this unmet need. This is a 3-arm multi-center randomized controlled trial (n = 1200) comparing MicroUS guided biopsy with MRI/US fusion and MRI/MicroUS "contour-less" fusion. This trial will investigate whether MicroUS alone, or in combination with mpMRI, provides effective guidance during prostate biopsy for the detection of clinically significant prostate cancer (csPCa) for biopsy naïve subjects. This study will also allow several secondary outcomes of interest to be assessed. These include the difference in the detection of csPCa with MRI/US fusion versus MRI/MicroUS fusion biopsy and the added value of each biopsy technique (MicroUS targeted, mpMRI targeted, and systematic). Additionally, economic health data will be collected as a part of the study to assess cost and time savings compared to mpMRI targeted biopsy.

Limitations

While MicroUS may enable the detection of some lesions not identified on mpMRI, it may have some limitations. First, increased the attenuation of the ultrasound beam at higher frequency can lead to limited depth of penetration, and this can therefore limit the diagnostic performance of the current generation MicroUS device in the assessment of the anterior prostate gland including the transition zone especially in large prostates. In addition, shadowing from the corpora amylacea when calcified can also limit the assessment of the anterior gland (see **Fig. 4**). Imaging enhancements to improve image quality in the anterior prostate and a modified PRI-MUS scale addressing regions outside the peripheral zone should address this discrepancy and provide further improvement in MicroUS performance.

Second, robust studies aiming to determine the learning curve of MicroUS and the interobserver agreement in the PRI-MUS score are still needed. Finally, despite presenting similar sensitivity to mpMRI for csPCa detection, MicroUS has been shown to be inferior to mpMRI for avoiding biopsy, due to lower specificity; nevertheless, most lesions visible on mpMRI are also visible on MicroUS, allowing real-time targeted biopsy.[15] Therefore, it may be best suited for use in conjunction with mpMRI, but results of the multicenter OPTIMUM trial will provide evidence on how best to utilize this new technology.

Future Perspectives

MicroUS has been proposed to address other challenging indications in prostate imaging, including the local staging of PCa and active surveillance of PCa. MicroUS has also the potential to add value to biparametric (bp) MRI, and may represent a promising guidance for focal therapy in the near future.

Knowledge of the existence and location of extraprostatic extension (EPE) allows for more confident decisions on treatment margin. A few studies have investigated MicroUS' ability to predict non-organ-confined disease and EPE of PCa. In 2020, Regis and colleagues first investigated MicroUS' ability to predict the presence of EPE before radical prostatectomy.[33] This study showed that a MicroUS based assessment for the prediction of EPE would yield a sensitivity of 87.5% (95% CI 74.3%–100%) and a specificity of 80.0% (95% CI 65.7%–94.3%). In 2022, Fasulo and colleagues also investigated MicroUS' ability to predict EPE of PCa prior to radical prostatectomy.[34] MicroUS correctly predicted the presence of EPE in 80% of the cases with confirmed EPE on surgery.

Active Surveillance is recommended by the main urologic clinical guidelines to manage patients with low-risk PCa.[2,3] Albers and colleagues has recently evaluated the potential role of MicroUS in active surveillance.[35] This study compared MicroUS' ability to detect disease progression for men within an active surveillance program from GG = 1 to GG $\geq$ 2, as compared to mpMRI. No difference between MicroUS and mpMRI was found in detecting GG $\geq$ 2 lesions. MicroUS (with PRI-MUS $\geq$ 3) had a higher sensitivity than mpMRI (with PI-RADS $\geq$ 3) in detecting GG $\geq$ 2 cancer (97% vs 85% respectively). The study concluded that microUS may be more sensitive than mpMRI in this patient population. More recently, Maffei and colleagues also evaluated the adoption of MicroUS in patients with low-risk PCa undergoing confirmatory biopsies at 1 year from AS initiation, and compared diagnostic performance of MicroUS to that of mpMRI-targeted biopsies.[36] In this study, MicroUS and mpMRI showed a sensitivity of 94.1% and 100% and an NPV of 88.9% and 100% respectively in detecting ISUP$\geq$2 patients, concluding that both modalities represent valuable imaging technologies with high sensitivity and NPV in detecting csPCa, thus allowing their use for event-triggered confirmatory biopsies in active surveillance patients. Further studies are warranted to support the use of MicroUS in the field of local staging and active surveillance.

Micro-US has also the potential to be an adjunct to bpMRI for PCa detection. Two metanalyses have shown no significant difference between bpMRI and mpMRI in performance.[37,38] The ongoing prospective PRIME Trial (ClinicalTrials.gov Identifier: NCT04571840) will answer whether bpMRI is non-inferior to mpMRI and will help to establish the role of bpMRI in the diagnostic pathway for the detection of csPCa. MicroUS has high sensitivity in detecting PCa in peripheral zone and the role of DCE (dynamic contrast-enhanced) sequence in mpMRI is limited to lesions in the peripheral zone. Therefore, MicroUS imaging and biopsy may complement bpMRI and provide for an ideal tool for the detection of csPCa.

Moreover, given the ability of precise and real-time visualization of the prostate lesions (especially in the peripheral zone), MicroUS may represent a promising tool for focal therapy guidance, and our Institution is initiating a pilot study testing MicroUS guided focal laser ablation.

SUMMARY

Available evidence has demonstrated MicroUS to be a potentially cost and time saving novel technology with comparable cancer detection rates to mpMRI, which allows real-time visualization for accurate targeted biopsy. It remains uncertain whether MicroUS should be used as a stand-alone modality or in combination with mpMRI for PCa detection. The ongoing OPTIMUM randomized controlled trial will provide further evidence for the best utilization of this novel technology in the diagnostic pathway for cancer detection. Early data also suggest this imaging technique may also have a role in local staging and active surveillance of PCa. MicroUS has also the potential to add value to bpMRI, and may represent a promising guidance for focal therapy.

CLINICS CARE POINTS

- Micro-Ultrasound (MicroUS) is a promising novel high-resolution ultrasound technology for prostate cancer detection and targeted biopsy.
- While existing literature supports MicroUS replacing conventional TRUS for prostate imaging and biopsy, its optimal use remains unclear, whether as a standalone method or in combination with multiparametric MRI to enhance prostate cancer detection.

> • Early data indicates that this new imaging modality may also be valuable for local staging and active surveillance of prostate cancer.

CONFLICTS OF INTEREST

A.B. Dias has nothing to disclose. S. Ghai was Institutional PI for the initial multi-institutional randomized controlled trial comparing first-generation transrectal high-resolution micro-ultrasound with conventional frequency transrectal ultrasound for prostate biopsy. The trial was funded by Exact Imaging.

REFERENCES

1. World Cancer Research Fund International. Worldwide Cancer Data. 2022. Available online: https://www.wcrf.org/cancer-trends/worldwide-cancer-data/(accessed on 3 April 2023).
2. EAU Guidelines. edn presented at the EAU Congress Milan 2023. Available at: https://uroweb.org/guidelines/prostate-cancer. Accessed April 2, 2023.
3. NCCN Clinical Practice Guidelines in Oncology (NCCN Guidelines®) for Prostate Cancer Early Detection V.1.2023. © National Comprehensive Cancer Network, Inc., 2023. Available online: https://www.NCCN.org (accessed on 2 April 2023).
4. Ahmed HU, El-Shater Bosaily A, Brown LC, et al. Diagnostic accuracy of multi-parametric MRI and TRUS biopsy in prostate cancer (PROMIS): a paired validating confirmatory study. Lancet 2017; 389(10071):815–22.
5. Rouvière O, Puech P, Renard-Penna R, et al. Use of prostate systematic and targeted biopsy on the basis of multiparametric MRI in biopsy-naive patients (MRI-FIRST): a prospective, multicentre, paired diagnostic study. Lancet Oncol 2019;20(1):100–9.
6. Klotz L, Chin J, Black PC, et al. Comparison of multiparametric mag-netic resonance imaging-targeted biopsy with systematic transrectal ul-trasonography biopsy for biopsy-naive men at risk for prostate cancer: a phase 3 randomized clinical trial. JAMA Oncol 2021;7(4):534–42.
7. Meijer D, van Leeuwen PJ, Roberts MJ, et al. External Validation and Addition of Prostate-specific Membrane Antigen Positron Emission Tomography to the Most Frequently Used Nomograms for the Prediction of Pelvic Lymph-node Metastases: an International Multicenter Study. Eur Urol 2021; 80(2):234–42.
8. Kasivisvanathan V, Rannikko AS, Borghi M, et al. MRI-Targeted or Standard Biopsy for Prostate Cancer Diagnosis. N Engl J Med 2018;378(19): 1767–77.
9. Giganti F, Allen C. Imaging quality and prostate MR: It is time to improve. Br J Radiol 2021;(1118):94.
10. Pavlovich CP, Cornish TC, Mullins JK, et al. High-resolution transrectal ultrasound: Pilot study of a novel technique for imaging clinically localized prostate cancer. Urol Oncol 2014;32(1):34.e27–32.
11. Ploussard G, Roubaud G, Barret E, et al. French AFU Cancer Committee Guidelines - Update 2022-2024: prostate cancer - Management of metastatic disease and castration resistance. Prog Urol 2022; 32(15):1373–419.
12. Klotz L, Lughezzani G, Maffei D, et al. Comparison of micro-ultrasound and multiparametric magnetic resonance imaging for prostate cancer: A multicenter, prospective analysis. Canadian Urological Association Journal 2020;15(1):11–6.
13. Cornud F, Lefevre A, Flam T, et al. MRI-directed high-frequency (29MhZ) TRUS-guided biopsies : initial results of a single-center study. Eur Radiol 2020;30(9):4838–46.
14. Lughezzani G, Saita A, Lazzeri M, et al. Comparison of the Diagnostic Accuracy of Micro-ultrasound and Magnetic Resonance Imaging/Ultrasound Fusion Targeted Biopsies for the Diagnosis of Clinically Significant Prostate Cancer. Eur Urol Oncol 2019;2(3): 329–32.
15. Ghai S, Perlis N, Atallah C, et al. Comparison of Micro-US and Multiparametric MRI for Prostate Cancer Detection in Biopsy-Naive Men. Radiology 2022; 305(2):390–8.
16. Hofbauer SL, Luger F, Harland N, et al. A non-inferiority comparative analysis of micro-ultrasonography and MRI-targeted biopsy in men at risk of prostate cancer. BJU Int 2022;129(5):648–54.
17. Sountoulides P, Pyrgidis N, Polyzos SA, et al. Micro-Ultrasound–Guided vs Multiparametric Magnetic Resonance Imaging-Targeted Biopsy in the Detection of Prostate Cancer: A Systematic Review and Meta-Analysis. J Urol 2021;205(5):1254–62.
18. Laurence Klotz CM. Can High Resolution Micro-Ultrasound Replace MRI in the Diagnosis of Prostate Cancer? Eur Urol Focus 2020;6:419–23.
19. Basso Dias A, Ghai S. Micro-Ultrasound: Current Role in Prostate Cancer Diagnosis and Future Possibilities. Cancers 2023;15(4).
20. Dias AB, O'Brien C, Correas jean M, et al. Multiparametric ultrasound and micro-ultrasound in prostate cancer: A comprehensive review. Br J Radiol 2022; 95(1131).
21. Koprulu S, Cevik I, Unlu N, et al. Size of the transrectal ultrasound probe makes no difference in pain perception during TRUS-Bx under adequate local anesthesia. Int Urol Nephrol 2012;44(1):29–33.
22. Ghai S, Eure G, Fradet V, et al. Assessing Cancer Risk on Novel 29 MHz Micro-Ultrasound Images of

the Prostate: Creation of the Micro-Ultrasound Protocol for Prostate Risk Identification. J Urol 2016; 196(2):562–9.

23. Ukimura O, Marien A, Palmer S, et al. Trans-rectal ultrasound visibility of prostate lesions identified by magnetic resonance imaging increases accuracy of image-fusion targeted biopsies. World J Urol 2015;33(11):1669.

24. Rohrbach D, Wodlinger B, Wen J, et al. High-Frequency Quantitative Ultrasound for Imaging Prostate Cancer Using a Novel Micro-Ultrasound Scanner. Ultrasound Med Biol 2018;44(7):1341–54.

25. Pavlovich CP, Hyndman ME, Eure G, et al. A multi-institutional randomized controlled trial comparing first-generation transrectal high-resolution micro-ultrasound with conventional frequency transrectal ultrasound for prostate biopsy. BJUI Compass 2021; 2(2):126–33.

26. Eure G, Fanney D, Lin J, et al. Comparison of conventional transrectal ultrasound, magnetic resonance imaging, and micro-ultrasound for visualizing prostate cancer in an active surveillance population: A feasibility study. Canadian Urological Association Journal 2019;13(3):E70.

27. Rodríguez Socarrás ME, Gomez Rivas J, Cuadros Rivera V, et al. Prostate Mapping for Cancer Diagnosis: The Madrid Protocol. Transperineal Prostate Biopsies Using Multiparametric Magnetic Resonance Imaging Fusion and Micro-Ultrasound Guided Biopsies. J Urol 2020;204(4):726–33.

28. Siddiqui MM, Rais-Bahrami S, Turkbey B, et al. Comparison of MR/ultrasound fusion-guided biopsy with ultrasound-guided biopsy for the diagnosis of prostate cancer. JAMA, J Am Med Assoc 2015;313(4): 390–7.

29. Lughezzani G, Maffei D, Saita A, et al. Diagnostic Accuracy of Microultrasound in Patients with a Suspicion of Prostate Cancer at Magnetic Resonance Imaging: A Single-institutional Prospective Study. Eur Urol Focus 2020;1–8.

30. You C, Li X, Du Y, et al. The Microultrasound-Guided Prostate Biopsy in Detection of Prostate Cancer: A Systematic Review and Meta-Analysis. J Endourol 2022;36(3):394–402.

31. Avolio PP, Lughezzani G, Fasulo V, et al. Assessing the Role of High-resolution Microultrasound Among Naïve Patients with Negative Multiparametric Magnetic Resonance Imaging and a Persistently High Suspicion of Prostate Cancer. Eur Urol Open Sci 2022;47:73–9.

32. Howick J, Chalmers I, Glasziou P, et al. The oxford levels of evidence 2. Oxford, UK: Centre for Evidence-Based Medicine; 2011.

33. Regis F, Casale P, Persico F, et al. Use of 29-MHz Micro-ultrasound for Local Staging of Prostate Cancer in Patients Scheduled for Radical Prostatectomy: A Feasibility Study. Eur Urol Open Sci 2020;19:20–3.

34. Fasulo V, Buffi NM, Regis F, et al. Use of high-resolution micro-ultrasound to predict extraprostatic extension of prostate cancer prior to surgery: a prospective single-institutional study. World J Urol 2022; 40(2):435–42.

35. Albers P, Wang B, Broomfield S, et al. Micro-ultrasound Versus Magnetic Resonance Imaging in Prostate Cancer Active Surveillance. Eur Urol Open Sci 2022;46:33–5.

36. Maffei D, Fasulo V, Avolio PP, et al. Diagnostic performance of microUltrasound at MRI-guided confirmatory biopsy in patients under active surveillance for low-risk prostate cancer. Prostate 2023;83(9): 886–95.

37. Woo S, Suh CH, Kim SY, et al. Head-to-Head Comparison Between Biparametric and Multiparametric MRI for the Diagnosis of Prostate Cancer: A Systematic Review and Meta-Analysis. AJR Am J Roentgenol 2018;211(5):W226–41.

38. Alabousi M, Salameh JP, Gusenbauer K, et al. Biparametric vs multiparametric prostate magnetic resonance imaging for the detection of prostate cancer in treatment-naïve patients: a diagnostic test accuracy systematic review and meta-analysis. BJU Int 2019;124(2):209–20.

Moving?

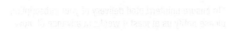